The Health and Fitness Handbook
A Family Guide

The Health and Fitness Handbook
A Family Guide

EDITED BY MIRIAM POLUNIN

SPHERE

SPHERE BOOKS LIMITED
30–32 Gray's Inn Road, London WC1X 8JL

First published by Windward and
Here's Health 1981.
The Health and Fitness Handbook was conceived,
edited and designed by Frances Lincoln Limited,
91 Clapham High Street, London SW4 7TA
in consultation with *Here's Health*,
30 Station Approach, West Byfleet, Surrey.
Copyright © Frances Lincoln Limited 1981
Published by Sphere Books Ltd 1983

SPHERE

Set in Monophoto Apollo
Printed and bound in Denmark by
Stibo Datagraphics Limited

Contents

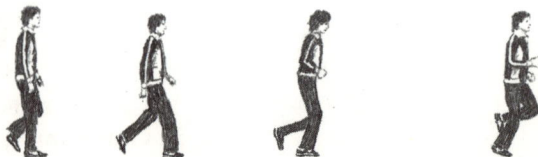

EATING FOR LIFE

MIND AND BODY

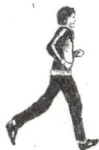

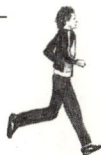

General Editor

MIRIAM POLUNIN is managing editor of *Here's Health*, Europe's largest-selling magazine on natural health. Three years in the Far East, mostly in Japan, awakened her interest in the effects of food on health, and she has spent the last nine years evaluating different patterns of eating, exercise and lifestyle. She gives courses on natural living for the magazine and is the author of *The Right Way to Eat* and *Minerals*.

Contributors

KOFI BUSIA is one of the top yoga teachers in the U.K. He studied yoga in England and at the Rama Mani Iyengar Institute in India, and is the founder of the Ashram in Oxford, where he gives yoga classes and courses for pupils of all levels.

LEON CHAITOW, N.D., D.O., M.B.N.O.A., is a practising osteopath and naturopath. He has researched for many years into the influence of nutritional, psychological and biochemical factors on health and disease. He lectures widely on these subjects and is the author of several books. He is also a regular contributor to *Here's Health*.

BARBARA DALE runs two body workshops in London, giving classes in bodywork, ballet and jazz dancing, relaxation, yoga and ante- and post-natal exercises. She is co-author of a book on exercise, *Simple Movement*, and contributed to *The Face and Body Book*.

HOPE JAMES, M.S.I.A.D., is a leading interior designer, specializing in space planning and function in the home.

MARGARET KENNEDY, M.C.S.P., trained in physiotherapy at the London Hospital, where she later worked. She now concentrates on geriatric physiotherapy.

SIMON MARTIN is the editor of *Here's Health*. An ardent fitness enthusiast, his main activities are running – including representative cross-country running – and practising a Japanese system of dynamic relaxation.

VALERIE NICHOLSON, N.D., D.O., M.B.N.O.A., is an osteopath and naturopath, and is currently researching into medical anthropology.

DAVID ROBINSON, Ph.D., worked in the Addiction Research Unit at the University of London, before becoming Senior Lecturer in Health Studies at the University of Hull. He is a regular World Health Organization consultant, and the author of a number of books on medical sociology and the addictions.

JON SANDIFER is a teacher and director of the East West Centre, London, where Shiatsu and Do-In are taught.

LESLIE WATSON, M.C.S.P., physiotherapist, is also an amateur long-distance runner, competing annually in the New York marathon. She broadcasts frequently on jogging and running, and on how to avoid sustaining injuries therefrom.

It's your life

'How well do you feel *today*?' has become my favourite question for people who tell me that taking care of their health is boring, that it's not worth the effort or that they'd far rather live 'a short life and a merry one'.

Choosing healthier living habits doesn't just enable you to live longer – it enables you to live better, without which longer life is not worth while. It's not only that it'll prevent an early heart attack, although that's a good reason for doing it. It's because it's a glorious feeling to feel well, day-to-day. It means that you have a built-in 'sunny side of the street' to walk down, that you have the energy and will to get the most out of yourself and your life.

This book can give you a flying start towards that powerful state of high-level health. It has been written by people who *do* the things they are writing about – and tell and teach other people. They know it works.

Your health is your responsibility, because the daily living habits you choose are the main factors in determining how well you are.

Yes, some people are born healthier than others. That doesn't affect the fact that most of us can develop better health. The major epidemics of this century are not accidents of fate – they are the diseases we have chosen by picking certain lifestyles: heart disease, stress illnesses, hypertension, some intestinal complaints, gallstones, maturity-onset diabetes, obesity, alcohol-related illnesses, lung cancer. . . .

This book concentrates on three main ways in which you can make a difference to your state of physical, and mental, health: what you eat, the exercise you take and the way you react to life. Physical, mental and spiritual health are not separable. They all affect each other. A healthy body favours a cheerful mind, and vice versa.

It has been my experience that people can build themselves the opposite of a vicious circle: a benevolent upwards spiral to feeling fitter than they had ever imagined. Simple changes in eating habits make them feel better, physically and mentally. They feel more like exercising and being energetic – which in turn lifts their morale and physical well-being a step further up. Their general good health, and added sense of self-improvement, increases their liking for themselves, which encourages them to take further positive steps.

In such a spiral, many everyday things that have been causing problems – physical, social, work-related – will sort themselves out. Just think, for example, how much better your life might be if you felt more relaxed: a fast result of exercise, relaxation techniques, better eating habits and following our advice on dealing with the stress that results from resisting reality. Irritating physical ailments – skin conditions, digestive upsets, headaches, asthma and more – are also likely to vanish with your newfound super-health.

Disease does not flourish in a healthy person. Your healthy body will resist infection, and recover more quickly if you succumb. Never look for a magic 'remedy' that you can swallow or rub on for illness: always look for what you've been doing to yourself to upset your

7

body's natural good health. Correct that, using professional help for crises, and your body will automatically right itself.

If you choose living and thinking habits that your body and mind can't cope with, don't be surprised that they react by losing their resistance to infection or stress or by slowly developing degenerative diseases.

What's more, many people handicap themselves with a feeling of helplessness often coupled with resentment. 'I'm a victim of circumstances' is an attitude that means you can avoid accepting responsibility for anything, and that makes it almost impossible to be healthy. That's because it seems to prove that you can't affect your own life – so it's not worth trying. It allows you to resent 'life' for giving you those circumstances – and resentment as basic as that precludes feeling in harmony with life. It's an attitude that can kill you. As long as you have it, you're giving your body a burden that will eventually contribute to illness. And even while you're 'well', it will go a long way to killing the life in your life.

Take responsibility – looking after yourself makes you more alive. It's not a self-indulgent fad : you are the most important asset you have. It's your life.

Miriam Polunin

FIT
FOR
LIFE

Why exercise?

Go to bed for a month and you will get up feeling exhausted. Freed from the battle with gravity and unable to move far in any direction, your muscles will atrophy and your joints stiffen up. Your circulation will become sluggish, starving tissues of vital oxygen and nutrients. You'll rise weak and stiff and pant at the slightest exertion; for days afterwards you'll feel fat, lethargic and probably depressed.

Yet the many thousands who take no exercise spend their lives in such a state – although everyone understands that a car deteriorates if the engine isn't in regular use, they tend to forget that, in the same way, the body, and the mind, work better the more they're used.

Exercise is a means of getting that necessary extra physical activity, and raising your general level of fitness in a way that is not only enjoyable, but gives you the strength, stamina and suppleness to get twice as much out of life. The point of fitness is not that it enables you to do 20 press-ups or run a mile – you're not going to spend your life doing that – but that it creates an energy reserve you can call on at any time.

The excuses

Some people come out with negative reasons to avoid exercise. Here are a few of the favourites – and the answers.

'It's dangerous . . . people can die exercising.' Making any demand of an unprepared body is dangerous, but regular exercise makes your body *less* likely to fold up when asked to do something extra. The exercise-related deaths that get publicity usually occur in people who ignored the sort of sensible precautions advocated on pages 22–24.

'I haven't got the time.' Most people can find time for a drink after work – you'll find the time for anything you really want to do.

'I can't be bothered.' It's easy to break the apathy barrier. Exercise with like-minded people who'll make you feel you *have* to turn up.

The case for exercise

In 1976, Britain's Department of Health and Social Security commissioned *The Case for Exercise*. It reviewed over 100 scientific papers to conclude that exercise could help to prevent or ameliorate heart disease and low back pain, to cure obesity, that it was of especial benefit to the elderly and those suffering from chronic diseases, and had 'a favourable effect on pregnancy and childbirth'. Subsequent research the world over has elaborated on its findings.

For heart disease, for instance, exercise has been proved valuable not only as a preventative measure, but also in convalescence. Men who take part in regular vigorous exercise seem less liable to coronary heart disease than those who don't – and that notwithstanding other risk factors such as obesity, smoking and hypertension, or high blood pressure. Indeed hypertension itself can be reduced by exercise. American scientists have suggested that marathon runners are immune from heart disease, and it is known that regular exercise lowers the cholesterol and general blood-fat levels, as well as increasing levels of high-density lipo-proteins that have a protective effect on the heart. This is in addition to direct effects on the health and efficiency of the heart muscle, lungs and circulation.

In obesity, it is now recognized that exercise does not work on a straight calorie-swap arrangement. You don't just eat a hamburger and then run enough to burn off the equivalent calories. Exercise affects the metabolic rate so that for a few hours afterwards you'll burn more calories and use up more of the body's stores of fat (even when resting) than if you had taken no exercise. Regular activity combined with a diet (see pages 160–62) is the most effective way to lose weight, because the body becomes more efficient.

Exercise demanding controlled breathing can benefit asthmatics and bronchitics. A campaign of a 12-minute walk and stair-climbing exercises produced a significant improvement in bronchitis patients, while asthmatics who swam regularly found the frequency of attacks and the amounts of drugs needed to control them were reduced.

Body and mind

One of the most exciting developments is in psychiatry, where regular exercise is now used to improve the self-esteem of mental patients and to reduce tension and anxiety. It has actually 'cured' some cases of depression, due to the release of hormone-like substances, including adrenalin and noradrenalin, that affect the emotions. Found at very low levels in depressives, they have been shown to be 600 per cent above normal in marathon runners during a race.

Since regular exercise promotes relaxation and a sense of well-being, it can help if you want to give up smoking, drinking alcohol or make other changes in your lifestyle. The stimulating effect of nicotine, for example, can be achieved without its life-threatening side-effects by vigorous exercise which, like smoking a cigarette, temporarily raises blood pressure and heart rate and releases energy in the form of free fatty acids into the bloodstream. If you have trouble sleeping you should find that regular exercise will help.

Exercise for life

Children who spend all their leisure time passively, maybe in front of the television, can suffer retarded mental and physical development; parents should try to build into a child the lifelong habit of exercise. Conversely, you're never too old to benefit from activity; indeed the athletic abilities of senior citizens can regularly be seen at veteran events. And since it results in a permanent increase in metabolic rate, and may lead to a better maintained body temperature, moderate exercise is the best remedy for hypothermia, the killer condition that particularly affects old people living on their own. But the less you exercise, the more you'll feel your age, and the more you'll be open to the degenerative diseases that can accompany the run-down of health and fitness in the later years. Exercising *now* could help you to a longer life, and an active, independent old age – and can certainly delay or avoid the need for institutional care.

But the big message missing from the welter of evidence that exercise is good for health is that it's *fun*. And, as the following pages will show, there are many enjoyable ways in which you can add extra activity to your life.

11

Check your posture

Perfect posture

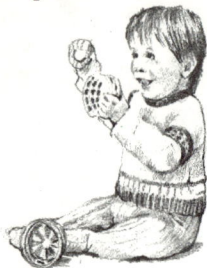

Good posture helps the body to function and wear well, makes you look slimmer and healthier and gives a feeling of freedom and ease – you have more energy if you're not burdened with the unnecessary tension that bad, uneven carriage creates. Good posture also conveys confidence, encouraging others to respond positively to you. Everyone starts off life well, but it's all too easy to slip into bad habits, such as round shoulders, and less easy to change them, especially if you're battling with badly designed furniture: see pages 18–21 for advice on how to adjust it. There are as many permutations of bad posture as there are people; this section will help you to recognize your own bad habits and shows you how to correct them.

Standing

The golden rule is to lengthen your spine, without trying to flatten its curves at the waist and neck. The discs between the vertebrae act as buffers as you move but if they're constantly cramped and strained, this suspension becomes damaged and the discs may be displaced. If one part of the spine tilts out of line, the rest has to curve to compensate, so it's important to keep the whole body in balance.

Head
Lift your head upwards. Imagine you're suspended by a string pulling up from the centre of the crown.

Chin
Try to hold it at roughly right angles to the throat. Nod your head up and down a few times to find the right position.

Ribs
Lift your ribcage upwards away from the hips, so your abdomen flattens, your chest opens and you can breathe freely.

Pelvis
Centre your pelvis; tilt it backwards and forwards and hold it balanced at the mid-point.

Knees
Try to keep them neither rigid nor bent, but at ease.

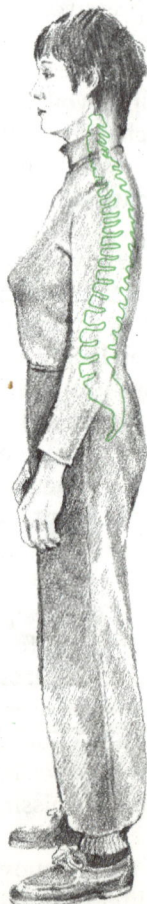

Neck
Lengthen the back of the neck; this comes naturally if you hold your chin and shoulders well.

Shoulders
Pull them down away from your ears and balance them directly above your hips. Try exercise 1, page 210, to help you get the feel of this.

Arms
Let them hang loosely at your sides.

Spine
Stretch the whole of your spine upwards; if you hold your pelvis correctly and keep the back of the neck long, your spine lengthens naturally. If you find it difficult to keep it long, strengthen it with the exercises on pages 38–41.

Feet
Stand with your feet slightly apart, your weight evenly balanced between the heels and the balls of the feet. Rock back and forth a few times to find the right balance. If you find this hard, see pages 44–45 for exercises to strengthen your ankles.

If the shoulders slouch (a), the spine rounds and shortens, the abdominal muscles become lazy so the abdomen sticks out, and breathing is inhibited. Practise the backward rolling movement in exercise 3, page 28, to balance the pelvis and the exercises on pages 34–35 to straighten up rounded shoulders.

Sway back (b) is a common fault, particularly in women in late pregnancy or who wear high heels and in men with a paunch. The bottom sticks out and the lower back is overarched, squeezing the spine and making the back tight and stiff. The pelvis is tilted down in front, so the abdomen pokes forwards and the muscles tend to become weak.

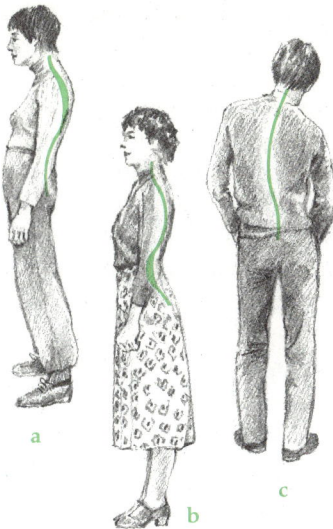

The buttocks are stretched instead of being tucked under the hips and the thighs can't work properly: so both the thighs and buttocks are often heavy. To correct all this, tuck the bottom under, centering the pelvis; try exercise 8, page 33, to help you do this.

Another common tendency is to pull the shoulders back, so the upper back becomes tense, and the back of the neck is shortened as the chin juts out in front.

Standing with your weight on one leg (c) pushes the weight-bearing hip up higher than the other. The opposite shoulder lifts and the head leans to one side, so the whole spine is curved wrongly.

Walking

The same principles apply here as to standing. Keep your head and body balanced as you walk. If your spine is lengthened and the pelvis centered, your legs are free to stride out, moving from the thighs, almost as though you were being propelled from behind. Strengthening your thighs and buttocks with the exercises on pages 42–43 will help. Keep your movements easy and your breathing free and rhythmical. Let your feet use all their tiny joints as you walk, putting the heel down first and then the toes. As your weight is transferred, the back foot should bend easily. Women should, ideally, especially if they have to do a lot of walking in the course of a day, wear comfortable, low-heeled shoes, as high heels distort posture.

If you must carry heavy bags, try to distribute the weight evenly on each side. If you habitually carry a bag or briefcase, change sides frequently and go through it to make sure that you really need all the extra weight.

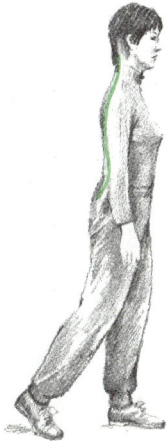

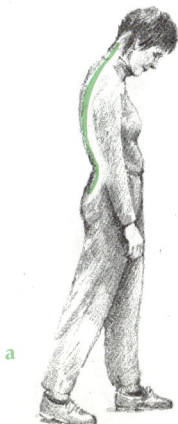

If you slouch (a), the feet plod forwards stiffly and heavily and are jolted unnecessarily. It's difficult to walk with long steps and there's a tendency to look down at the feet.

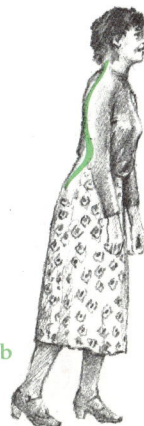

When the back is overarched (b), the buttocks and thighs are underworked, the knees are strained and the feet land on the ground stiffly, tending to kick up dust or mud behind. The top half of the body lurches forwards, instead of remaining poised over the back foot until the weight is transferred. It's difficult to take big strides.

13

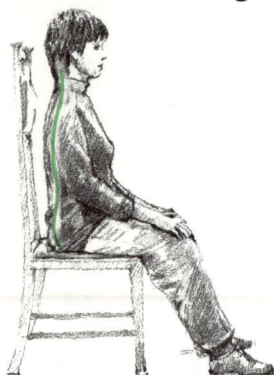

Sitting   When sitting, make good use of the support your body is getting. Sit back into the chair, lengthen your spine and, if possible, allow it to be fully supported. Sit with your hips square on to the direction you are facing, with your thighs lying straight forwards from your hips. Have your feet flat on the floor and try not to pull your feet back under your chair as this tenses up the calf muscles and prevents good circulation: this is especially important if you suffer from varicose veins. When you're sitting at a table or desk, hinge forwards from the hips to work instead of rounding your spine.

Crossing the arms and legs (c) or, worse, double-crossing the legs cramps and twists the body so that breathing is restricted and the spine is strained and shortened.

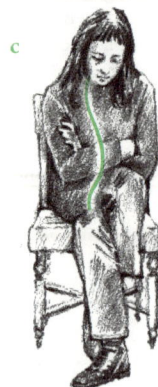

Slumping forwards (a) rounds and shortens the spine. If the chin juts forwards, the back of the neck also shortens. Crossing your legs shifts all your weight to one side.

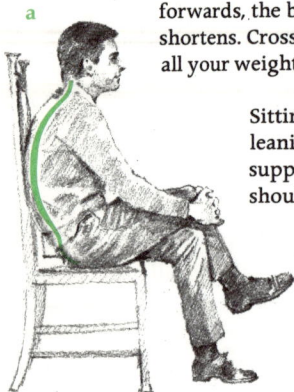

Sitting on the edge of the chair and leaning back (b) gives the spine no support and curves the neck and shoulders forwards.

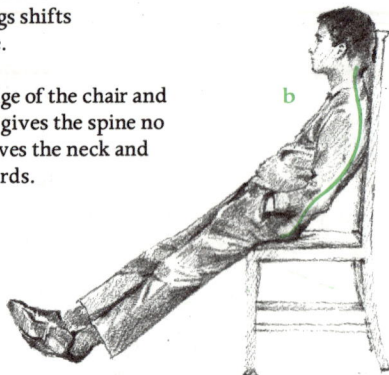

Many people sit badly when driving, as tension builds up easily. Try not to hunch forwards over the wheel, rounding the spine and shortening the neck (a). Sit well back into your seat, using it for maximum support, and keep the back of the neck long and the head in balance (b); hold the wheel gently.

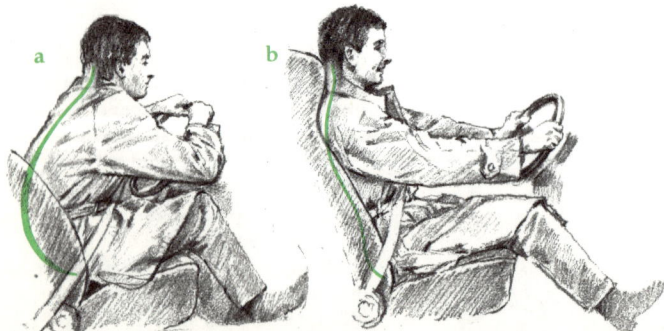

When standing up, have the feet one in front of the other to give a wide, stable base. Don't use the arms, but instead push off with the feet and thighs, hinging forwards from the hips only as much as you need to (a). Don't lunge forwards, slumping your shoulders (b), or let your chin or bottom stick out (c).

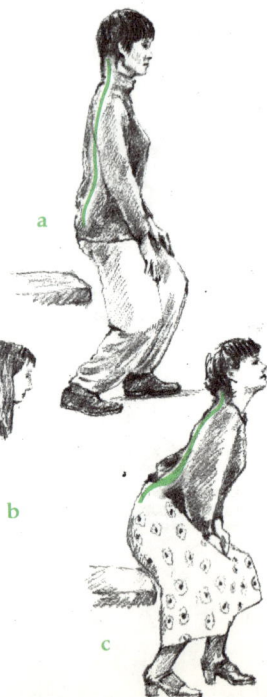

Lying

The golden rule, as before, is to keep the spine lengthened and in a straight line. So try to lie without twisting to either side or hunching your shoulders and at least start the night lying in a good position – it should help you to get to sleep more easily as well as protecting your spine. Don't use too many pillows as this curves the spine in whichever position you lie.

If you suffer from backache or have a sway back, try placing a pillow or two under your thighs when lying on your back. A pillow placed lengthways between your legs is also helpful if you feel discomfort in the upper hip when lying on your side – this is a particularly comfortable position for women during pregnancy.

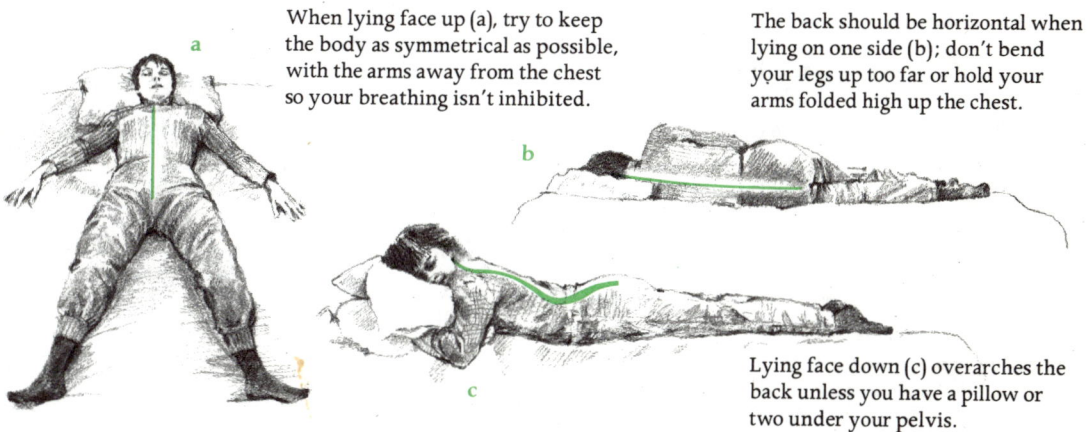

When lying face up (a), try to keep the body as symmetrical as possible, with the arms away from the chest so your breathing isn't inhibited.

The back should be horizontal when lying on one side (b); don't bend your legs up too far or hold your arms folded high up the chest.

Lying face down (c) overarches the back unless you have a pillow or two under your pelvis.

The Alexander principle

Matthias Alexander originated much of modern thinking on posture. An Australian who started life as an actor, his career came to an abrupt halt when he lost his voice on the stage. After long hours spent studying himself, he discovered that the cause of the problem was his tendency to pull his head backwards, shortening the back of his neck. Simply by lifting his head and lengthening his spine upwards, he managed to cure his speech difficulty.

He became so interested in the general applications of this discovery that he devoted the rest of his life to research and teaching. The core of his theory is that it is essential to use your body properly in order to allow it to function well. By unlearning the bad postural habits created by past tension you become free to cope with present demands. Great energy is released by keeping the spine, including the neck, lengthened – this is the basic principle of moving and resting correctly. Advice on how to lengthen the spine is given above, but for instruction in the Alexander technique go to a qualified teacher, who can help not only to improve posture but to release stress and to relieve a variety of physical ailments, from asthma to rheumatism.

Everyday movements

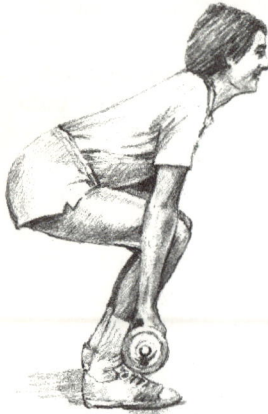

Using your body correctly when going about everyday activities helps to prevent problems with muscles, joints and especially the spine. If you have back pain already, it is essential to learn to move properly to prevent the problem becoming worse. These are the general rules that apply to many common everyday movements, such as lifting, bending, pushing and reaching.

● Keep your spine lengthened and bend forwards from the hips, which form the natural hinge of the trunk. Use the bigger joints and stronger muscles of the hips and thighs rather than the numerous delicate joints of the spine, which are easily strained.

● When lifting a weight, stand with your feet apart to provide a stable base and bend your knees to pick it up.

● Stand as close as you can to any object to be manoeuvred.

● Carry any weight as near as possible to your own centre of gravity – the hips.

● Never twist at the same time as lifting a weight.

● Avoid lifting heavy weights above waist level as it's all too easy to overarch the back as you brace yourself to take the load.

● Push rather than pull whenever you can, with your hips square on to the object, using your body weight to help you.

● Protect your knees with a pad or mat when kneeling.

Below are some examples of how to apply these rules.

The weight-lifter obeys all the rules. He bends his knees and lifts the bar close to his hips; then he uses the muscles of his arms and legs to raise it up high rather than straining his back.

Scrubbing or weeding
Don't reach down while standing – kneel on all fours. If you're working close in to your body, sit back on your heels and hinge forwards from the hips.

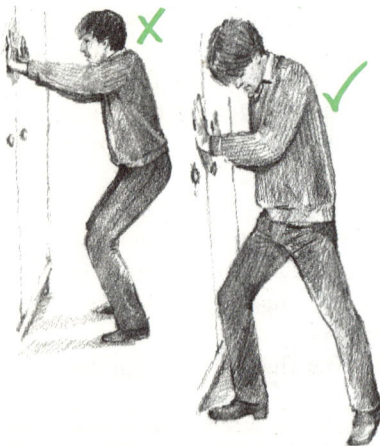

Moving a heavy weight
Stand close to the object and push, leaning forwards from the hips and using your body weight; if possible, push with your back.

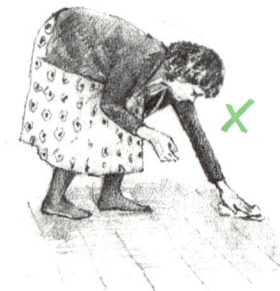

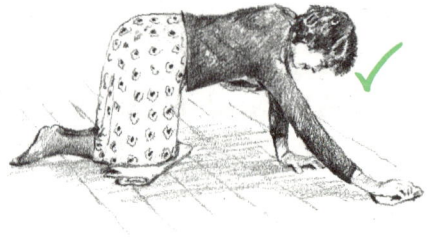

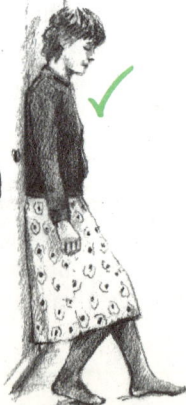

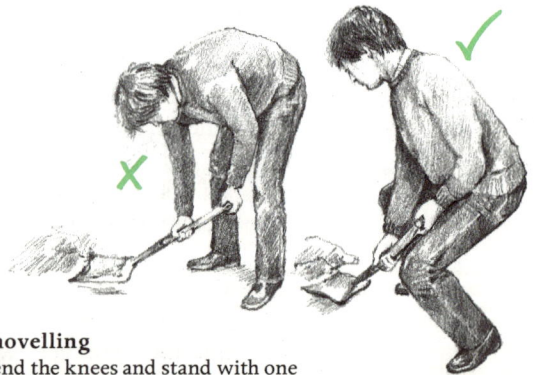

Shovelling
Bend the knees and stand with one foot in front of the other, to allow you to manoeuvre the weight of the shovel easily.

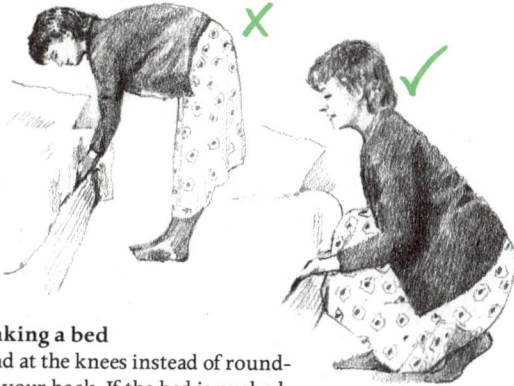

Making a bed
Bend at the knees instead of rounding your back. If the bed is pushed against a wall, pull it out to tuck in the sheets and blankets instead of reaching across (see page 21).

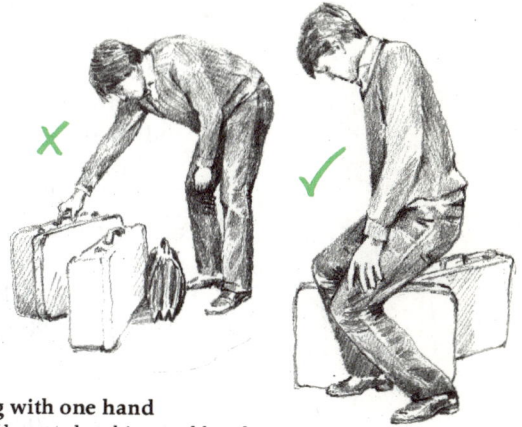

Lifting with one hand
Stand close to the object and bend at the knees instead of reaching over with a rounded back.

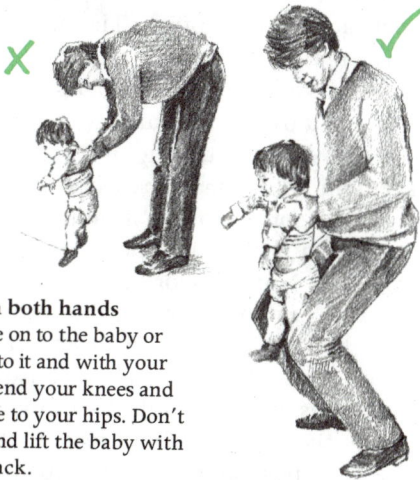

Lifting with both hands
Stand square on to the baby or object, near to it and with your feet apart. Bend your knees and lift it up close to your hips. Don't reach over and lift the baby with a rounded back.

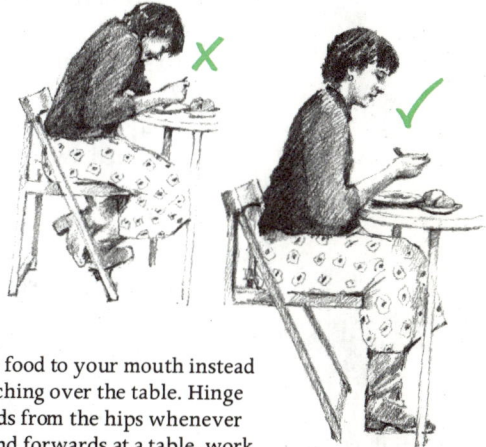

Eating
Lift the food to your mouth instead of slouching over the table. Hinge forwards from the hips whenever you bend forwards at a table, work surface or desk.

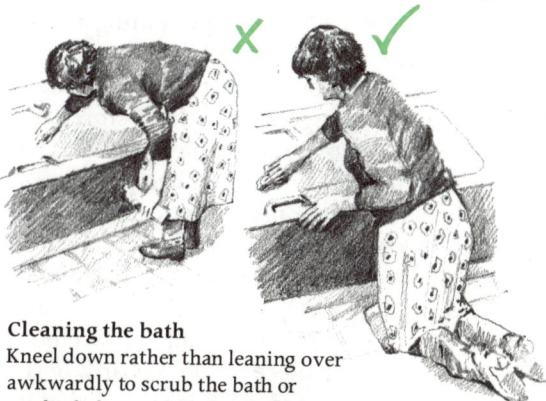

Cleaning the bath
Kneel down rather than leaning over awkwardly to scrub the bath or wash a baby. Fold the bath mat to protect your knees and lean your hips against the bath so you're free to stretch and bend.

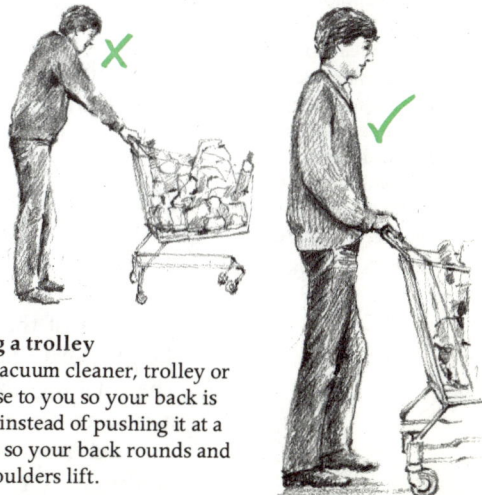

Pushing a trolley
Hold a vacuum cleaner, trolley or mop close to you so your back is straight instead of pushing it at a distance so your back rounds and your shoulders lift.

Organizing the environment

Your body is constantly moving, so a position taken up in any one place – on a chair, at a bench, in bed – is always changing. Just as people come in different sizes – even with the same overall height there are innumerable variations in length of legs, width of shoulders and so on – the body's ability to move its joints for extra reach or visibility is also individual.

Above all, you owe it to yourself to maintain correct posture as much as you can. This means that sometimes you'll need to assess your surroundings, especially those in which you spend a lot of time, then alter them so that you can be more comfortable and more efficient. The following pages give some guidelines to follow, and offer suggestions on the types of changes you can make.

Work

Wherever you are working, your equipment should be laid out so that you can always maintain good posture, see everything you need, and do your work most efficiently.

To stand comfortably at a work surface (see left), you need room for your feet to project beneath it for stability. The optimum height for a counter top depends on the work being done, but generally 75 mm [3 in] below the elbow is considered the most comfortable. The body should not be bent forward over a low surface, nor the forearm strained by working above the elbow. Strip lights over the worktop stop shadows from a centre light falling on to the work surface.

Most standing work involves some moving around. When this is not the case, studies have shown that people prefer to work seated, when good seating is provided. Normal working or writing height depends upon the comfortable seated height of the individual and should be just below elbow height. If a desk or other surface is too high, lower it if you can, or else raise the seat height and use some kind of footrest – telephone directories will do. A tall stool should be fitted with a footrest that supports the whole of both feet. If the desk or worktop is too low, add a thickness of blockboard to it. If further height is needed, fix wooden blocks beneath the board, gluing a layer of sheet rubber to their undersides, to prevent the board moving.

In the kitchen, appliances should be set out so that the fewest steps are required between sink, stove and refrigerator or food store, and there should be enough work space. A stove should have a put-down surface on either side and uninterrupted work space between it and the sink. Since varying levels in a small area make for accidents, and continuous worktops are easier to keep clean, a compromise must be found between the optimum height of the base of the sink (not lower than the flat of your hand held parallel to the floor while standing), and that of the stove and linking worktop (75 mm [3 in] below elbow height). Add height to a low surface with a piece of blockboard, or do the washing up in a bowl on the draining board, draining the dishes in a rack above. For convenience, keep cutlery and utensils in a compartmented tray or drawer, store plates and saucers upright in racks within easy reach, and hang cups and mugs on hooks under shelves.

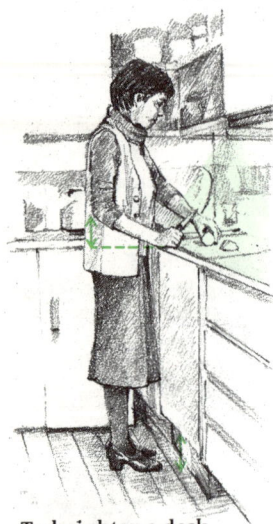

To heighten a desk Use a piece of blockboard. For more height still, glue or nail wooden blocks to its underside, placing them at each corner and, depending on the board size, diagonally across the middle. For stability, glue sheet rubber to the block bases.

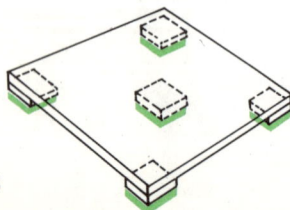

1 The height of a workbench should suit the type of work involved: high for light handling or instrument reading, so that the back can be kept straight (a). For work requiring pressure, like carpentry or ironing, the surface should be lower (b), to enable you to press down.

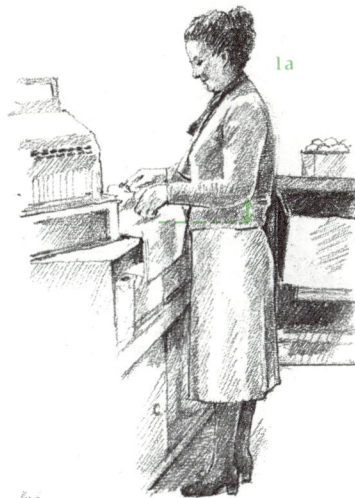

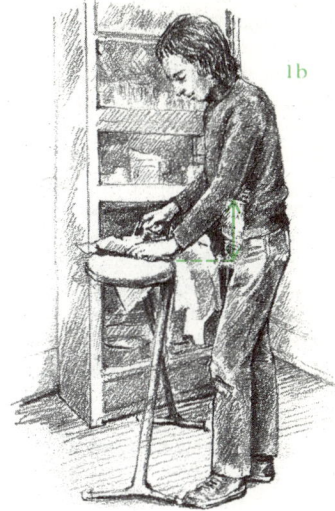

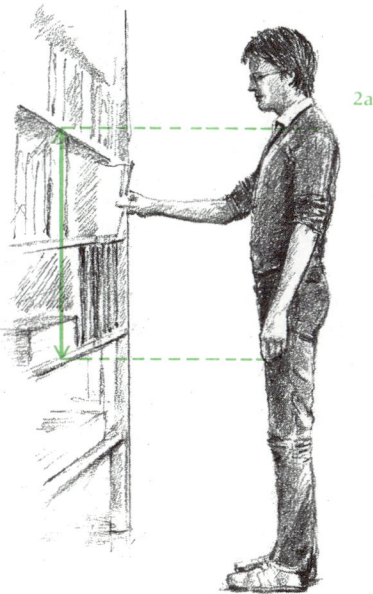

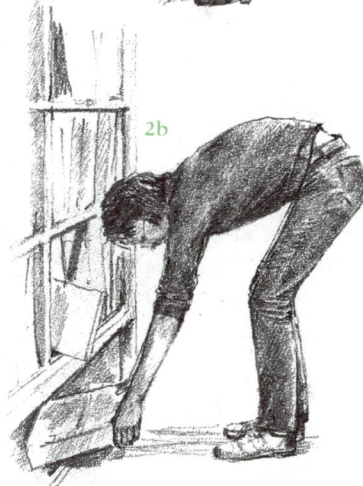

2 Storage and shelves in a work area should be within easy reach. Place heavy goods and those most frequently used on the middle shelves, between your shoulder level and finger level with your hands by your side (a). This will prevent your bending down too often to fetch big items (b); nor will you be tempted to stand precariously on some nearby object and strain upwards.

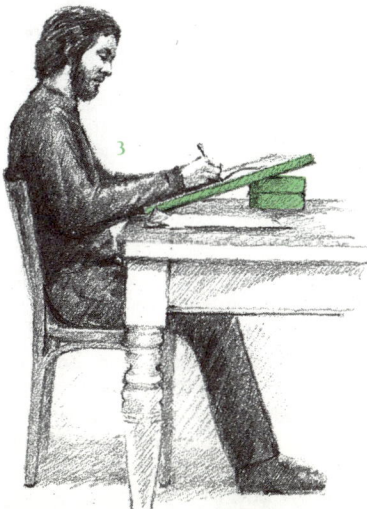

3 Writing or drawing for a long period can be made easier by using a sloped surface to support the work and the forearm. Make a slope by propping up a board on books, or on bricks wrapped in brown paper to stop them scratching the surface.

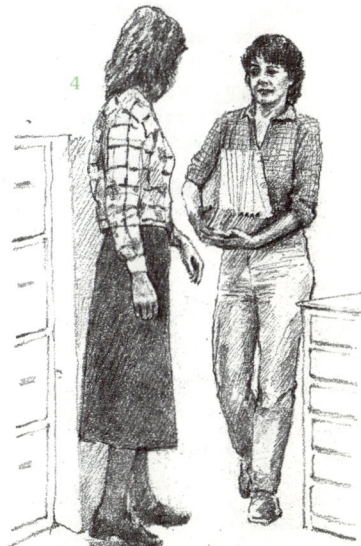

4 In busy areas there should be sufficient room between furniture or other fixed objects for one person carrying something and another passing to go through together – approximately 1.2 m [4 ft]. If the gap is too narrow, as here, inconvenience and even accidents may result.

19

5 A chair should support buttocks and thighs and allow your feet to rest flat on the floor. The seat should not be so deep that its front presses into the backs of the knees, nor so shallow that your thighs are unsupported. The backrest should cushion the lumbar region but leave room for your buttocks. For a straight back when reading, prop up your work at an angle (a) and make sure light shines directly on it.

When using a typewriter or visual display unit, your hands should come halfway up the keyboard with the forearms horizontal (b). Thus such equipment should often be about 50 mm [2 in] lower than normal working or writing height. If a chair is too high, support your feet.

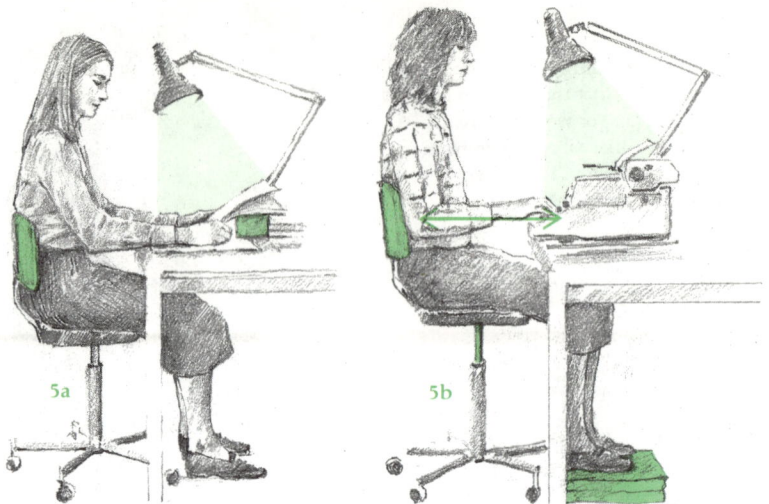

5a

5b

Travelling

As always when seated your feet should be flat on the floor, the buttocks, thighs and lumbar region properly supported. On trains and aircraft, stow hand luggage and parcels away to leave as much space for body movement as possible. Sit well back into the seat and, if your feet don't have good floor contact, use a parcel or flat case as a footrest. Whatever the means of transport, getting up and moving your position will help to avoid strain. So will wearing suitable, comfortable clothes and easy fitting shoes.

1 Don't push a car seat too far forward so you're jammed up against the steering wheel (a). It should be adjusted to provide good contact with the floor pedals without bending the knees too much. A slightly angled upright back position gives easy handling of the steering wheel, with access to the dashboard controls, all with the safety belt on (b). If the seat still isn't right, try placing a small cushion or rolled-up coat behind the lumbar region. Maintain correct posture (see page 14) and set the mirrors to suit your new seated position.

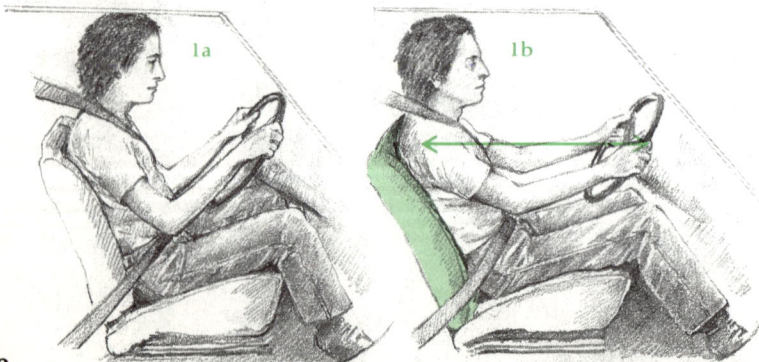

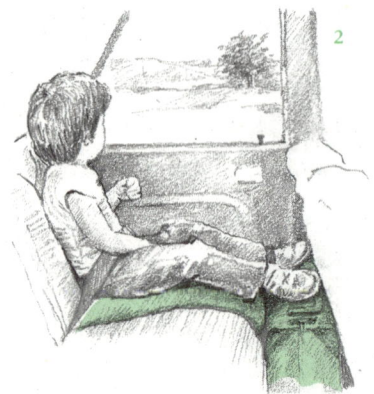

2

1a

1b

2 Children may require extra seat height to see out. Provide it by a covered foam slab or folded blanket, and raise the floor level with a small suitcase or filled bag positioned firmly under the feet.

3 A headrest should support the curve under the bulge at the back of the head. If it's in the wrong place – making the head come forward (a) – and can't be adjusted, sit slightly forward with a cushion, rolled-up garment or soft parcel behind your back to support your lumbar region and keep your head upright (b).

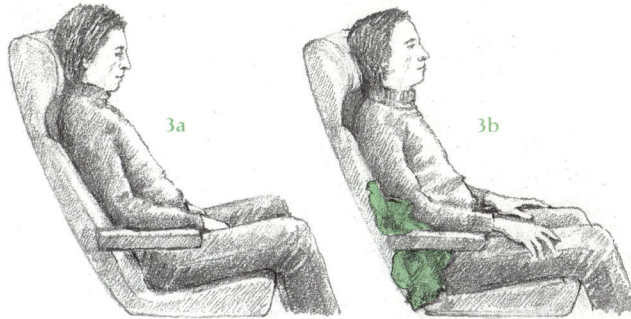

Relaxation and rest

Test an armchair to see that it gives adequate support for your buttocks and thighs, back and shoulders, and head too if preferred. For greater comfort try a footstool to raise your feet and keep your legs straight. When you read, light should fall directly on the page, to prevent any strain from unconsciously reaching towards the light source; if you have an adjustable lamp move it to find the most satisfactory position. A side table for use with the armchair should be of the same height as the seat.

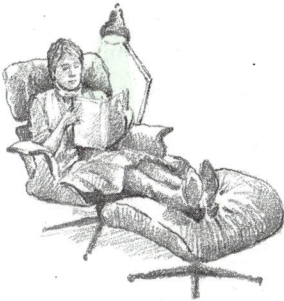

A bed should give comfort and support. It should be at least 20 cm [8 in] longer than standing height and as wide as the width from elbow to elbow held at shoulder height to give room for movement. Choose a mattress that gives a little at the hips and shoulders and fills out the hollows. If you cannot slide your hand between the bed and the small of your back, the mattress is probably too soft. Placing a full-size board, with ventilation holes cut in it, under the mattress will give better support. A lightweight person finding a bed too hard can make it more comfortable by placing a soft layer, such as a quilt, under the bottom sheet, although a firm mattress will soften with use. Using a duvet instead of sheets and blankets takes a lot of hard work out of bed-making – particularly useful if you have back trouble. For easy cleaning and making, a bed should not be too low and should have a minimum of 60 cm [2 ft] space around it. If you read in bed, make sure that the light is positioned to fall directly on the page.

1 A bed should be firm and without the lengthway or crossway sags that can lead to back troubles.

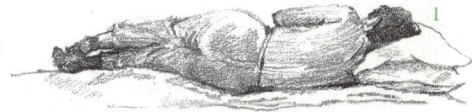

2 For extra comfort when lying on one side, balance your body by placing a pillow or cushion between your legs.

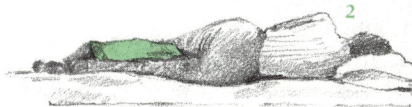

3 The arms of the chair should not hamper you when reading or knitting, nor make it hard to stand up – also a problem if the seat is too low. If the seat is too deep or too high, so that your feet are unsupported, your upper body will strain to adjust the balance.

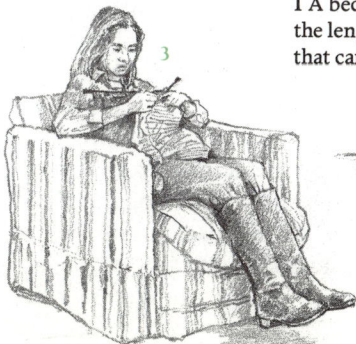

21

Before you start

Once you've decided that you need more exercise, the next step is to test how fit you are *now*. Exercise is only the term used for getting a fair share of natural activity back into your life. You don't have to struggle for it: bodies were designed to be used – they are at their best when in motion, so the more you move, the more comfortable you feel. Once you've made the initial effort to get over your own lethargy, you'll find it gets steadily easier and the benefits you'll experience will encourage you to keep it up.

Professional check-ups

We've all heard stories of people dropping dead during work-outs or when jogging. Many of these are indeed just stories but from the documented cases it's clear that heart attacks and irritating injuries occur during exercise because people think they're fitter than they are. It's nothing to get anxious about as long as you check your fitness first if you don't exercise regularly.

Dr. Kenneth Cooper, the founder of the Aerobics Institute in the United States, has started thousands of people on fitness campaigns based on activities – such as walking, running, swimming and cycling – that strengthen heart, lungs and circulation. He has a superb safety record, and his recommendations, graded according to age, are simple. You may start exercising if:

Under 30: you've had an all-clear medical check-up in the past year.

Between 30 and 39: you've had a check-up within the last three months that included a resting electrocardiogram (ECG) measuring the electrical activity of the heart.

Between 40 and 59: you've had a check-up within the last three months that included a resting ECG and an exercise stress test (an ECG while exercising on a stationary bicycle or treadmill).

Over 59: you've had a detailed examination including both types of ECG immediately before you start.

Be honest with yourself, and if there's any doubt in your mind, and especially if you're over 30, get a *qualified* opinion.

If you're having medical treatment you should check with whoever is looking after you before you begin exercising. Bear in mind, too, that when you start unaccustomed exercise you're adding another stress to your body. So consider what sort of pressure you're already under; stress, whether it comes from your work or a tension-filled home environment, means you should proceed with caution. You should also be careful if you smoke, drink a good deal of alcohol, have a history of heart disease in the family, suffer from hypertension, or are very much overweight.

If you already exercise regularly there's no harm in spending further time at it. But if you're over 30 don't switch suddenly to a more violent activity without a check-up. Watch out for any of the signs that you're overdoing things: a pulse rate that refuses to fall below 100 beats a minute, pains in the chest, dizziness, feeling sick or having stomach ache or digestive upsets, difficulty in breathing or a constricted chest.

Checking your pulse

The simplest way to assess your current state of fitness is to take your pulse. When you do, what you feel is the wave of blood travelling through one of the arteries that carry blood from the heart. What you are after is a 'resting pulse', so take it first thing in the morning before it has had a chance to be increased, as it can be, by exertion, mental excitement, tension, or stimulants such as alcohol, nicotine, coffee or tea. Count the number of beats per minute: rates vary greatly but the average for men is between 70 and 85 a minute; a woman's pulse tends to be slightly faster – 75 to 90. Whichever your sex, if your pulse is up in the 100s when you're sitting, lying or standing still, there is cause for alarm. If it is in the 90s, you're fairly unfit, and your heart is having to work harder than it should to keep up with demand.

Generally speaking, the slower your pulse the better. It provides a sensitive barometer of your fitness – and when this increases, the pulse slows down, becoming stronger and more regular, indicating that your heart is becoming more efficient and that you're developing a reserve of power.

Whatever your age, if your resting pulse rate seems very high, or if you have any doubts about the state of your heart and lungs, you must have a *personal* examination by a qualified health professional.

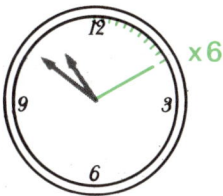

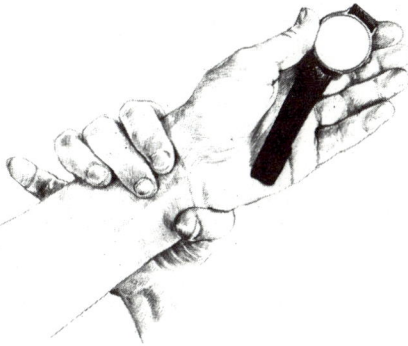

To take your pulse use a watch that shows seconds. Hold it in your left hand, palm up, and grasp the left wrist with your right hand. With the first two fingers of the right hand, find the pulse in your wrist under the base of the thumb. Or find the pulse at the neck: lay two fingers to one side of the Adam's apple.

Count the number of beats per minute: for convenience, count for ten seconds and multiply by six. This gives you your pulse rate.

Safe pulse rate

The next step is to take your pulse during exercise (for instance, running on the spot in the fitness test, over), since it's the easiest reliable way to gauge whether you're overdoing things. It's particularly vital when you're embarking on exercise after a long period of inertia – although you may *feel* strong enough to undertake violent activity, you could be straining your heart and lungs. So before you start, work out your safe pulse rate, and try not to exceed it.

The maximum rate at which the heart can beat declines with age, from 200 beats a minute at 20 to about 150 at the age of 70. During exercise, your pulse rate should not rise above 75 per cent of your maximum. The following useful guidelines for finding your personal safe pulse rate were developed by Alistair Murray at the City Gym in London: from 200 subtract your age, and then a further handicap of 40 for being unfit. Thus a 50-year-old would subtract 50 plus 40, to

23

get a safe pulse rate of 110. Try not to go too far over your safe pulse rate – if you find that you've done so, cut down the strenuousness of your activity. If you haven't reached it, make your exercise more vigorous, in order to get a positive benefit from it. As you get fitter, you can reduce your handicap slowly, a single beat at a time. As a rough guide, if you're under 30 you should eventually be able to cut it out altogether; between 30 and 40, aim to reduce it to about five; between 40 and 50 don't go under 15; if you're over 50, keep it to 20.

If you're very unfit, your pulse rate may rocket up as soon as you start exercising; if it does, just take a rest between each exercise to bring it down. As you get into shape you'll be able to cut down and finally eliminate these pauses.

Don't stop suddenly during vigorous exercise to check your pulse – keep moving, and get the pulse quickly before it has had a chance to fall too much. At first, and after particularly taxing work-outs, you may find it remains high for quite a while, but as you get fitter it will slow down very soon after exercise. You can use this as a progress guide: take your pulse just as you finish exercise, and then again a minute and a half later. The fall in the rate during that time will become more marked, the fitter you get.

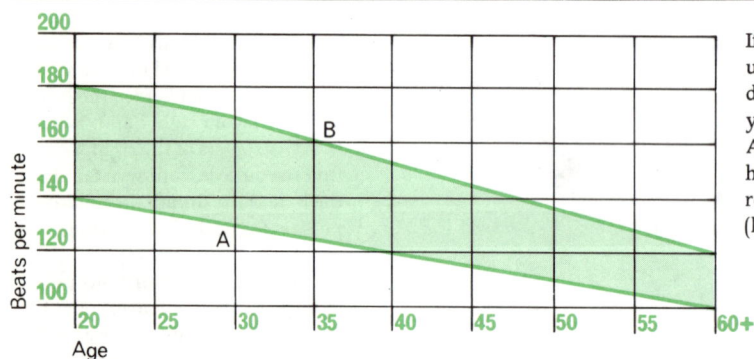

If you know that you're completely unfit, find your safe pulse rate by deducting from the maximum of 200 your age, plus a handicap of 40 (line A). As you get fitter cut down your handicap beat by beat until you reach the top rate for your age (line B).

Test your fitness

All activity depends on the heart's ability to shunt oxygen-carrying blood round the body, but the heart itself relies on the other muscles to help pump the used blood back to be filtered of waste products and revitalized with fresh oxygen. So they must be in good shape, too.

Strong muscles don't mean unsightly bulges; they mean the ability to carry heavy suitcases easily or to deal with household emergencies; they mean a lean, firm shape that diet alone cannot deliver. Take the quick fitness test opposite to see whether you have the arm-, waist-, and leg-power to cope efficiently with daily life. The test will show not only your current state of fitness but also indicate the areas needing particular improvement. The worse your results the more gently you should start out. Note the results, and repeat the test in three months' time: if you've adopted the right exercise routine you should really see the difference in your performance.

FITNESS TEST

Running on the spot tests not only leg muscles but also heart and lungs, so if you've any doubts about the latter and haven't had a recent medical examination, skip this exercise. With arms dangling loosely at your sides, raise alternate knees. Try it for two minutes to start with. The higher you step and the longer you can keep at it, the fitter you are. If you have to gasp for breath, your chest hurts, you feel dizzy or sick, STOP immediately.

A similar test, a little less demanding, is exercise 11, page 33. Step up and down for one minute with the left leg; then with the right.

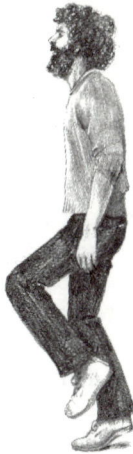

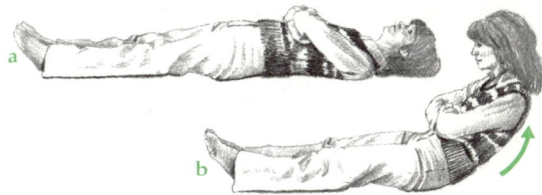

How flexible are you? Sit on the floor, legs straight in front. Reach slowly towards your toes – don't force the stretch. Reach the point where you feel comfortable, and hold your legs. If you can hook your hands over your toes (a), that's good; if you reach the ankles (b), not bad; if you grab somewhere between ankle and knee (c), that's not very good at all.

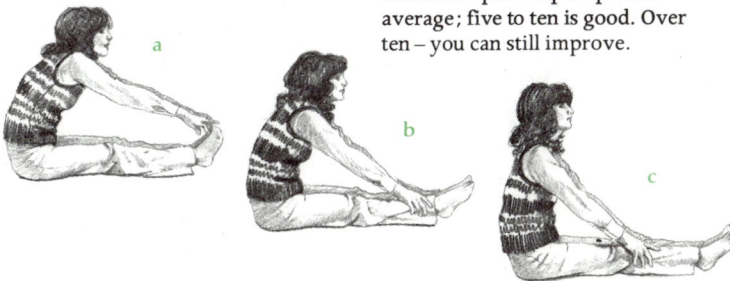

To test the strength of your abdominal muscles, lie on your back with legs out straight and arms folded on your chest (a). Try to raise your back, *rolling* it smoothly up from the floor, head going up first (b). Don't try to keep your back straight. All the way up, time after time – you're in good shape; half way up easily is average; barely off the ground . . . ?

Test the strength of your arm, shoulder and chest muscles with table press-ups. With body straight and feet slightly apart, place both hands on a table, or other firm, horizontal surface, standing comfortably away from it (a). Keeping the body straight, bend your arms (b), so that your chest comes forward to touch the table (c). Straighten your arms again. From one to five press-ups is poor to average; five to ten is good. Over ten – you can still improve.

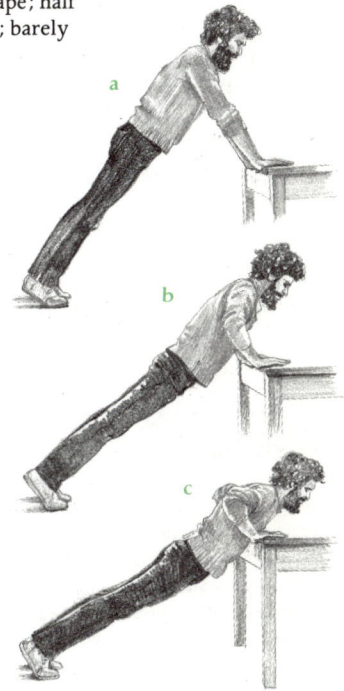

Selecting an exercise routine

The following pages give a wide variety of fitness routines for you to choose from. Pick something you like doing – all that matters is that you do it regularly enough to have a positive effect on your health. Find a routine to suit your lifestyle and the time available.

If you're not at your best first thing in the morning, exercise in the middle of the day or in the evening. Don't exercise for an hour or so after a meal, though – you may feel sick and you could get cramp. There's no need to dress up in tracksuits or leotards – wear whatever feels comfortable; it shouldn't impede movement, so avoid tight waistbands or girdles. Don't wear plastic or rubberized clothing as it can raise body temperature dangerously.

Everyday exercise

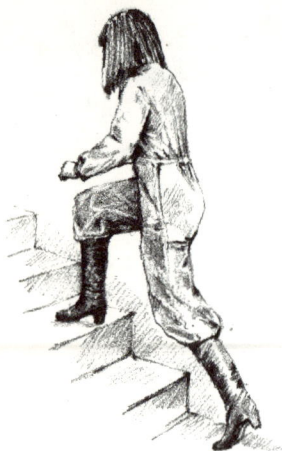

Climbing stairs is an excellent form of exercise – let your legs do the work instead of pulling yourself up on the banister.

If you can't bear formal exercise, this is the section for you. These exercises can be fitted into your daily routine, so you don't have to set aside part of your day or change into special clothes. They won't strengthen your heart and lungs significantly (see pages 67–68) but you'll become more flexible and you should also feel less tense.

Maximize the opportunities for exercise. Walk or cycle instead of sitting in a car, bus or train and use housework and gardening as an opportunity to stretch and twist. Walk upstairs, preferably two steps at a time, so that you work your hip joints, buttocks and thighs and also exercise your heart and lungs. Sitting on the floor helps to loosen the hips; people in Eastern countries where squatting or sitting on the floor is common tend to become less stiff in the hips in later years. Do some of the floor exercises while sitting watching television.

The body becomes tired of being held in one position for too long, so compensate for too much of one kind of activity with its opposite. For example, stand up and walk about for a while at regular intervals when you have to sit for long periods; when working with the arms forwards, pull them back from time to time. These changes keep the body in balance and refresh you. Some large companies in Scandinavia have introduced *pausgymnastik*, or regular morning and afternoon exercise breaks, and even five minutes of calisthenics can help to banish muscular aches and pains.

The selection of exercises on the next four pages is safe for beginners, even if you can't easily do the exercises on page 25. Repeat each exercise as often as you like *without straining*. You can also adapt some of those on pages 32–45, 210 and 212–13 for everyday use.

ON THE BED

1 Counteracts rounded shoulders, opens the chest and helps release tension in the lower back. Lie facing up with your shoulders on the edge of the bed. Lower your head and let it hang down, stretching your arms back and letting them flop. Hold; come up slowly.

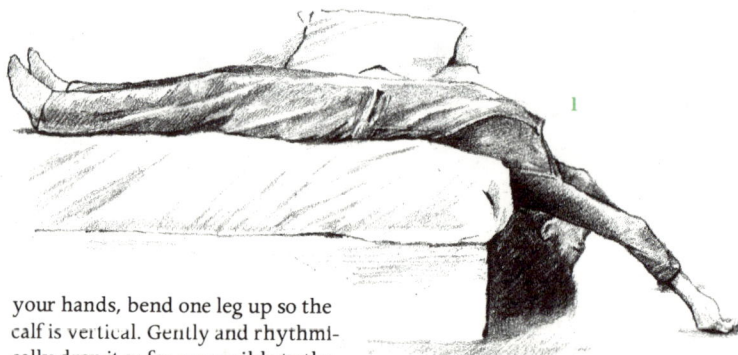

2 Try this to keep your hips mobile. Lie face down on your bed or the floor, with a pillow or cushion under your hips; use two if your back is weak. Resting your forehead on your hands, bend one leg up so the calf is vertical. Gently and rhythmically drop it as far as possible to the right (a) and to the left (b). Repeat with the other leg.

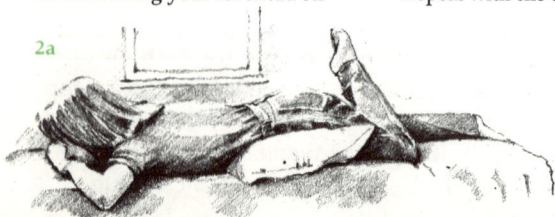

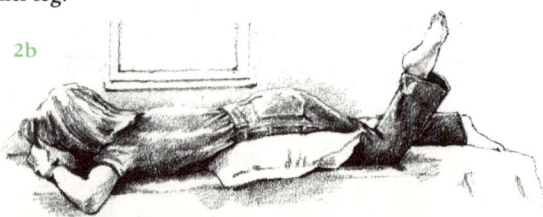

ON THE FLOOR

1 Strengthens the back and buttocks. Lie facing up, arms at your sides, with your legs propped up on a low piece of furniture (a) – resting in this position helps the circulation in the legs. Push the hips upwards as far as you comfortably can (b), and hold for a few moments.

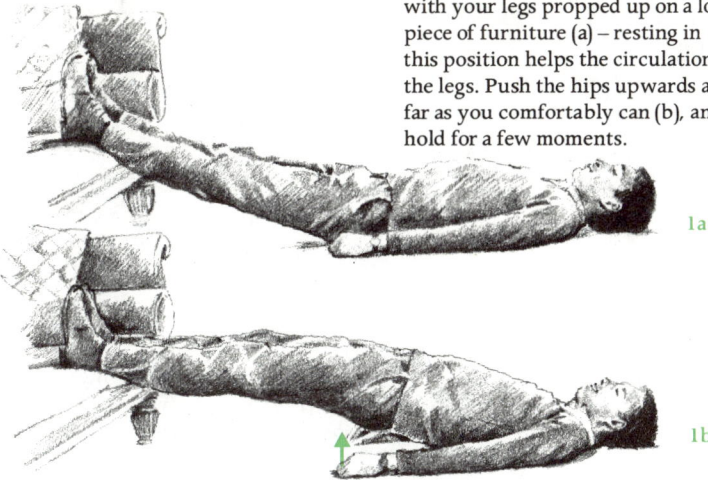

2 Mobilizes the lower back and hips. Sitting on the floor, with your legs straight out and arms folded, roll from side to side, lifting your left hip up towards the left ribs as you roll to the right (a) and the right hip up towards the right ribs as you roll to the left (b).

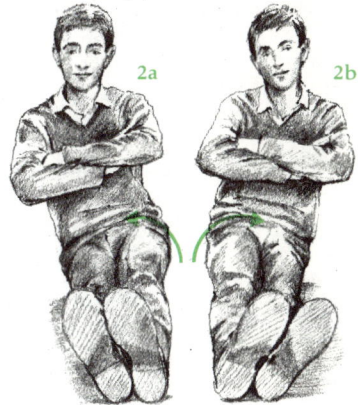

1a

1b

2a   2b

3 Stretching the backs of the calves and ankles helps to prevent cramp and curled up toes and aids circulation in the calves and feet. Women will find it particularly useful during pregnancy when cramps can be severe and for counteracting the bad effects of high heels on calves and feet. Sit with both legs straight out in front and hold the right knee down with the right hand. Grasp the right foot with the left hand and gently pull the foot inwards several times (a). Repeat with the left foot.

If this is a strain, sit with your hands behind you and ask a partner to put one hand on your knee and to pull your foot in towards you with the other (b). He should then press lightly on the knee and gently pull the foot inwards a few more times.

4 Twisting mobilizes the spine and works the diagonal abdominal and back muscles. Sitting well, with crossed legs, place your right hand on the left knee and your left hand behind you; turn both head and chest round as far to the left as possible. Hold; repeat to the right.

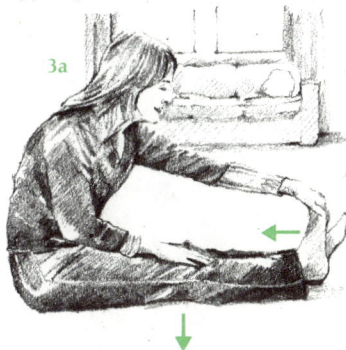

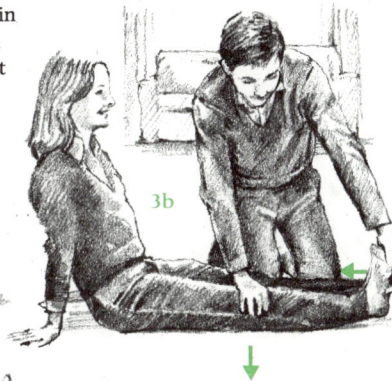

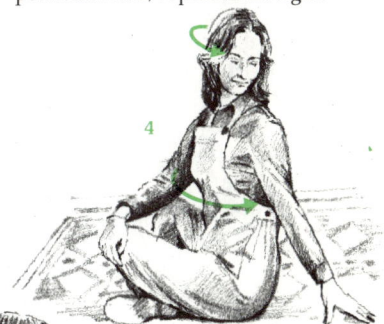

3a

3b

4

5

5 To mobilize your hip joints and lower back. Sit with your legs straight out in front and your arms folded, and walk forwards and back on your bottom. Try to straighten your back when sitting in this position (see page 38).

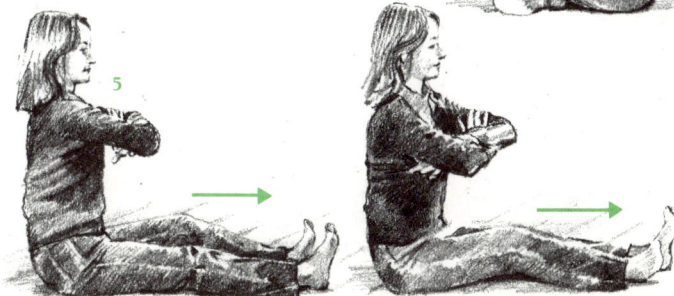

27

Everyday exercise

SITTING ON A CHAIR

1 Loosens the shoulder joints. With your hands on your shoulders to keep them down, circle your elbows up, back (a), down (b) and forwards. Circle in the opposite direction, unless you have rounded shoulders. You can try this sitting on the floor too.

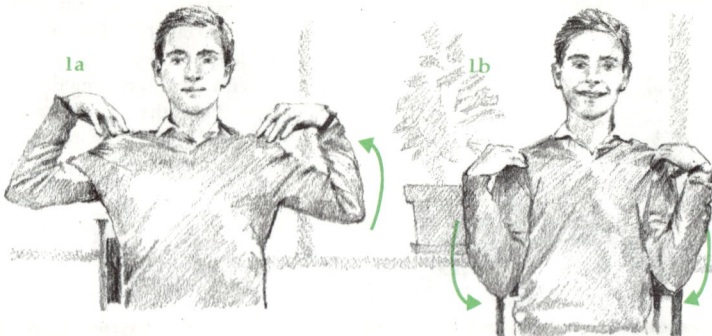

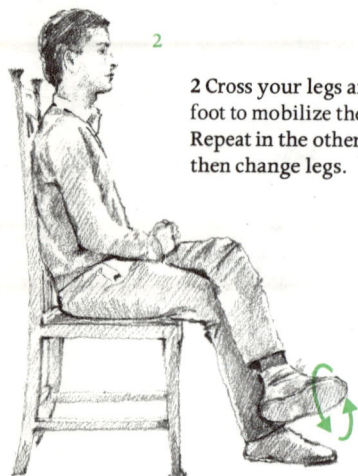

1a

1b

2

2 Cross your legs and circle the top foot to mobilize the ankle joint. Repeat in the other direction, and then change legs.

3 To prevent stiffness in the lower back when sitting, move to the front of the chair and roll the pelvis, tilting the pubic bone down (a) and up (b).

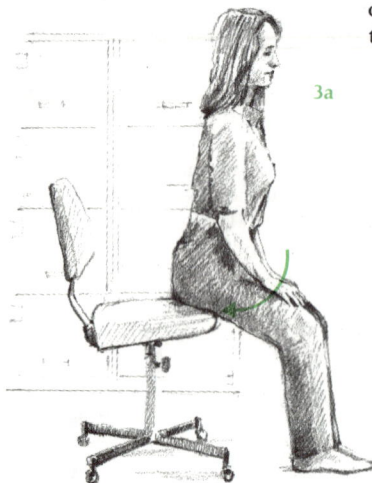

3a

3b

4 For a good stretch between the shoulder blades. Clasp your hands, turn the palms away from you, let your back round and tuck your chin in, as you push your hands away from you, stretching the arms. Try this sitting on the floor or standing as well.

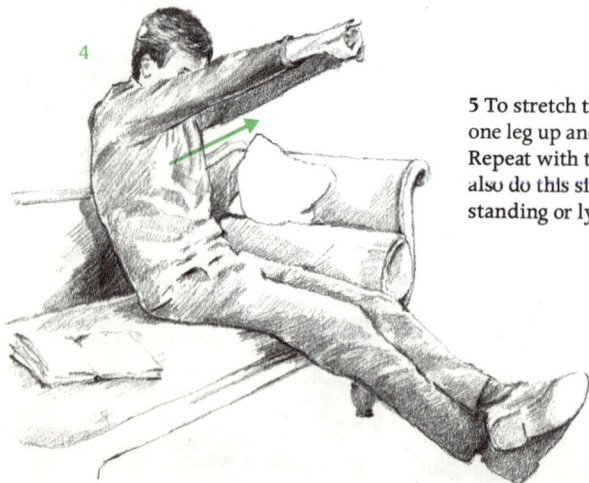

4

5

5 To stretch the lower back, bend one leg up and hug it to you. Repeat with the other leg. You can also do this sitting on the floor, standing or lying on your back.

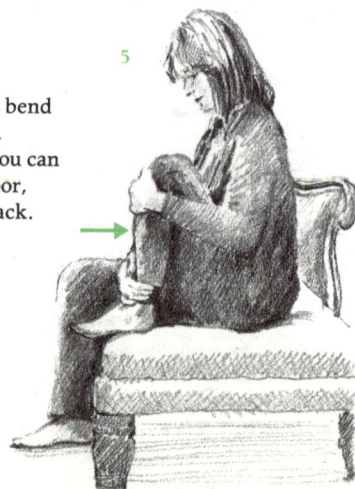

STANDING

1 To strengthen the calves and stimulate circulation in the calves and feet. When standing, on the phone or when ironing for example, rise up and down on your feet.

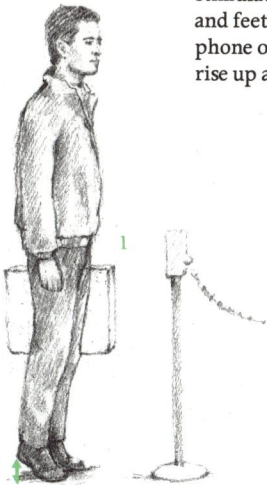

2 To stretch the backs of your legs and spine. Avoid this if your back is weak. Rest your wrists on a worktop or table and lower forwards from the hips, keeping your legs and back straight. Drop your head and pull your shoulder blades together, squeezing the upper back. Lift your head and come up slowly.

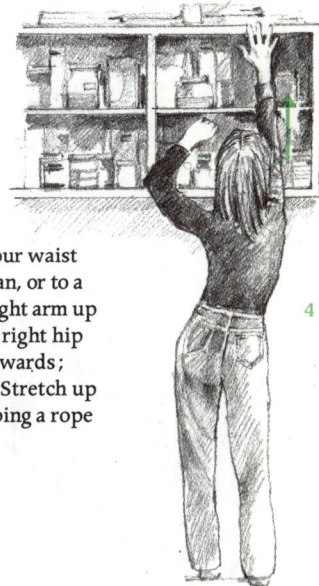

3 A useful exercise to do when working, to release tension and stimulate circulation in the shoulders, and to lift the ribs. Stand under a doorway, far enough back so you have to stretch to reach it, and hold the frame. Lean forwards, with your weight on your arms and breathe deeply. Push your heels down to stretch the calves.

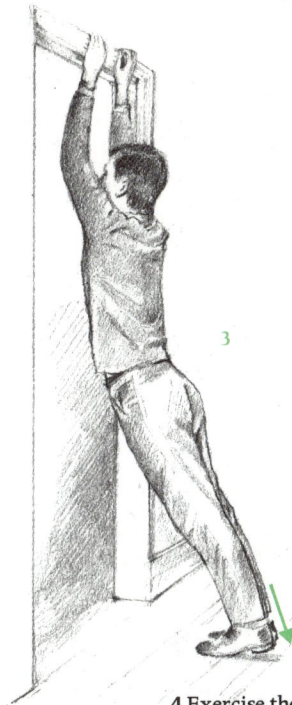

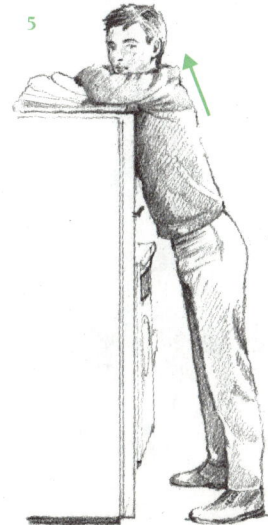

4 Exercise the sides of your waist when reaching up to clean, or to a high shelf. Stretch the right arm up with your weight on the right hip so the left hip moves outwards; repeat with the left arm. Stretch up alternate arms as if climbing a rope ladder.

5 To squeeze and strengthen the upper back; this is useful after carrying heavy bags. Fold your arms and prop them up on a high surface, so the shoulders are lifted.

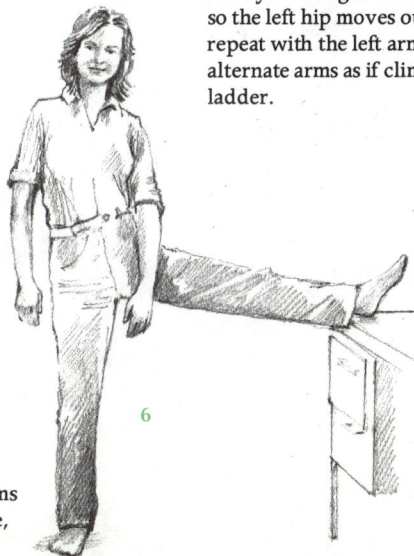

6 To loosen the hips and inside legs, lift the left leg to the side and rest it for a while on a prop such as a stool or desk. Raise the leg only as high as you need for a gentle stretch – you shouldn't feel any pain. Repeat with the right leg. To stretch the backs of the legs, try lifting each leg up in front in the same way.

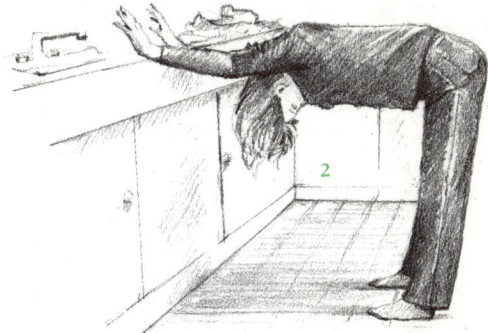

29

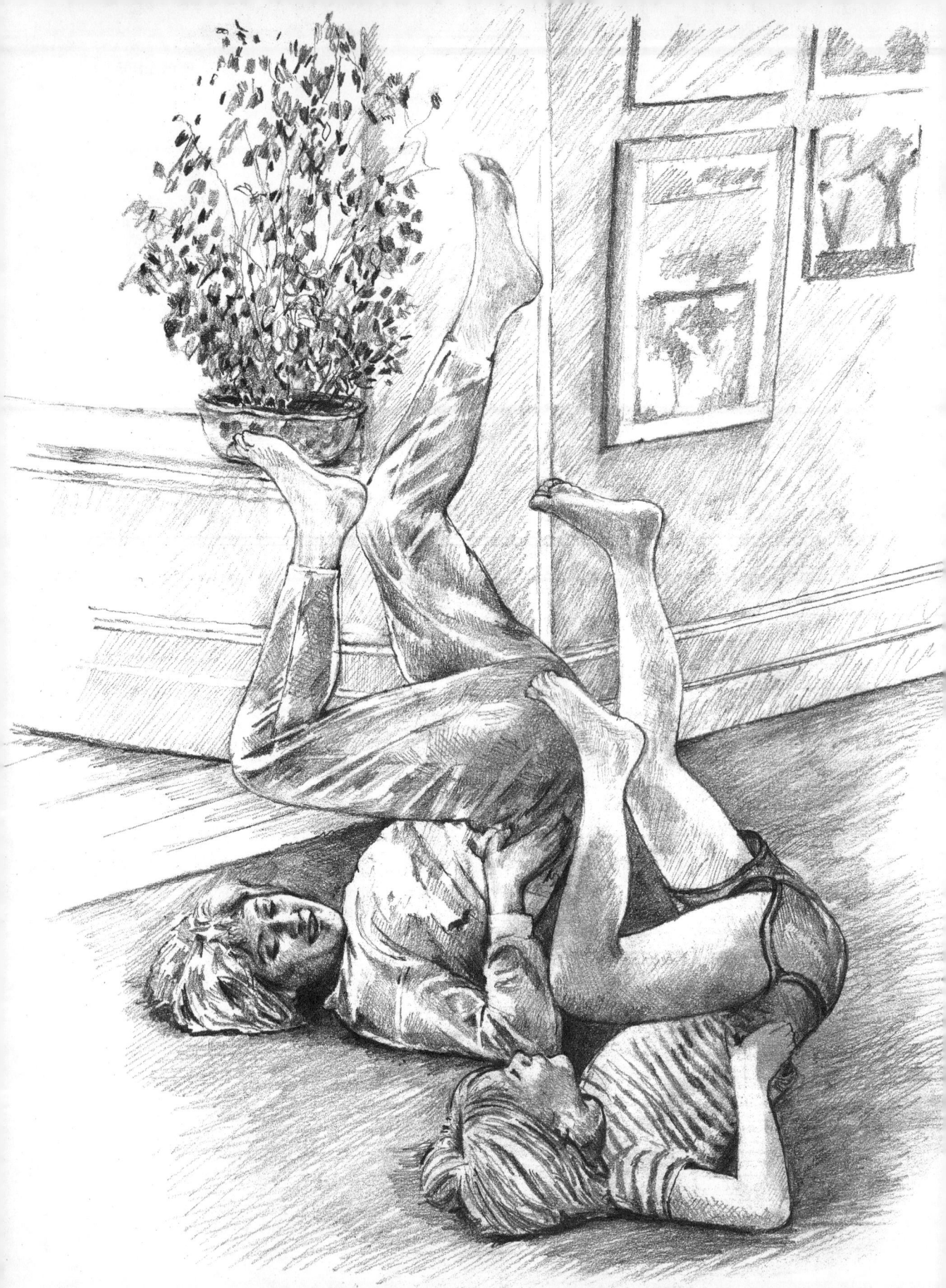

BODYWORK

There are three types of exercise in this section. The basic work-out on pages 32–45 is designed to strengthen, streamline and mobilize the whole body. Even if you've not done any exercise for a long time you can safely begin with this routine: if you're in any doubt about your level of fitness, do consult your doctor before starting though. It's based on the work of Bess Mensendieck, an American doctor who specialized in muscle function and devised her own system of exercises, isolating the various parts of the body in order to concentrate on working each area precisely, yet gently. So, in addition to gaining overall flexibility, you can pick out exercises for problem areas. If your time is at a premium, just do the Daily minimum on pages 32–33.

The next part of the section, a selection of all-over conditioning exercises, on pages 46–51, is for those who are fitter and want a more demanding routine, using up more energy (and calories). You should feel at ease with the exercises on page 25 and with the basic work-out before you start.

Lastly, using weights (see pages 52–55) or exercise machines (see pages 56–59) adds extra resistance to each movement, helping to build up muscles and so improving your physique.

Remember that you're training not straining your muscles. You should feel stretched but pain is always a danger signal – stop whatever you're doing if it hurts. Breathe freely as you move, and always breathe out when bending forwards or contracting the abdomen to avoid squeezing your full lungs and so building up pressure and straining your abdomen and back. At first, try to work little and often, building up gradually. It's better to do an exercise only once or hold a position briefly and get the correct messages across to your body than to tire yourself and perform badly.

Daily minimum

For those with strictly limited time to spend on exercise, the Daily minimum routine on the next two pages is the answer. A basic sequence to keep you in shape, it can be fitted into your day whenever is most convenient. The morning is an excellent time to do it, since many people, especially the over-thirties or those with back problems, tend to wake up feeling stiff. None of the exercises takes up much space, so they can easily be done in a small bathroom and many can even be done in the shower. Indeed, think of them in the same way as brushing your teeth or washing your face, as an integral part of your daily routine. Just as those activities make you feel fresh, so will the exercises. Don't push yourself too hard – do them only as many times as feels reasonably comfortable. If you do each one ten times in the suggested sequence, the whole thing takes ten minutes at most.

Once you know it – and the sequence is very easy to remember – you may like to do your Daily minimum to music. You could also add a few of the exercises from pages 34–45.

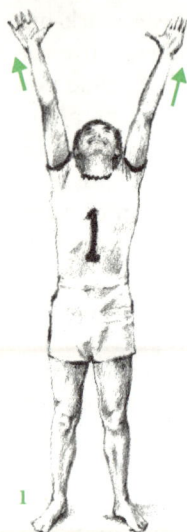

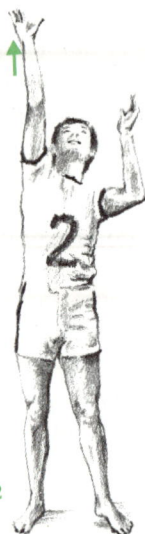

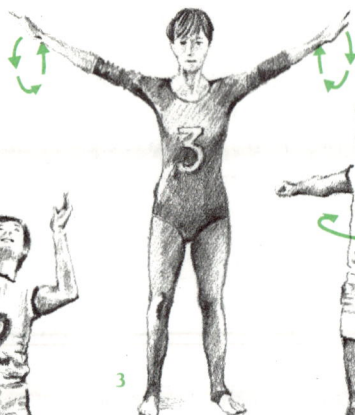

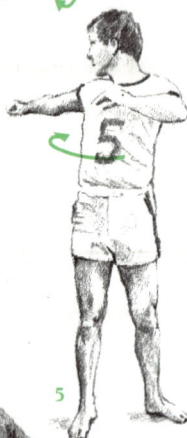

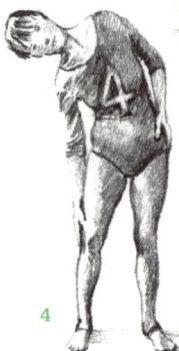

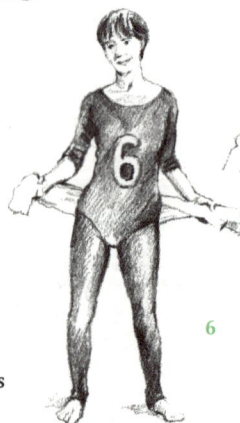

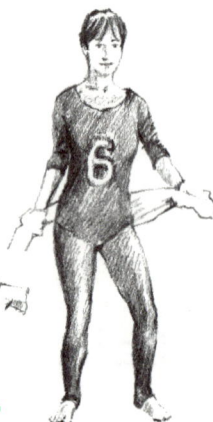

3 Lower the arms to shoulder level and, keeping the elbows straight, make small circles backwards with both arms. Two or three times is enough at first.

5 To mobilize the spine and strengthen abdomen and back muscles, lift the arms to shoulder level and twist your head and chest round to the right, arms following, and then to the left. Swing the arms and let the chest twist as far as it can. Keep your eyes on a particular mark behind you each time to prevent dizziness – this is known as spotting. Both hips should remain facing the front – easy if you keep your bottom tucked under. If you have back trouble or if space is limited, do the twist with your arms down.

It's a good exercise to do in the shower because you get the relaxing hot water on each shoulder as you twist. Afterwards, let the hot water run on the nape of your neck, to reduce tension there.

1 Stand with your feet comfortably apart. Tuck your bottom under gripping your buttocks together. Stretch upwards as far as you can, breathing in deeply. Look up, too, and try to lengthen the centre of the body, so any feeling of heaviness disappears. For a good squeeze between the shoulder blades, try this stretch in a doorway – stand on tiptoe if you are not tall enough to reach the frame (see page 29). Loosen up the shoulder area by letting your body come forwards gently as you stretch.

2 Go on stretching up, first with one arm, then the other – feel the stretch at either side of the body as you pull upwards.

4 Drop the arms and bend sideways from the waist – first to one side and then the other. Keep looking straight to the front and make sure your ear is lined up over your shoulder. Make the bends easy and heavy, breathing out as you bend over and squash your ribs, in as you straighten up in between. Don't let the hips sway from side to side; keep them in place by tucking your bottom well under.

6 This tightens the oblique abdominal muscles, improves the mobility of the lower back and hips and gets the blood flowing. Holding a towel across your lower back, bend your knees and wiggle your pelvis from side to side. This twist can easily be done while you dry yourself after a bath or shower; doing it with a towel also strengthens the arms. Once you've mastered the correct twisting action you can dispense with the towel.

7 To mobilize lower back and hips, tighten abdominal muscles at the sides and help your balance, rock the pelvis from side to side by lifting alternate hips. Lift the right hip up to the right ribs, then do the same to the left.

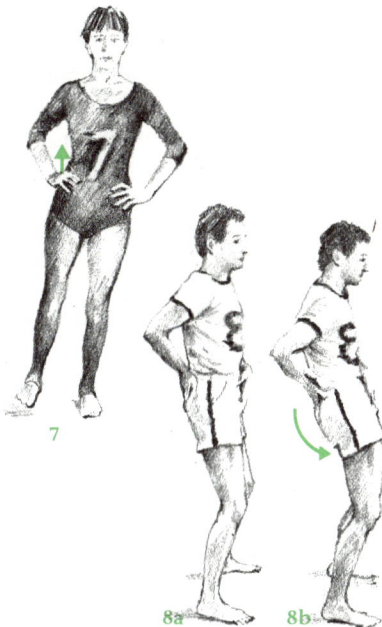

10 Good for heart and lungs, arms and chest muscles, and for stretching Achilles tendons and backs of calves. Stand away from a wall, lean slightly towards it and place your palms flat on it (a). Breathing out, bend your arms and lean forwards, keeping your body in a straight line (b). Breathe in again and straighten your arms, pushing away from the wall.

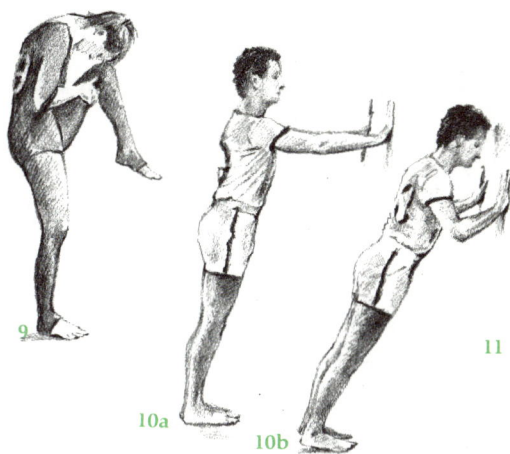

11 Stepping on and off a chair or bench is good for heart and lungs, and strengthens the buttocks and thighs. Lean the body slightly forwards from the hips and step up with the left leg, then the right leg and straighten up completely, with feet together. Step down, left leg first. Straighten up once more. Repeat, changing the leading leg from time to time.

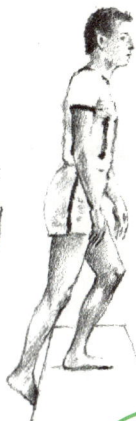

8 This pelvic tilt works the pelvis forwards, tightening the abdominal muscles, then backwards to strengthen the back muscles. Stand with your knees slightly bent and place one hand at the front of the pelvis and one behind (a). Breathe in. Breathing out, push the pelvis forwards (b), then, breathing in, push it right back.

9 This stretches the spine and improves balance. First stand well (see page 12) and take a good breath in. Breathing out, lift your left leg, slipping your hand under the knee, and lower your forehead to touch the knee. Let the standing leg bend slightly. Breathe in as you straighten up, and out as you lift the right leg in the same way. Repeat with alternate legs, standing upright in between. If your balance is bad at first, do the exercise standing against a wall.

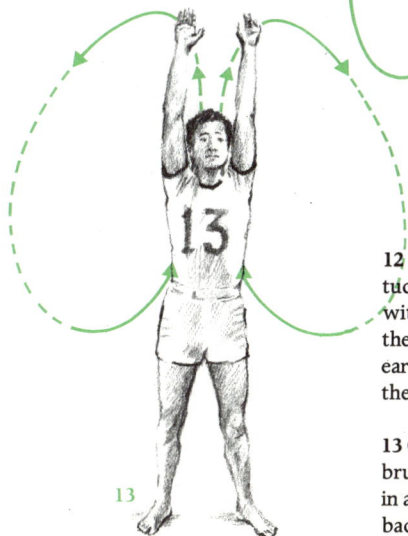

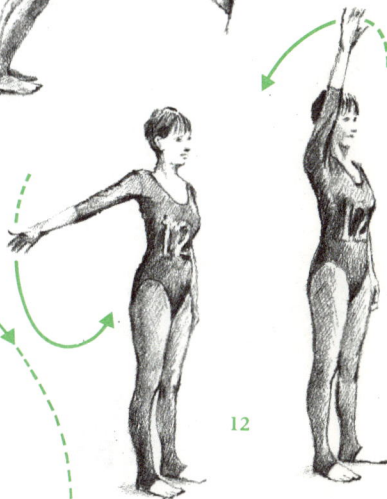

12 Stand with legs apart, bottom tucked under. Make a large circle with the right arm, taking it up to the front, brushing it past the right ear and on back and down. Repeat, then switch to the left arm.

13 Circle both arms up and back, brushing them past the ears. Breathe in as the arms lift, out as they come back and down.

33

Chest and shoulders

The shoulders are the most mobile joints in the whole body: this is why it's so easy to dislocate them – it's especially dangerous to swing or pull a child by the arms. However, this looseness has advantages: the shoulder blades can move about 5 cm [2 in] and pulling them together opens up the chest in front, which encourages good breathing as well as good posture and helps to banish round shoulders. Movement in the shoulders also helps to relieve tension in the upper back.

Strong chest and shoulder muscles are essential for lifting, pushing and pulling, and for carrying heavy loads: these exercises gently develop strength and mobility. Repeat them as often as you like without causing strain; for exercises 5, 6 and 7, build up to about 12 repetitions only. For more strenuous muscle-building routines, see the weight-training exercises on pages 52–55.

1 Strengthens the chest muscles. Stand with arms outstretched sideways, hands loosely fisted and facing forwards (a). Breathe in; breathing out, swing both arms strongly across your chest (b). Breathe in as you swing your arms outwards. Swing to and fro, alternating the upper arm and breathing rhythmically. Repeat with the arms swinging across and up in front of the face (c) and then down in front of the hips (d). *Bonus: strengthens arms, exercises heart and lungs.*

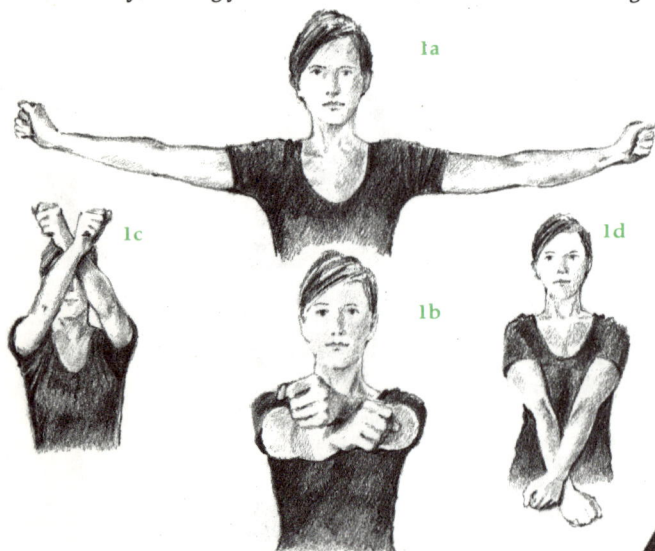

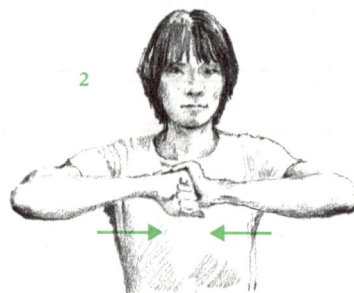

2 Strengthens the chest muscles. Make a loose fist with the right hand and cup the left around it; lift the elbows so your arms are at chest level. Press the hands against each other for a few moments. If you stand in front of a mirror, you can see your chest muscles tighten. Repeat with the right hand clasped round the left.

3 For a stretch between the shoulder blades. Hold your arms straight out in front of you and cross the right elbow over the left (a). Bring the left hand up under the right and gradually lift the arms up in front of you until you feel a stretch between the shoulder blades (b); hold for a while and release. Repeat with left arm uppermost.

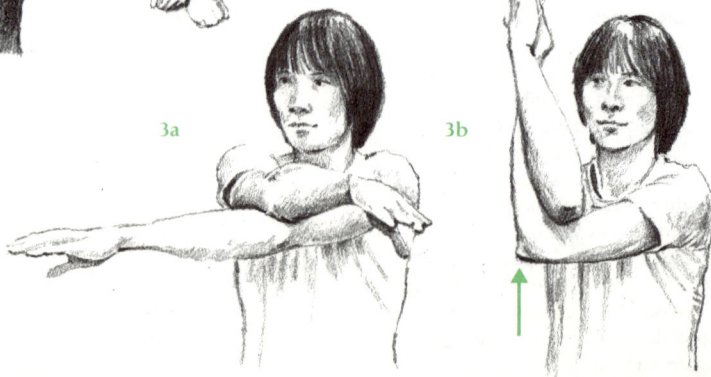

34

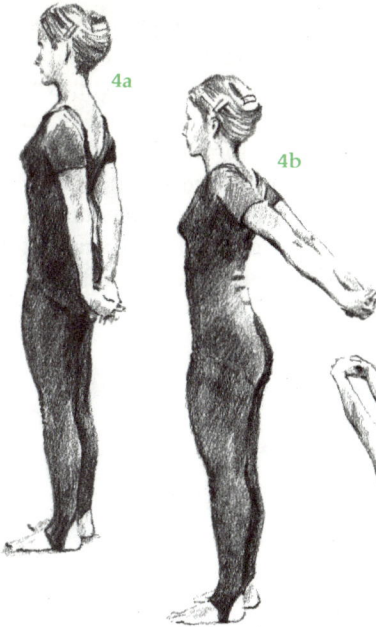

4 To open and lift the chest and squeeze between the shoulder blades. Stand well, with feet slightly apart. Clasp your hands behind you, keeping your arms straight (a). Gently lift them up (b), without bending forwards. If you have no back problems, bend forwards, keeping your hands clasped and letting your head hang, and raise your arms as high as possible (c). Breathe in and straighten up, lifting your head first, so your back straightens as you come up.

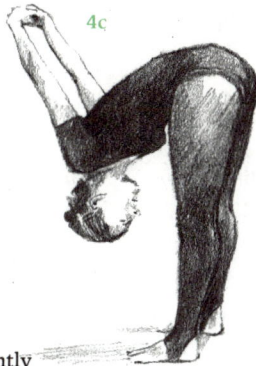

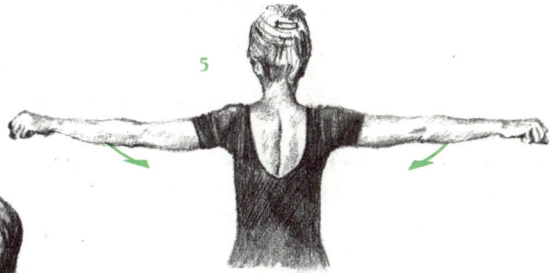

5 Strengthens the upper back and shoulders and opens the chest. Stretch your arms out sideways at shoulder level and make a loose fist with each hand. Pull your shoulder blades together and, holding them in, push your arms backwards in short, sharp swings.

6 Strengthens the chest muscles. These half push-ups are sufficiently strong for most women. Lie face down, palms flat beside your shoulders (a). Breathe in; breathing out, push up, bending at the knees (b). Breathe in as you lower to the floor. *Bonus: strengthens arms, exercises heart and lungs.*

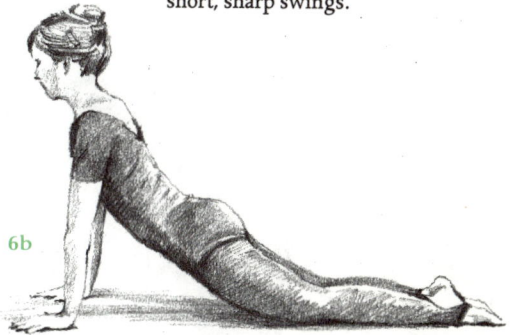

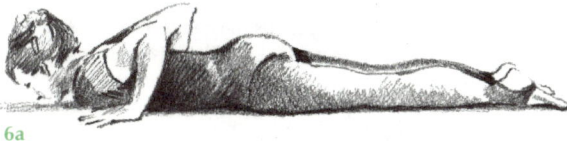

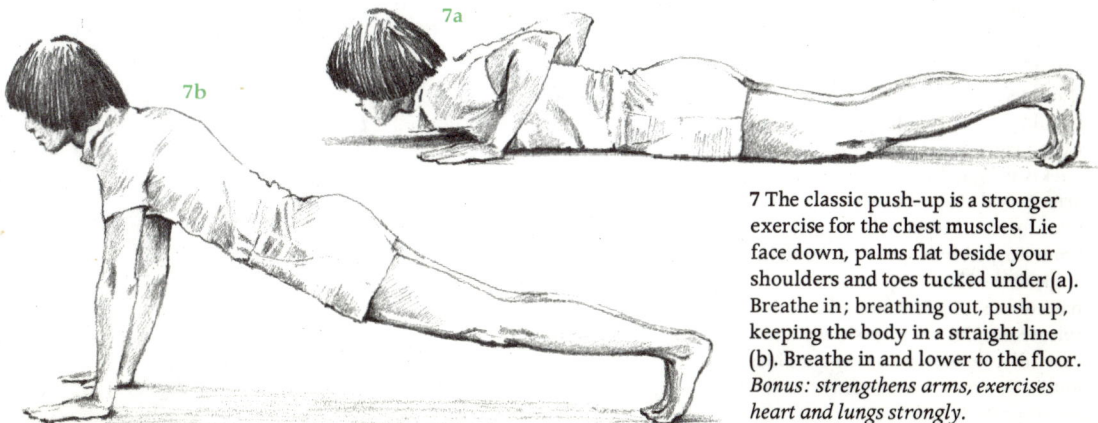

7 The classic push-up is a stronger exercise for the chest muscles. Lie face down, palms flat beside your shoulders and toes tucked under (a). Breathe in; breathing out, push up, keeping the body in a straight line (b). Breathe in and lower to the floor. *Bonus: strengthens arms, exercises heart and lungs strongly.*

35

Arms and hands

These exercises are designed to mobilize the joints of the elbows, wrists and fingers and to strengthen and tighten the muscles. Flexible joints are essential for comfort and are useful for all kinds of movements, from putting on a jacket to reaching up to a shelf. As almost all activities involve working with the arms bent forwards and with rounded fingers, it's important to stretch out the fingers and to pull the arms up and back. If you're prone to flabby upper arms, a common problem for women, exercising can help to tighten and firm them. All the exercises can be done sitting or standing; repeat them as often as is reasonably comfortable.

1 A gentle rotation for the shoulder and elbow joints. Hold your arms out a little way from the body, palms facing upwards (a). Try to turn the little fingers up and backwards. Bend the elbows and turn the arms over, rotating your wrists so that the palms still face up. Restraighten the elbows and turn the arms as much as possible (b), trying to turn the thumbs forwards. Bend the elbows as you return to (a): the movement should be flowing, rather like an Indian dancer.

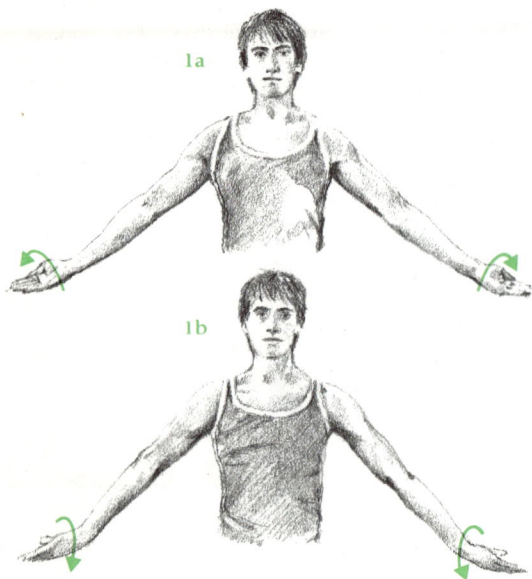

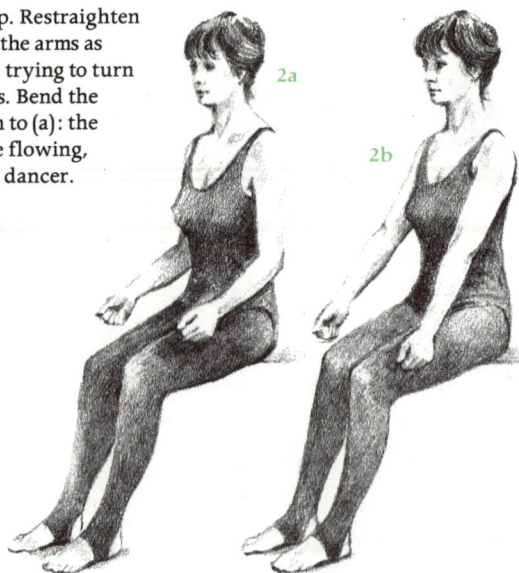

2 Tightens the backs of the upper arms. Make a loose fist with each hand and bend your arms slightly (a). Punch forwards and downwards strongly with both arms (b).

3 A stronger rotation for the shoulder joints. Lift your arms to shoulder level, bending them up to form a right angle and press backwards (a). Keeping the upper arms raised at shoulder level, turn your forearms so that the fingers point downwards, holding the right angle at the elbow (b). Press backwards for a few moments and release. Do this exercise slowly and carefully, never forcing the shoulder joints. You may manage only one or two repeats at first.

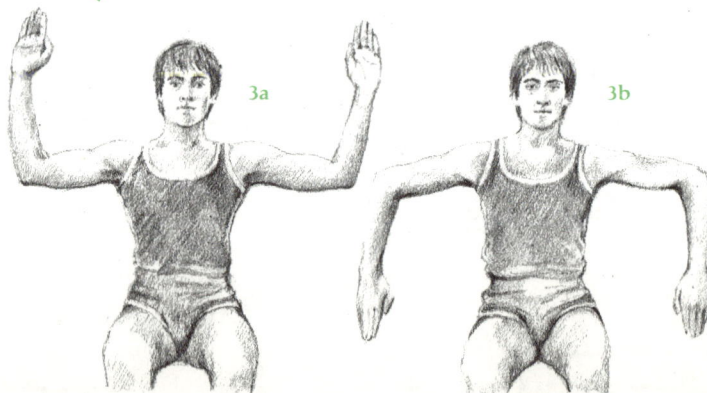

4 A stronger exercise for tightening the backs of the upper arms. Sit with arms bent forwards, hands in loose fists (a). Straighten the arms backwards, punching them back as far as possible (b). The backs of the upper arms may well feel stiff afterwards; if so, repeat the exercise and the stiffness will lessen.

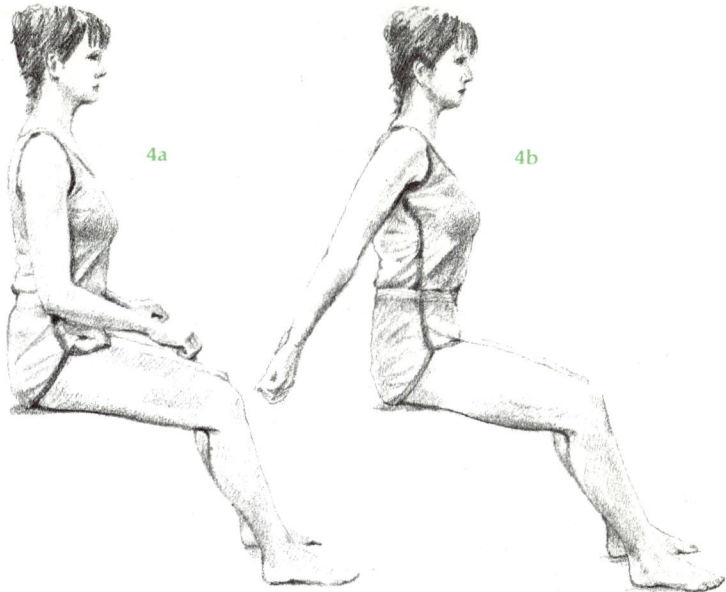

4a

4b

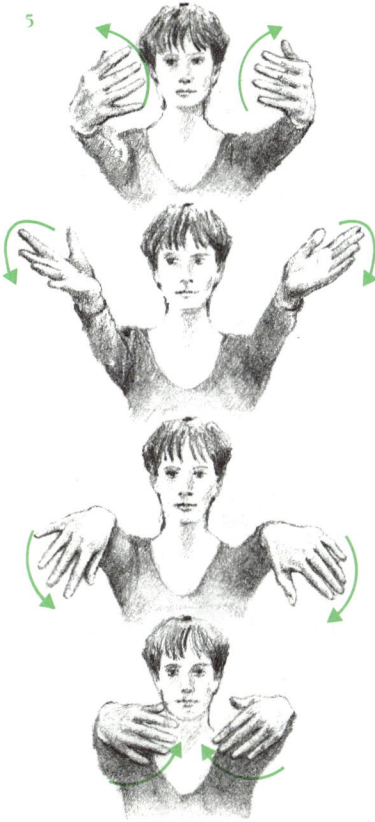

5

5 For mobility of the wrist joints. Hold the arms straight out in front so the elbow joints are locked and the wrists have to do all the work. Rotate your hands, drawing circles in the air. Make this a flowing, easy movement. Repeat in the opposite direction.

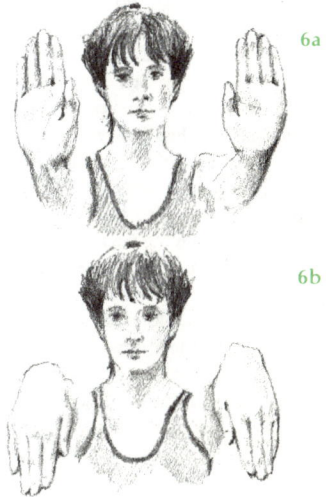

6a

6b

6 For mobility in the wrists. With arms straight out in front, elbows locked, lift your hands up and back as far as possible, fingers stretching upwards (a). Push the hands down, so the fingers point to the floor (b).

7 Stretches the finger joints and helps to maintain their mobility. Practise this whenever you can: it's especially useful if you tend to clench your fists (see Relaxing your muscles, pages 208–209). Rest the wrists on a support such as your thighs, chair arms or steering wheel (a). Stretch the fingers and thumbs up and out, making as much space as possible between them (b). Let them go, so they fall back on to the support.

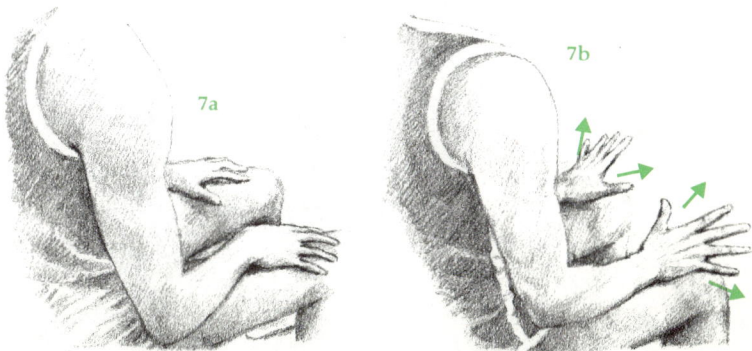

7a

7b

37

Abdomen and back

The way you hold and move your trunk is of great importance to how you look and the condition of the spine. The muscles of the back and abdomen both support the trunk and so, to prevent backache and for a flat, firm abdomen, they must be strong and properly used.

The strengthening of the abdominal and back muscles must be a slow and gentle process, however, if it's to be effective in improving the everyday use of the body – and this is what's important. You must gradually train the muscles to support your trunk more efficiently, so lifting and lightening the burden on the spine and making it more mobile.

Start with exercises 1 to 5, and don't move on to exercises 6 to 11 until you feel you have mastered the first five; never begin with the harder exercises. Don't force yourself to hold a position or repeat an exercise more often than is reasonably comfortable.

1 To straighten the spine and so strengthen the back and abdomen. Sit with an upright back, sideways on to a mirror or ask a friend to help. Look to see if your back is really straight; you may find that it's rounded. Straighten up (a); bend the legs if necessary and try to re-straighten them gradually. If you can't quite straighten your back, put a belt or folded towel round your feet and, holding on to it, lift your ribcage upwards (b). This strengthens and lifts the back. *Bonus: stretches the backs of the legs.* For beginners, placing the fists behind you gives extra support for the back. Do not let your shoulders lift but bend the elbows and pull them together, as in (c). If you still find it difficult to straighten your back, try practising this exercise sitting against a wall or against a sofa for support.

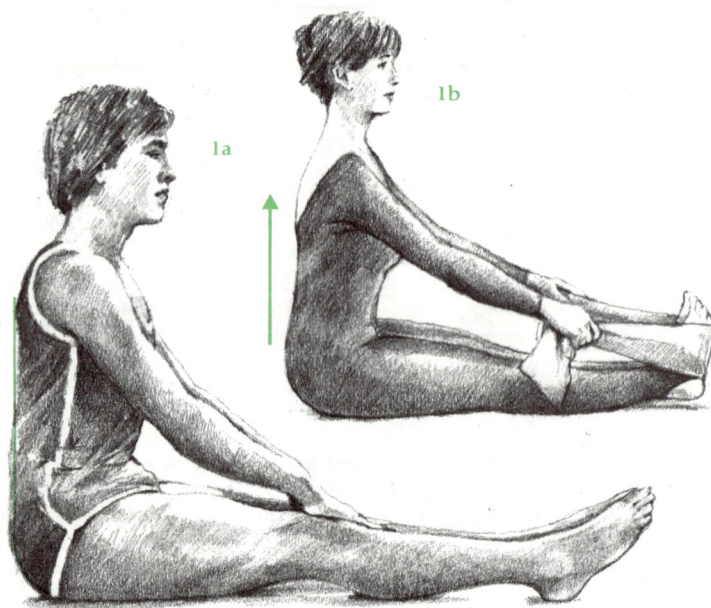

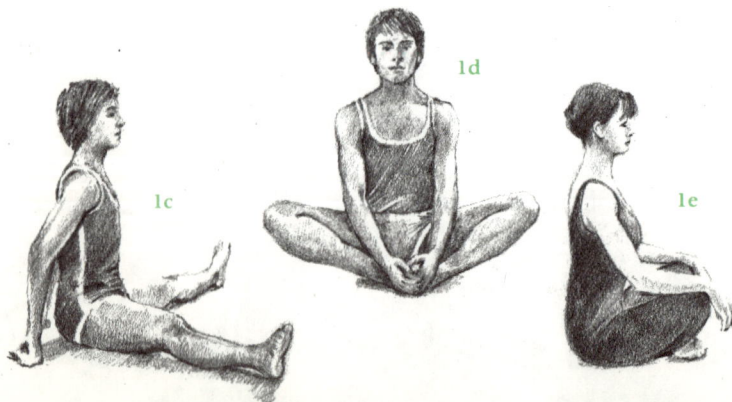

For a change, try straightening your back while sitting with your legs straight and apart (c). *Bonus: stretches the inside thighs.* Or sit with the soles of the feet pressed together. Hold on to the feet or ankles while lifting your ribcage and straightening your back (d). *Bonus: loosens the hip joints and the thighs.* Or straighten your back while sitting with crossed legs. Make sure that the same leg is not always in front as you practise this movement (e).

2a

2b

2c

2d

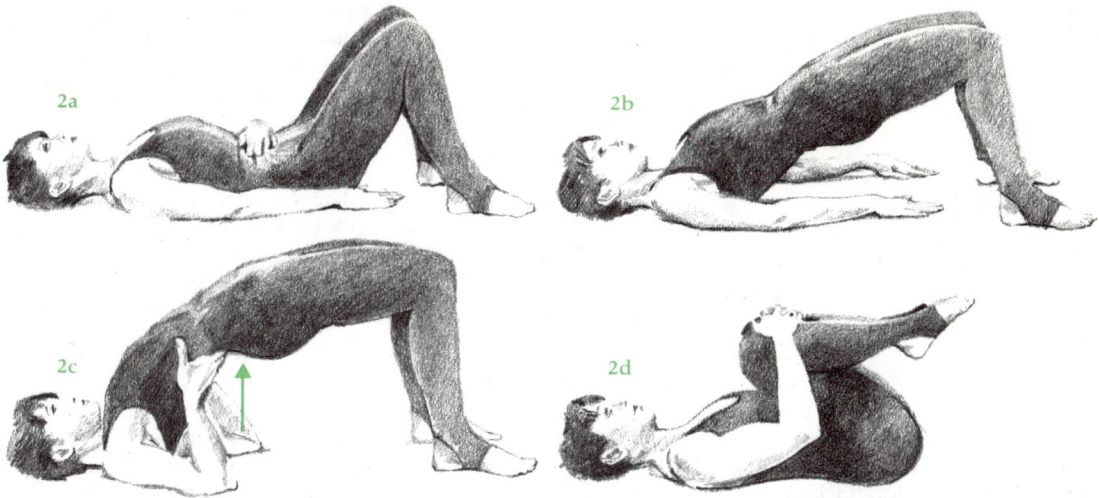

2 Strengthens the abdominal and back muscles. Lie facing up with knees bent and feet apart. Breathe in; breathe out, tilting your pubic bone up and sucking your abdomen in, so the back of your waist presses into the floor (a). With your arms by your sides, palms down, push your hips up (b). Place your hands under your waist and lift the hips up as far as you can (c). If possible, take your hands away and stay lifted for a few moments. Return to the floor, going through the pelvic tilt position. Still lying on your back, give your spine a stretch by bending your knees up to your chest and clasping your hands round them (d).

3 Tightens up the abdominal muscles. Lie facing up, hands resting on your thighs. Breathe out as you flex your feet up and lift your head to look at your toes. At the same time, pull your abdomen in and reach towards your toes. Breathe in as you relax the feet and return your head to the floor.

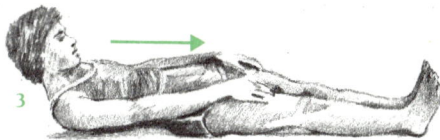

3

4 Mobilizes the back and strengthens the abdomen and back. Kneel on all fours. Breathe in and arch the middle of the back down as far as possible, looking up (a). Breathe out and round the middle of the back up, tucking the head in and pulling in the abdomen (b).

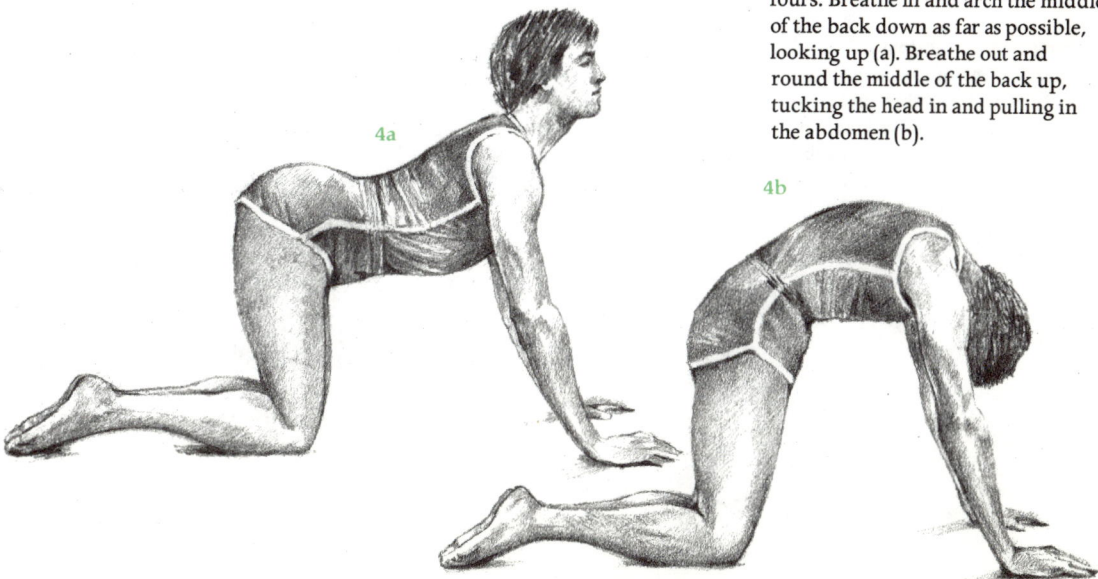

4a

4b

39

▷

5a

5b

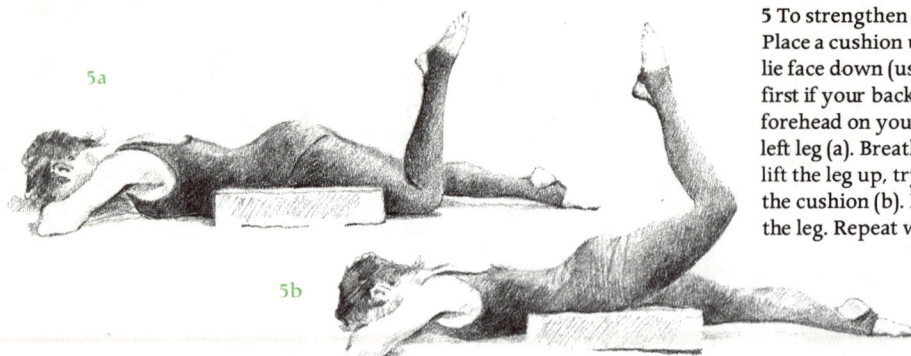

5 To strengthen the lower back. Place a cushion under the hips and lie face down (use two cushions at first if your back is weak); rest your forehead on your hands. Bend your left leg (a). Breathe in; breathing out, lift the leg up, trying to raise it off the cushion (b). Breathe in and lower the leg. Repeat with the right leg.

6 Tightens the abdominal muscles. Lie facing up, knees bent and feet apart (a). Breathing out, lift your head and shoulders only, reaching forwards and pulling your abdomen in (b). Breathing in, lie back.

Breathing out, lift your head and shoulders to the right, reaching forwards so your shoulders and arms pull towards the right knee (c). Feel a squeeze in the left side. Breathing in, lie back. Repeat to the left and to

the centre, breathing out as you lift up and in as you lie back. Resting your head on the floor, roll it gently from side to side to ease any tension that may have built up in the neck muscles during the exercise.

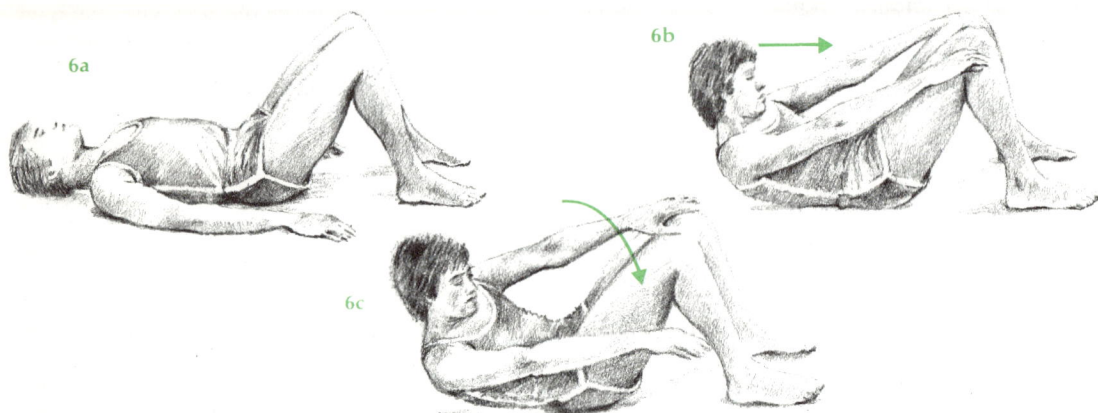

6a

6b

6c

7 Strengthens the abdominal muscles. Lie on your back with knees bent, feet together, and breathe in. Breathe out as you half sit up, lifting only the upper back off the floor and letting your head roll back if possible. Breathe in as you lower your back on to the floor.

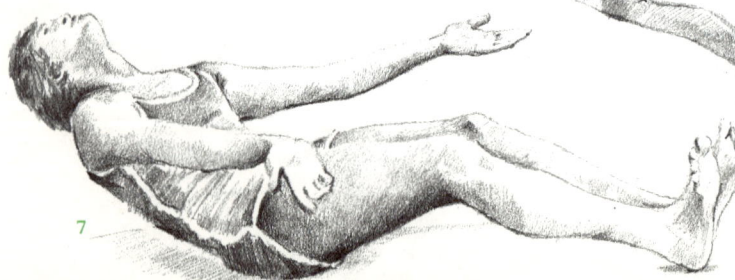

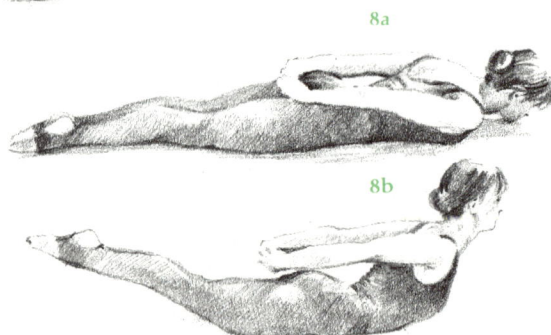

8a

8b

7

8 Strengthens the back. Lie facing down, hands clasped behind you and feet together (a). Breathe in and lift your head, shoulders and legs (b). Hold as long as possible. Breathe out and lower to the floor.

9 To strengthen the abdomen. Lie facing up, a cushion under your hips, legs bent, feet together (a). Bend both legs to your chest (b).

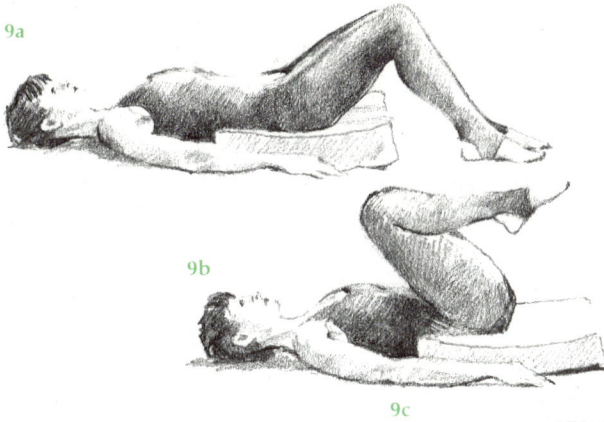

Straighten the legs, stretching them upwards as much as possible and pulling the abdomen in strongly (c). Hold for a few moments. Return to

(b) and take a deep breath before straightening the legs up again. Repeat. When this movement has become easy, lower the left leg towards you and the right leg away from you (d), breathing out, but go no further than shown, as you may strain your back. Breathing in, bring the legs together and repeat the scissoring movements with the right leg pulled towards you, the left away from you.

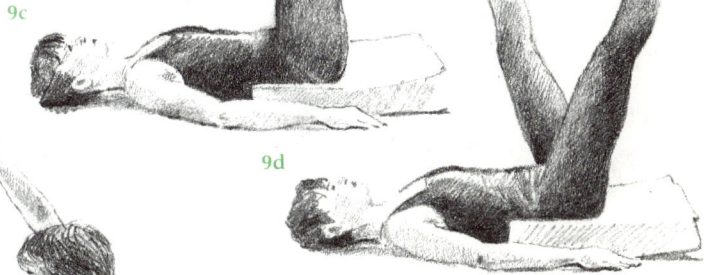

9a

9b

9c

9d

10 Strengthens the diagonal muscles of the back. Lie facing down, arms stretched out in front of you. Breathe in and lift your head, chest, right arm and left leg. Breathing out, lower to the floor. Repeat with the other arm and leg.

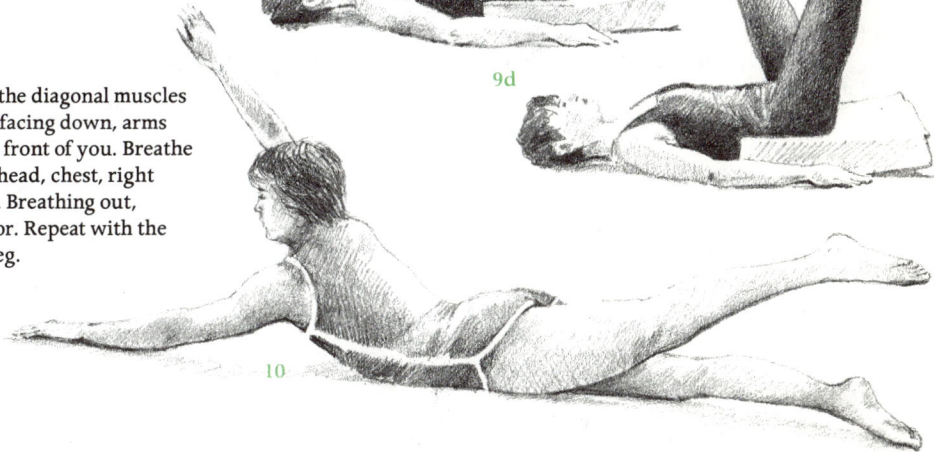

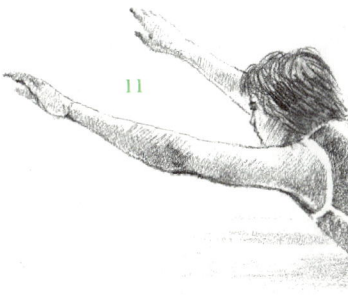

10

11 Strengthens the back. Lie facing down, arms stretched out in front of you. Breathe in and lift your head, chest, both arms and both legs. Breathe out as you lower to the floor.

11

12 To stretch out the back: always do this for a few minutes after any strenuous back work. Kneel and curl into a ball, tucking your head down, hands resting by your feet, with the palms facing up.

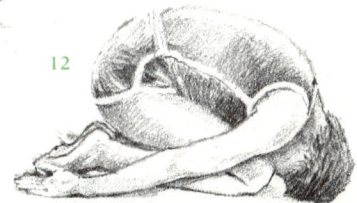

12

Bottom and hips

Both mobility and strength are essential for this area: the hip joints need to be moved in every direction to keep them flexible and the buttock muscles must be worked to keep them in shape. Everyday movements, such as climbing stairs, are helpful (see page 26).

Too much flesh on the hips and buttocks is a problem that mainly affects women, but whereas female hips are intended to be rounded, fat buttocks are not part of the blueprint for either men or women. The buttocks belong behind you, forming a tight, firm bottom to help support the trunk. Diet is essential to slim away excess fat, but exercise and good posture (see pages 12–15) can tighten up contours and help to correct bulges at the sides of the legs. Repeat each exercise up to 12 times, or until you've had enough.

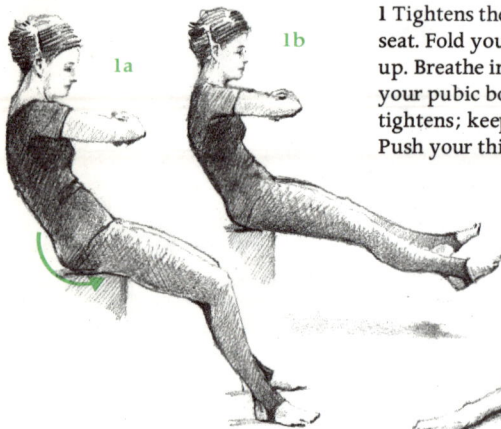

1 Tightens the buttocks. Sit on a hard seat. Fold your arms and hold them up. Breathe in; breathing out, tilt your pubic bone up so the abdomen tightens; keep it tilted throughout. Push your thighs down so your bottom lifts, squeezing the buttocks together tightly (a). Repeat, sometimes slowly, sometimes quickly. If you have no back trouble, lift your legs at the same time, keeping the pelvis tilted (b).

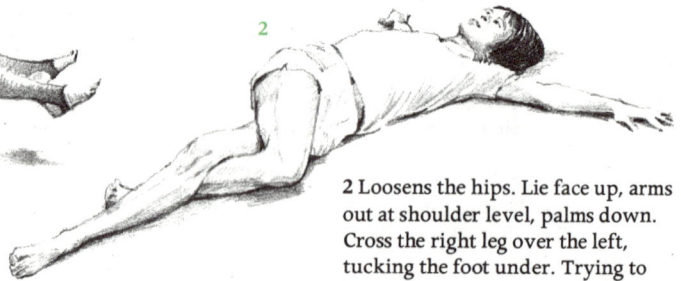

2 Loosens the hips. Lie face up, arms out at shoulder level, palms down. Cross the right leg over the left, tucking the foot under. Trying to keep your shoulders on the floor, drop the right knee to the left and hold. Repeat with the left leg.

3 To strengthen and mobilize the hips. Stand facing a wall or worktop, fingertips on it for balance, feet together. Lift the right hip (a). With the foot flexed up and knee facing forwards, slowly lift the leg to the right, until it squeezes the hip (b). Slowly lower the leg until the foot touches the floor and lift again. Repeat. Turn the right leg outwards. Lift it diagonally back, with the foot flexed (c), and lower it. Repeat. Letting the foot hang loosely, raise and lower the right leg backwards (d). Repeat the entire sequence with the left leg. Afterwards, bend forwards from the hips with knees bent to stretch out the lower back area; if your back is weak, try exercise 12 on page 41 instead.

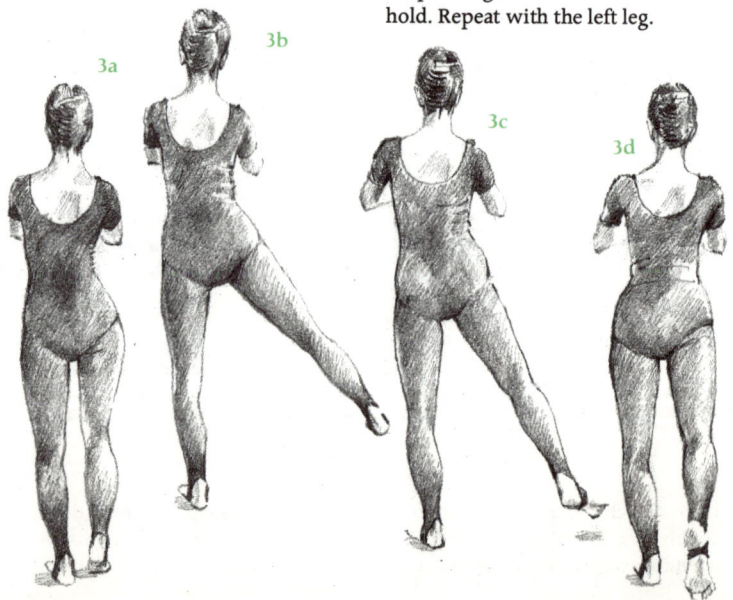

4a

4b

4c

5a

5b

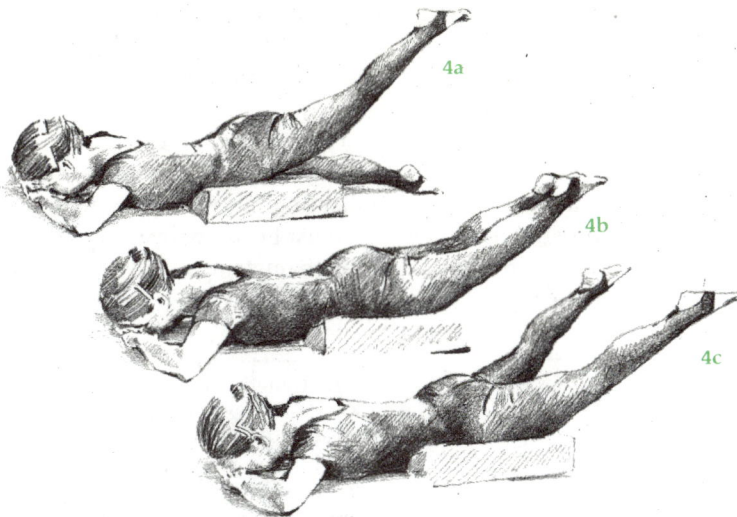

4 To tighten the buttocks. With a cushion under your hips, lie face down (use two at first if your back is weak); rest your forehead on your hands. Feel all your weight in your chest, so the elbows lift easily. Breathe in; breathing out, raise the left leg slowly, lifting the thigh up off the cushion if you can (a). Breathing in, lower the leg slowly. Repeat and switch to the right leg. If you find this movement easy, repeat with both legs, first together (b), then apart (c). *Bonus: mobilizes and strengthens the lower back.*

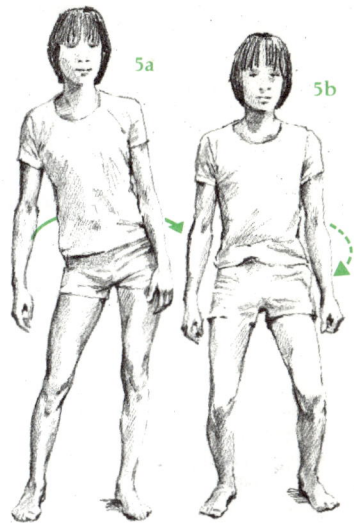

5 To increase mobility in the hips and work the buttocks. Standing with feet apart, knees bent, circle the hips to the left (a), forwards (b), to the right and backwards. Repeat, reversing the direction. Try this exercise kneeling down as well.

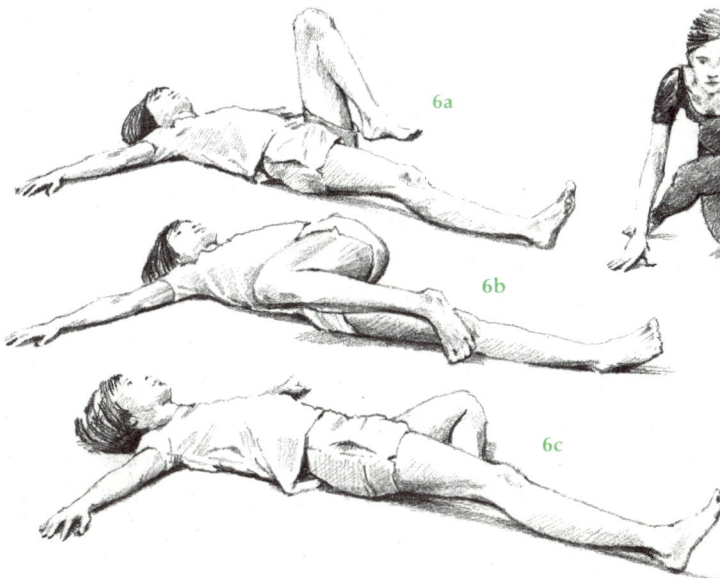

6a

6b

7a

7b

6c

6 To mobilize the hips and work the buttocks. Lie facing up, arms out to the sides, palms facing down. Keeping your shoulders on the floor throughout, bend up the left leg (a) and lower it across your body (b). Raise it to the centre and lower it outwards (c). Return it to the centre and slide the foot along the floor, straightening the leg. Repeat with the right leg. *Bonus: mobilizes the lower back.*

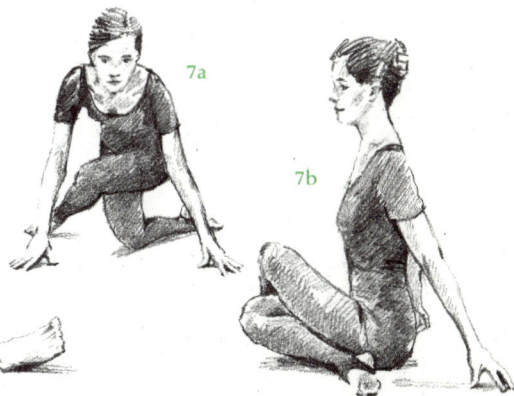

7 Loosens the hips and thighs. Be gentle as the stretch may be strong at first. Kneel down, put your hands on the floor in front of you and cross the left leg over the right (a). Separate the feet so you can sit between them and walk your hands back, taking your weight on them. If this is easy, lower your bottom and sit with a straight back (b). Hold either position for a while, without straining. Repeat, crossing your legs the other way.

43

Legs and feet

Strong and flexible legs and feet are essential not only for mobility but for a general feeling of well-being. As well as making the joints more mobile, these exercises stretch and strengthen all the muscles and help to tighten flabby inner thighs.

It's important to strengthen the quadriceps, the large muscles at the front of the thighs, as these enclose and protect the knee-caps; strong quadriceps also prevent fat collecting above the knees, a problem for some women. The hamstrings must be loose for the quadriceps to work properly and unless your hamstrings and Achilles tendons are flexible you may damage them with a sudden movement. Repeat each exercise until you begin to tire.

1 Tightens the inner thighs. Stand with legs apart, feet parallel (a). Press your legs inwards strongly so the feet roll in slightly and the inner thigh muscles tighten (b). Hold for a few moments.

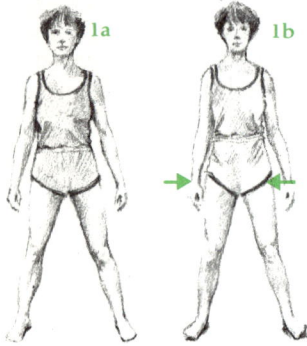

2 To strengthen the quadriceps. Kneel with legs apart, arms stretched forwards (a). Breathe in; breathing out, tilt your pubic bone up in front and lean back as far as possible, breathing normally (b, c). Feel your thighs working to prevent you falling back. Breathe in as you straighten up.

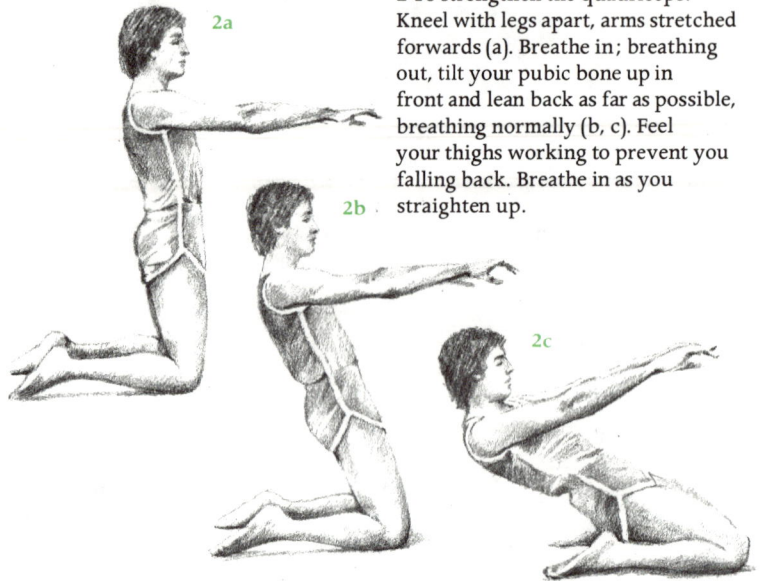

3 This helps to strengthen the quadriceps. Stand a little way from a wall, fingertips resting on it for balance, and rise up on to the balls of your feet (a). Breathe in; breathing out, tilt your pubic bone up in front and bend the knees, leaning back at the same time (b). You will feel a tightening above the knees. Breathe normally, retain the pelvic tilt and do some small extra knee bends.

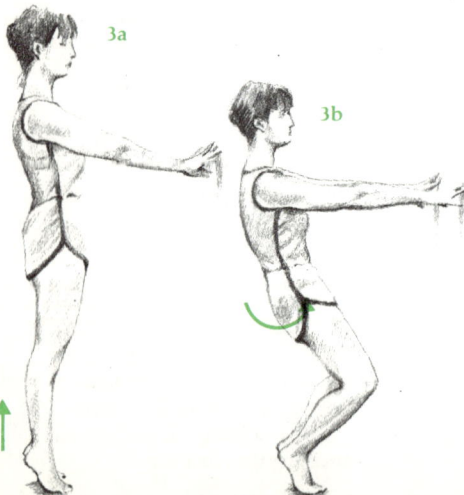

4 To strengthen the calves and stimulate the circulation in them. Stand with feet together, facing a wall, fingertips resting on it for balance. Rise up on to the balls of your feet, keeping the heels together. Lower your heels half way to the floor and lift again.

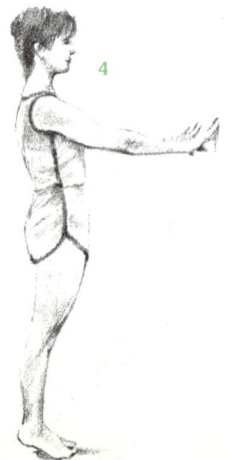

44

5 Stretches the quadriceps and also works on balance. Stand on one leg and bend the other up behind you, catching it with both hands. Try to bring the heel in to touch the buttocks. If this is easy, tilt your pubic bone up as well. Repeat with the other leg.

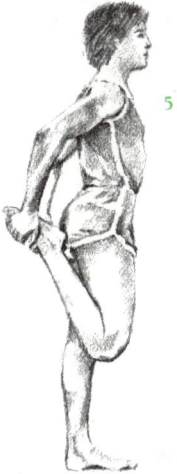

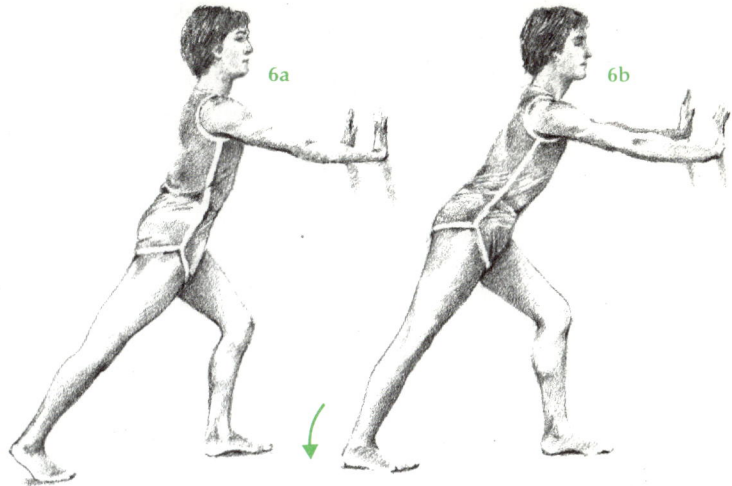

6 Stretches the backs of the calves and the Achilles tendons. This is important for sports players and joggers, who need pliable Achilles tendons, and also for women who wear high heels, as they tend to shorten the muscles at the backs of the calves, sometimes causing cramp. Stand facing a wall, hands on it for balance (a). Step forwards with the left foot, bending the knee. Press the right heel down (b). If this is hard, bounce gently on the left leg. Repeat with the other leg.

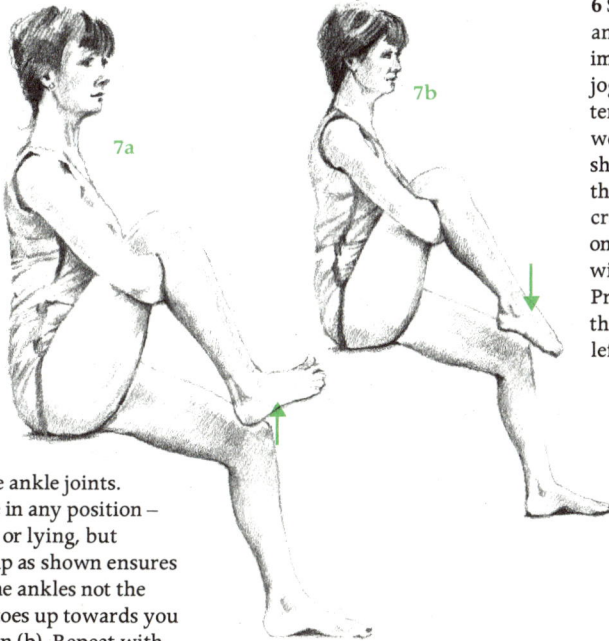

7 To mobilize the ankle joints. This can be done in any position – standing, sitting or lying, but holding the leg up as shown ensures that you work the ankles not the calves. Flex the toes up towards you (a) and then down (b). Repeat with the other foot.

8 To strengthen and stretch the feet. Sit with heels resting on the floor and feet flexed up. Curl the toes under and squeeze tightly (a).

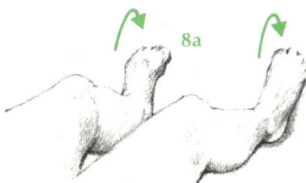

Stretch the toes out as much as possible (b). Don't worry if there isn't much movement; flexibility will slowly develop.

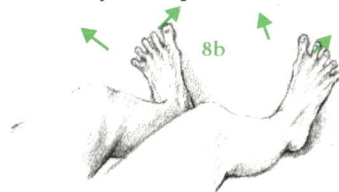

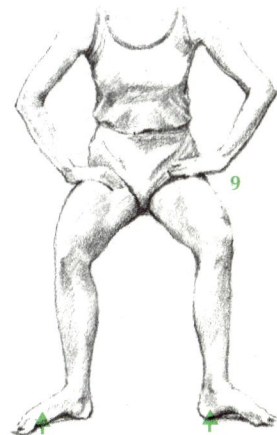

9 To strengthen the arches of the feet. Sit with feet flat on the floor. Without raising the feet, draw the toes in towards the heel so the centre of the foot lifts; hold for a few moments.

Super-conditioners

These exercises are designed to strengthen and stretch your whole body and to condition the heart and lungs: each one benefits several areas at the same time. They should be attempted only when you're sure that your posture is good (see pages 12–15) and that you're fit and flexible – you should be able to pass the fitness test on page 25 and do at least the Daily minimum from the work-out on pages 32–45 without undue strain. It's all too easy to pull a muscle if you launch into these exercises without knowing your limits. Warm up beforehand with the short routine on pages 70–71.

The harder you work the more important it is to be relaxed. These exercises should be fun, with a swing and flow to them – try doing them to lively music. Breathe well and don't hold your breath. If your back is weak or stiff, don't attempt the forward-bending exercises. Otherwise, repeat each exercise *but never persist until it becomes a strain.*

STANDING EXERCISES

1 Stand with feet apart, arms outstretched (a). Push your ribs to the left, stretching out the left arm (b). Return to (a) and push your ribs to the right, stretching out the right arm (c). Return to the starting position.

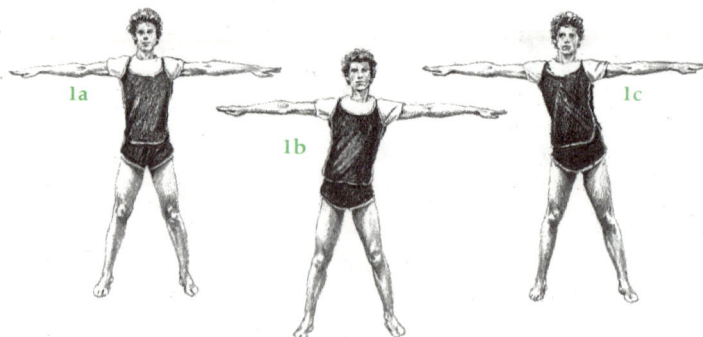

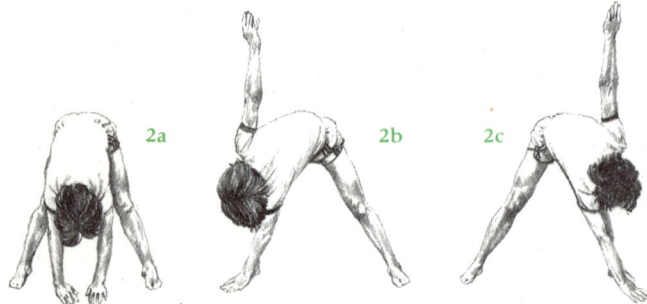

2 With feet apart, bend from the hips, letting your head and hands hang loosely (a). Reach for your right foot with your left hand, stretching your right arm up behind you and looking to the right (b). Swing to the left, changing arms and looking to the left (c).

3 Stand with feet apart, arms outstretched (a). Turn to the right, lifting your left arm up (b). Swing it down to touch your right foot (c). Swing back to (a) and repeat to the other side in a continuous movement.

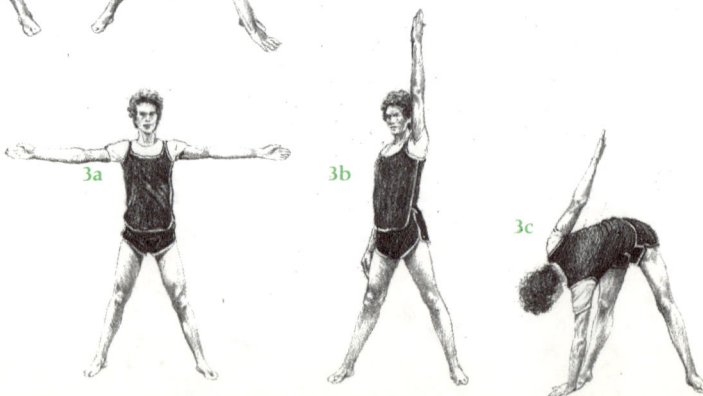

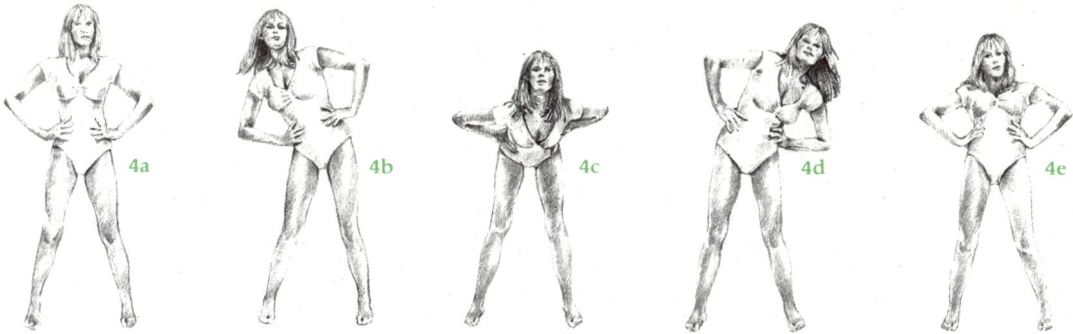

4 Stand with your hands on your hips, feet apart (a). Bend from the waist to the right (b), forwards (c), to the left (d) and backwards (e) in a smooth circular movement. Change to the opposite direction.

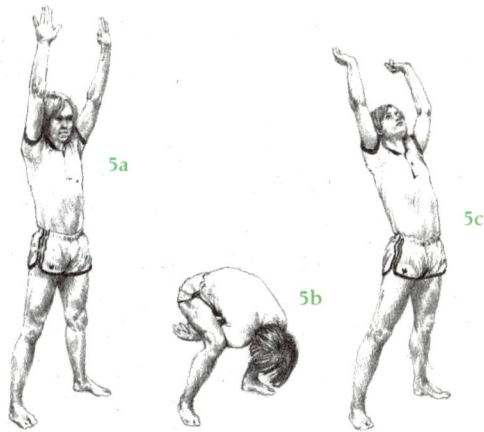

5 Stand with feet apart, arms stretched upwards (a). Drop forwards, letting your knees bend and swinging your arms through your legs (b). Straighten up, lifting your arms up and stretch back a little (c).

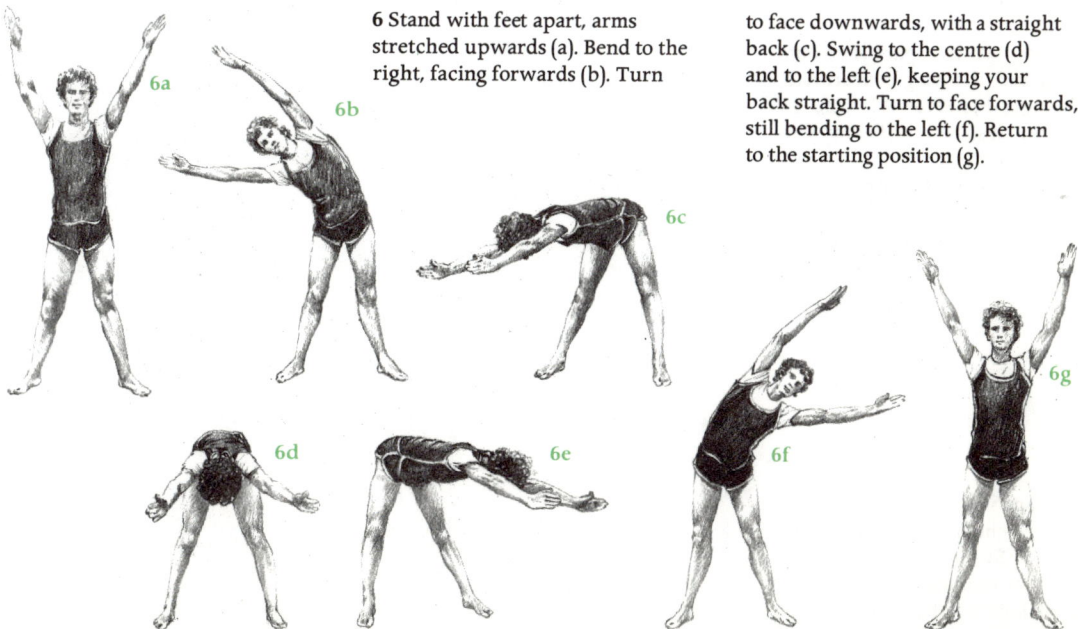

6 Stand with feet apart, arms stretched upwards (a). Bend to the right, facing forwards (b). Turn to face downwards, with a straight back (c). Swing to the centre (d) and to the left (e), keeping your back straight. Turn to face forwards, still bending to the left (f). Return to the starting position (g).

47

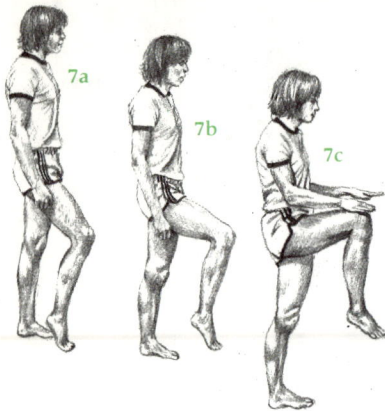

7 Standing well, lift your right heel and press the ball of the right foot into the floor (a). Repeat and change to the left foot. Spring from one foot to the other (b), going through the ball of the foot, as in (a). Bend your arms, hands pointing to the front, elbows by your lower ribs and spring from foot to foot, lifting your right thigh up to your right hand (c), and your left thigh up to your left hand.

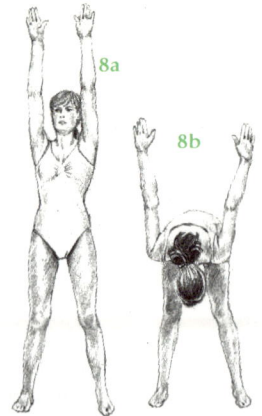

8 Stand with feet apart, arms stretched upwards (a). Bend forwards from the hips and swing your arms up behind you (b). Return to the starting position.

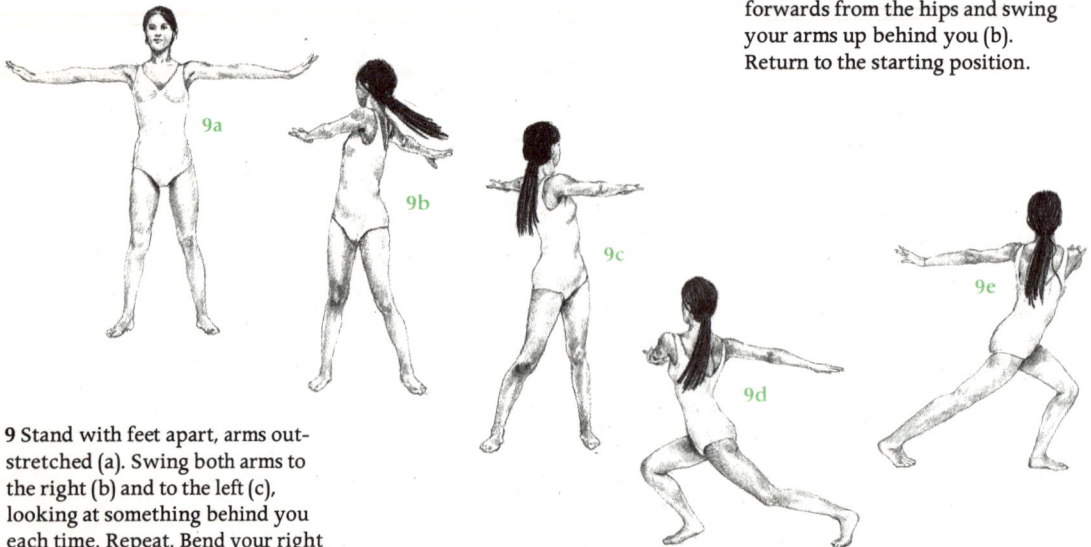

9 Stand with feet apart, arms out-stretched (a). Swing both arms to the right (b) and to the left (c), looking at something behind you each time. Repeat. Bend your right leg as you swing to the right (d) and your left leg as you swing to the left (e) so you can turn further.

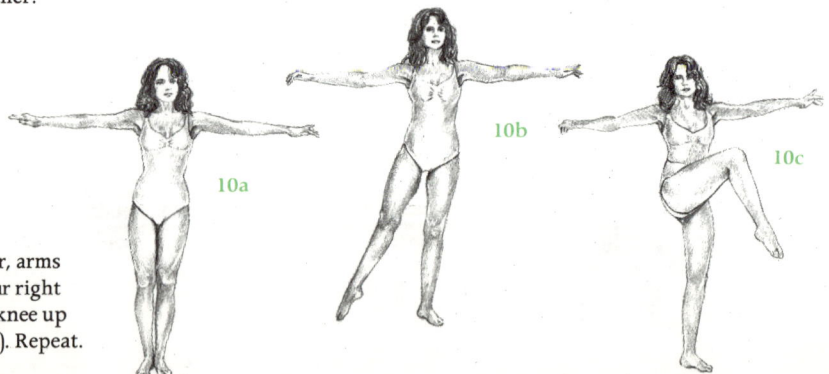

10 Stand with feet together, arms outstretched (a). Point your right toes (b). Swing your right knee up towards your left elbow (c). Repeat. Switch to the other side.

11a 11b 11c 11d

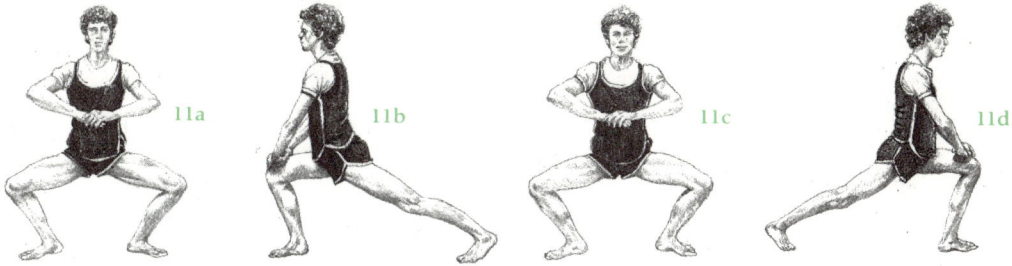

11 Stand with feet apart, hands resting one on the other. Turn your legs out and bend your knees (a). Bounce up, turn and lunge to the right, straightening your left leg and resting your hands on your right knee (b). Return to the centre (c) and lunge to the left (d).

12a 12b 12c

12 Standing with feet slightly apart, leap up and bend your legs as you come down, hands on the floor for balance on either side of your legs (a). Jump up (b) and bend your legs to the left, returning your hands to the same position so your chest faces forwards (c). Repeat to the centre and to the right.

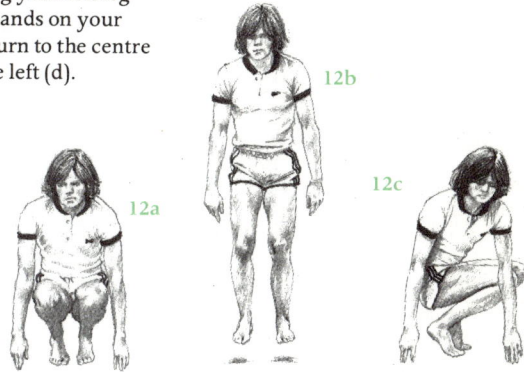

FLOOR EXERCISES

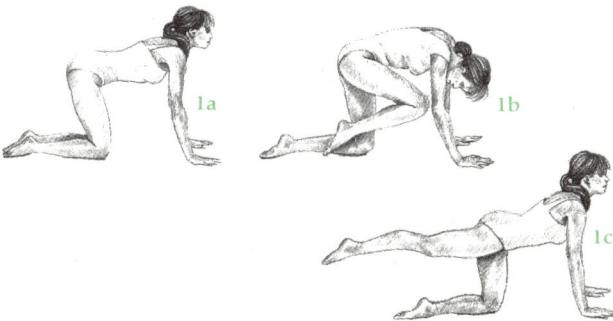

1a 1b 1c 1d 1e

1 Kneel on all fours (a). Lift your right knee up towards your nose (b), round your spine and curl your head in to meet your knee. Stretch the right leg back strongly, looking up (c). Bending your arms, lower your chest to the floor (d) and lift again, straightening your arms (e). Repeat with the left leg.

2 Lie on one side, propped up on one elbow, legs together (a). Lift the upper leg (b), keeping the knee facing forwards; lower it. Swing the leg back (c) and return to the starting position. Repeat with the other leg.

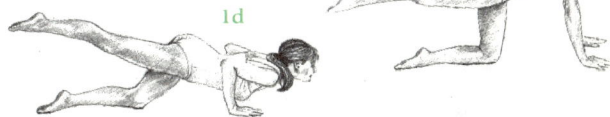

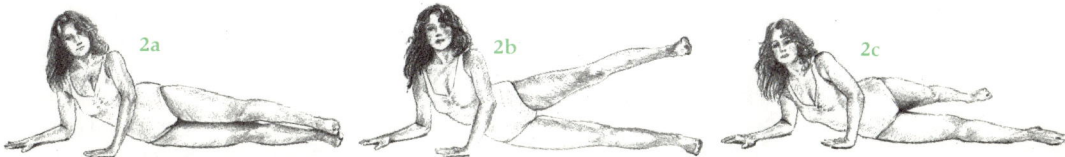

2a 2b 2c

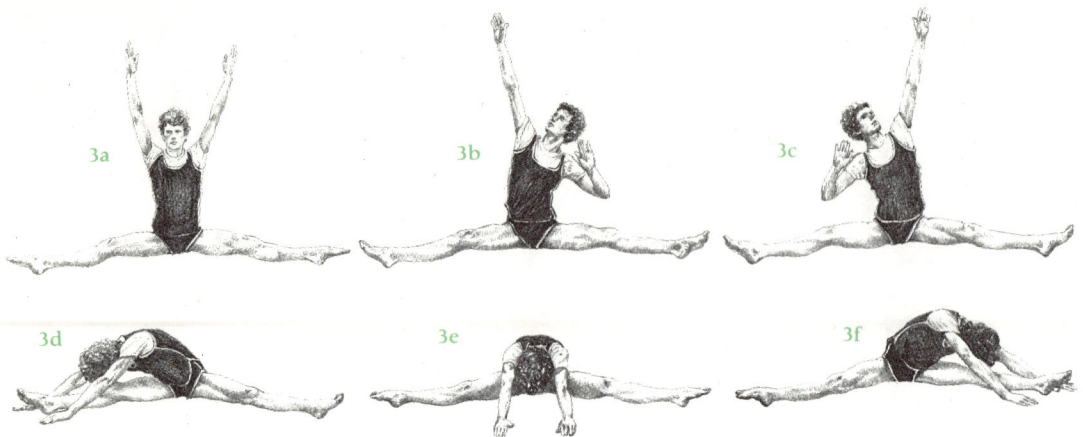

3 Sit with legs wide apart, arms stretched upwards (a). Reach up with the right arm (b) and the left (c). Repeat. Stretch forwards with both arms to the right leg (d), to the centre (e) and to the left leg (f); return to the starting position.

4 Lie on one side, propped up on one elbow, legs together (a). Bend your left leg up (b) and straighten it upwards (c). Return to (b) and slide the left foot down to the starting position. Repeat. Turn to lie on the other side and repeat.

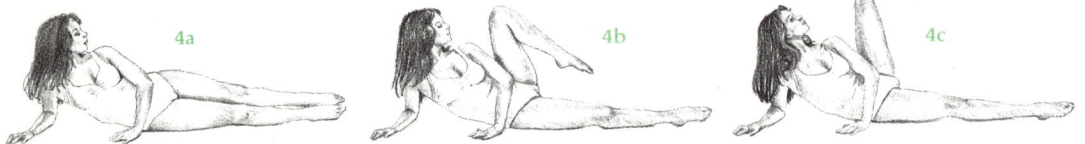

5 Lie facing up, propped up on both elbows, legs together (a). Bend your right leg up to your chest (b) and stretch it upwards (c). Bend it and slide the foot along the floor, returning to the starting position. Repeat with the left leg.

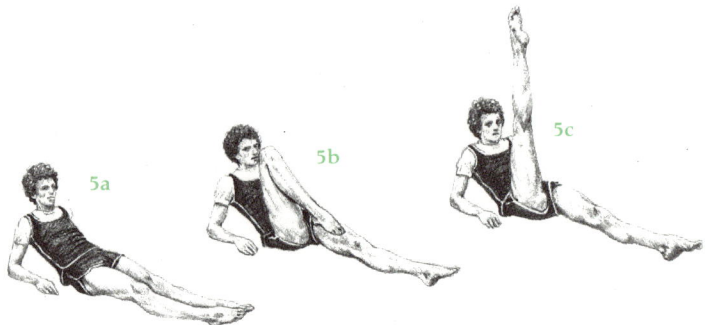

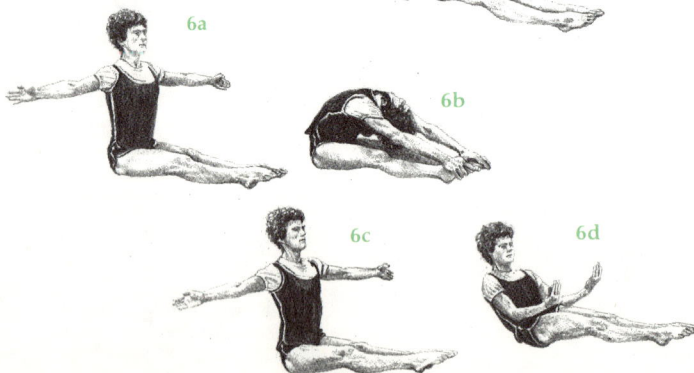

6 Sit with legs together, arms outstretched (a). Breathing out, bend forwards from the hips, reaching as far down your legs as you can (b). Breathe in as you straighten up, arms outstretched (c). Breathing out, lean backwards slowly, rounding the spine and bending your arms up in front (d). Breathe in and return to the starting position.

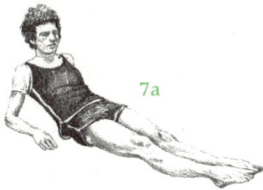

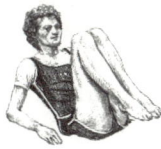

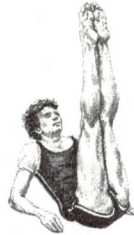

7 Lie facing up, propped up on both elbows, legs together (a). Bend both legs up to your chest (b) and straighten them upwards (c). Bend them and slide your feet along the floor to return to the starting position.

8 Lie facing up, arms outstretched. Bend your legs and lift them up vertically (a). If uncomfortable, place a cushion under your hips. Lower your right leg sideways to the floor (b). Lower the left leg to join it, holding your shoulders down (c). Lift the left leg up as in (b) and then the right leg to return to the starting position. Repeat to the other side.

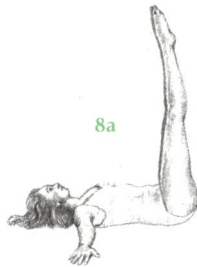

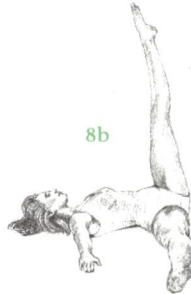

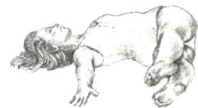

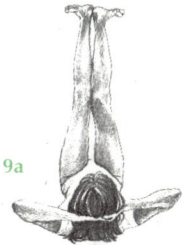

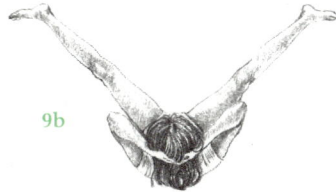

9 Lie facing up, hands clasped behind your head. Bend your legs and lift them up vertically. If uncomfortable, place a cushion under your hips. Lift your head and shoulders off the floor (a). Holding your head up, drop your legs apart (b) and draw them together. Repeat. Bend your legs and lie back down.

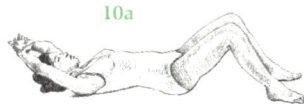

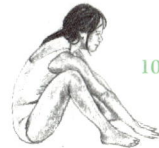

10 Lie facing up, hands clasped above your head, legs bent, feet on the floor (a). Breathe in; breathing out, sit up and reach forwards with both hands, letting your back round (b). Breathing in, roll back on to the floor, keeping your back round as long as you can.

11 Lie facing up, arms outstretched. Bend your left leg up (a). Stretch it to the right, holding down your shoulders; touch the floor with your toes (b). Bend the leg up to the centre. Stretch it to the left (c), touching the floor with your toes. Repeat with the right leg.

12 Lie facing up and lift up on to your shoulders, supporting your trunk with your hands on your hips. Circle your legs in a continuous bicycling movement (a, b). Stop if this strains the back of your neck or upper back.

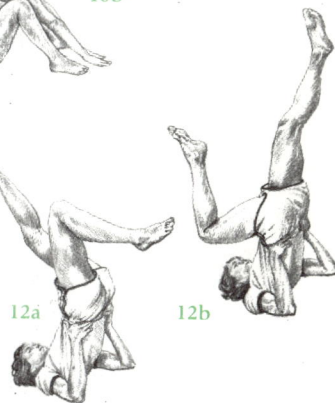

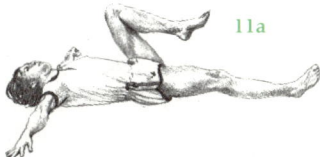

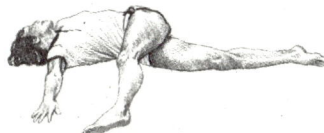

Training with weights

Weight-training is for both men and women, of all ages. Don't confuse it with the weight-*lifting* you may have seen on television where gigantic athletes hoist floor-splintering barbells above their heads. Weight-training uses far lighter loads – no heavier than a big dictionary to start with – moved ten or more times, rather than hoisted in one straining heave. It can't turn you into a muscle-bound freak (unless you step up the heaviness of the weights to excess); it *will* give you a firm and healthy figure. Women need have no fear of developing enormous bulging muscles, since muscle bulk depends on the male hormone testosterone, of which they have very little. The female hormone oestrogen, moreover, slows down the development of muscle mass; a woman generally has around 20–30 per cent more fat than a man, and only half the amount of muscle.

Benefits

There's nothing unnatural about weight-training – after all, we lift heavy objects every day. In training you develop your capacity by gradually overloading your body – either by lifting something a little heavier than before, or by raising a weight once or twice more. This sort of progressive resistance training forces muscle growth and burns up local stores of fat.

Weight-training can give you a lean figure, trimmed of excess fat – use it to concentrate on specific problem areas. It doesn't strengthen just muscles: by using light weights and high numbers of movements, or 'repetitions', you train your heart and lungs as well – although not as much as by doing aerobic sports. You'll also have stronger ligaments, tendons and connecting tissue, increased flexibility, quicker reflexes and improved coordination. If you take part in other sports, or simply plan to lead a more active life, weight-training can improve your performance and protect against injury. You get the mental benefits of greater self-confidence and a better self-image.

Losing weight

Muscle tissue is heavier than fat, so if you start weight-training because you're too heavy, don't be dejected if you put on more weight. Exchanging fat for muscle may make you weigh more, but you'll look leaner and firmer, and be stronger and fitter.

Equipment

Health clubs and centres have a range of barbells and dumb-bells; they can also be bought for use at home. The barbell is a long bar with weights on either end: these come in different sizes so that the heaviness of the barbell can be adjusted. Dumb-bells are smaller, one-handed versions of the barbell; you can use them singly or two at a time. The barbell enables you to lift greater weights.

Barbells and dumb-bells are the easiest weights to use, but you can improvise quite well with everyday items such as large books or unopened cans. Adjustable weights can be produced by using shopping bags containing various heavy items. Plastic detergent containers are another possibility; fill them with water to start with, and as you progress increase their weight with sand, which is heavier.

barbell

dumb-bell

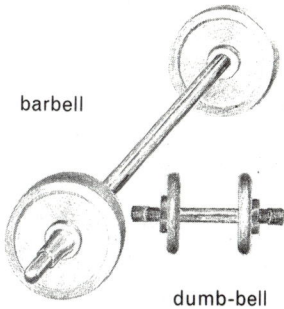

Wear warm clothing to train in: loose, but not floppy, it must not snag on your weights. You can weight-train at home, indoors, or outdoors if the weather is fine. Indoors, the room you choose should be well-ventilated but not cold. Make sure you have clear space all around you, with plenty of room to move, and don't forget overhead clearance. Pay particular attention to the floor. It should be even and free of any snags that might trip you up. Don't stand on carpets or rugs that could slide from under you, and whether you go barefoot or wear shoes, make sure you can't slip. If possible, train in front of a mirror; it'll help you to check that you're moving correctly. A total beginner would do well to visit a sports centre or club just once to see correct weight-training style.

When to train

Don't train every day. For the best results put aside three sessions each of about an hour a week. Allow at least a day between them so that the body can rest and repair itself as it adjusts to its increased level of activity.

Beginners' training routine

These exercises are basic, reach the major muscle groups and can be done with any type of weight. In each exercise, find your correct weight by first trying the movement 10–15 times with any handy items – say two heavy books. If you can do this without straining, use their combined weight as the one to start with.

Before you train, warm your muscles and raise your pulse rate: run on the spot (see page 25) and do warm-up exercises 1, 2, 3, 5, 8 and 9 on pages 70–71. Spend only a few minutes on this, since exercise 1 below is itself a general body toner.

Each exercise is divided into sets, so take a rest between sets if you need to; cut the rests down as your fitness improves.

Don't forget to breathe during a movement. Breathe *out*, forcing the air out of your lungs, when you reach the hardest part of each action.

Concentrate on the *style* of the exercise. When you lift weights keep your back straight, whatever the movement. Never round it to pick weights up from the floor. If you need to strain to finish a movement, or stray out of strict style, the weight is too heavy. Reduce it. If you mishandle even a light weight

you could injure yourself, so follow the exercise instructions and illustrations carefully.

1 The power clean strengthens the legs, back and forearms. Use a light weight, or even an empty bar, until you've mastered the quick, all-in-one movement. With the barbell on the floor in front, stand with feet about 30 cm [1 ft] apart, shins just touching the bar. Keeping your back flat, bend your knees; grasp

the bar with hands shoulderwidth apart and knuckles to the front (a). Keep your head up and your back straight. In one movement quickly straighten your legs, and using the momentum of this leg-push, bend your arms to raise the bar until it touches your chest (b). Return the weight to the floor in two movements, pausing when the weight is at about knee-level, and keeping a straight back (c). Do three sets of ten repetitions.

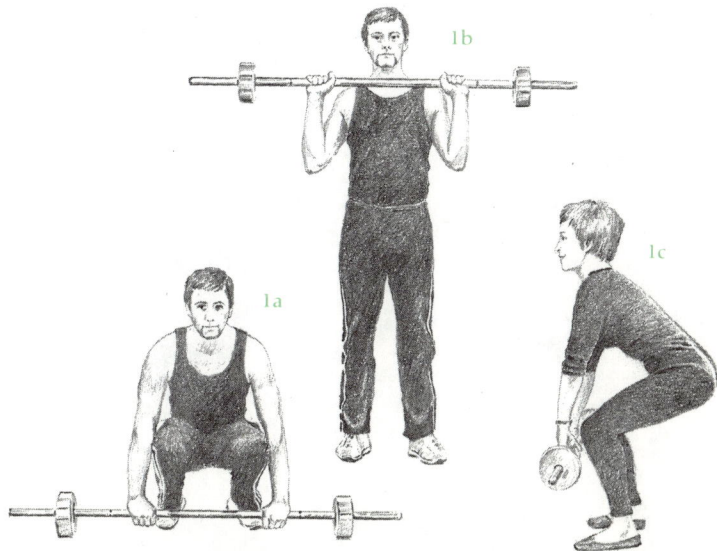

53

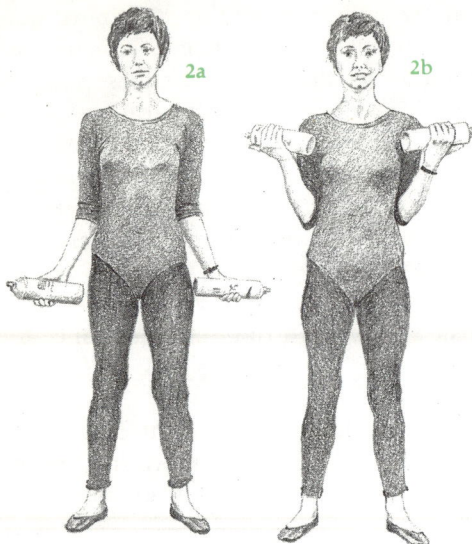

2a   2b

3 Strengthening the muscles of the calves with calf raises improves the power and shape of the legs. Stand with your toes on a board or firm book 7 cm [3 in] high, heels on the floor, grasping either a barbell at your chest OR dumb-bells (or improvised weights) with arms by your sides (a). Rock forwards raising yourself on to tiptoe (b). Rock back. Keep up the gentle tiptoe movement as long as feels comfortable. Work up to 50 or 100 repetitions.

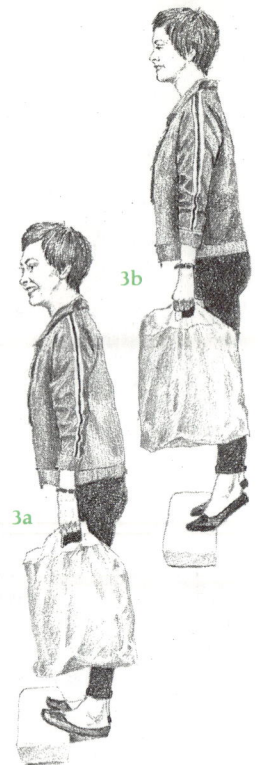

3b

3a

2 The curl strengthens the forearms and the pectoral muscles. It produces quick results and works for everyone: in men it produces a stronger bicep; in women it firms the muscles that support the breasts. Stand with elbows by your sides, holding a barbell OR dumb-bells (or improvised weights) with knuckles to the back (a). In a single movement bend your elbows and 'curl' the weights into your chest (b). Lower them slowly back to the starting position. Do three sets of ten repetitions.

4 Both sexes can gather fat round hips and waist and will benefit from this exercise and exercise 5, which strengthen abdominal muscles. Don't overdo them to start with or they may make you feel sore.

Use an empty bar (a broom handle will substitute). Stand with feet apart, toes slightly turned out. Hold the bar across your shoulders behind your neck, knuckles facing the back (a). Keeping hips and legs still, twist your body round as far as possible to the left (b), and then to the right (c). Do three sets of 20 repetitions (ten to each side).

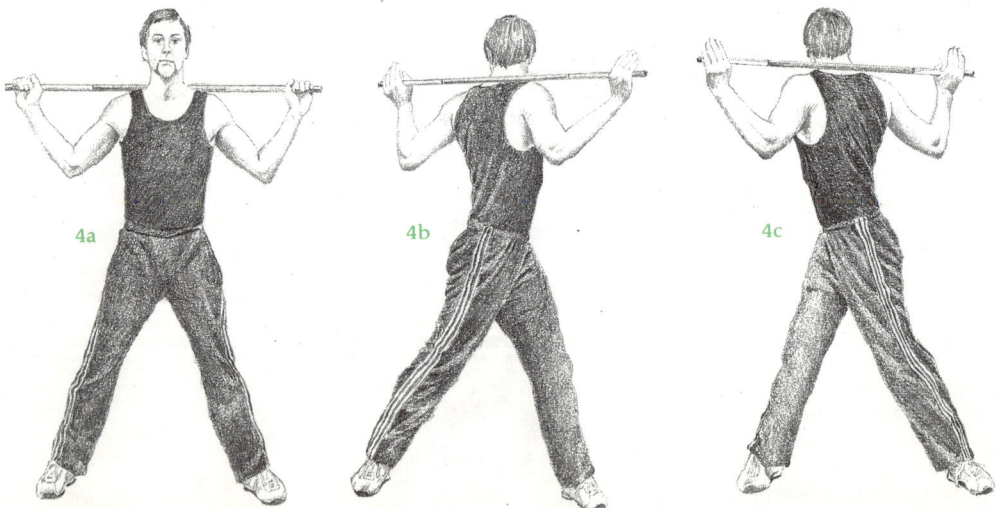

4a   4b   4c

5 Use dumb-bells OR an empty bar. Stand with feet apart. Hold the bar across your shoulders behind your neck, knuckles to the back, OR dumb-bells by your sides, knuckles outwards. With a straight back, tuck your bottom in and bend sideways at the waist (a). Straighten up; bend to the other side (b, c). Do three sets of 20 repetitions (ten each side).

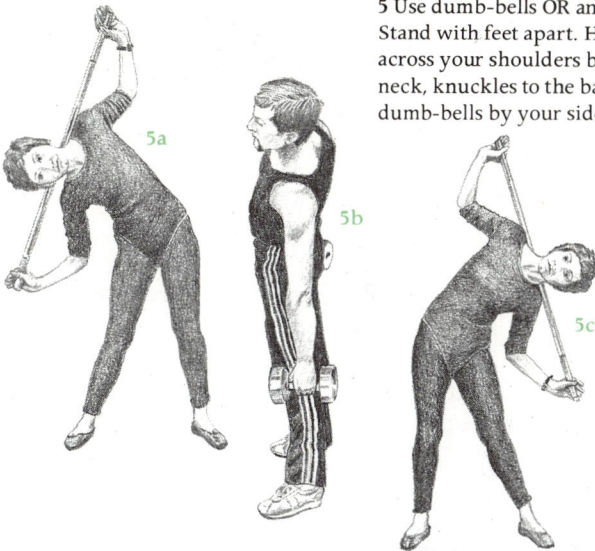

6 The bench press strengthens the arms and pectoral muscles, giving men a shapely chest and support for the breasts in women. Lie face up on a bench or similar firm horizontal surface. Hold dumb-bells OR barbell at chest level, hands shoulderwidth apart, knuckles facing upwards (a). Push the weights away from your chest until your arms are straight (b), then slowly return to (a). Do three sets of ten repetitions.

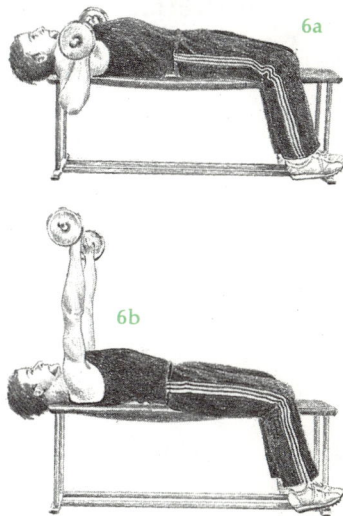

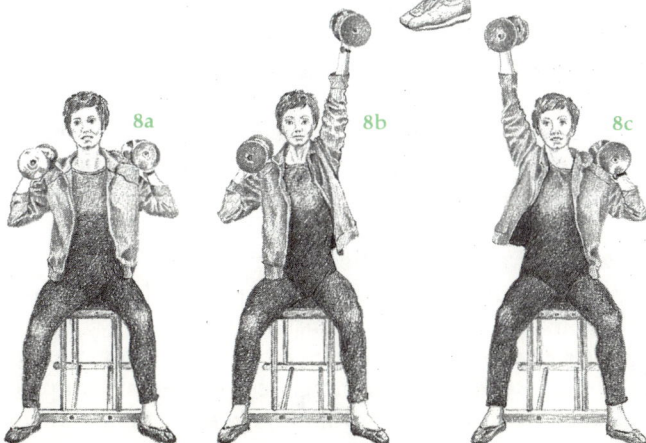

7 The front squat strengthens the legs, back and arms. Use either a barbell, raising it to chest level (a) by doing a power clean (see 1), OR dumb-bells held with the knuckles facing outwards and raised to the sides of your shoulders. Keeping your back straight, bend a little at the knees, going just half way down – as if beginning to sit in an imaginary chair and then thinking better of it (b). Return to the starting position with barbell held at chest level or dumb-bells at shoulders. Do three sets of 15 repetitions.

This gentler version of the standard 'squat' avoids strain on the back and knees.

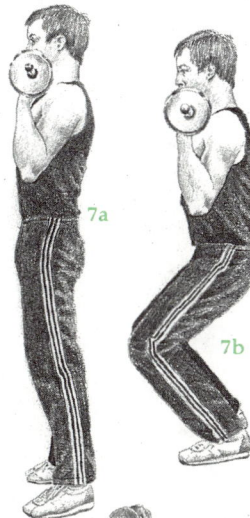

8 The alternative press or seated military press strengthens the neck, back and upper arms – especially the triceps at the backs of the upper arms, a common flab site. Sit upright on a steady seat. Raise dumb-bells to shoulder height (a) OR barbell to front of chest. If using dumb-bells, straighten alternate arms above head (b, c). If using a barbell, push the weight above your head by straightening both arms. Doing this exercise seated safeguards your back but you can do it standing if you use very light weights. Do three sets of ten repetitions.

Exercise machines

You can't cheat at exercise. The gadgets that promise 'instant' fitness just give exercise machines a bad name. There are many valuable aids to fitness but you have to be prepared to put effort into them. They're useful when your enthusiasm is flagging or when it's too wet or cold to get out for aerobic activity, and can be used to augment a general exercise scheme by working on specific areas. Exercise machines fall into two types: passive and active. The latter subdivide into isometric and isotonic.

Passive machines

The idea of getting fit while doing nothing more strenuous than reading a book appeals to many. Unfortunately, it just doesn't work. Passive exercisers that stimulate the muscles with small electric charges have no more than a temporary effect, although they can be relaxing. Vibrator belts are beneficial for toning muscles only when used along with more demanding exercise.

Isometric exercisers

Isometric devices act by making muscles contract, but without any movement at joints. One famous piece of exercise equipment, the Bullworker, is designed on isometric principles and undoubtedly does succeed in strengthening and firming up muscles. It scores over other isometric systems in that it encourages progressive resistance, by making it easy to measure your improving strength; as this increases, movement becomes correspondingly harder. However, if you have a tendency towards hypertension avoid the Bullworker and all isometric devices since they can stress the heart and lead to a build-up of blood pressure. Since isometric activity doesn't exercise muscles over a full range of movement, some experts claim that the big, shapely muscles it builds are no use when you want to *apply* strength. It won't develop your endurance, nor benefit the heart or lungs.

Isotonic exercisers

In isotonic activity, such as weight-training (see pages 52–55), the exertion of the muscles *is* accompanied by movement of the joints. The machines most commonly found in gyms and health clubs work on the same principles as the dumb-bell and barbell. They are, however, safer and easier to handle, they can isolate particular muscle groups for concentrated training, and they enable you to manage a heavier weight.

The basic machine in any gym is a version of the multi-gym. The most sophisticated ones can occupy six weight-trainers at a time, each of them using a different station at the machine. The weight can be changed to suit each individual by inserting or removing keys. The units can also be found as free-standing machines.

In the U.S.A. the multi-gym has been superseded by Nautilus equipment; it also makes you work against weights, but has a pulley system that enables resistance to be provided *throughout* a movement. After you've raised a weight, for instance, conventional equipment allows you to relax as you lower it – Nautilus keeps you working on the way down, too.

Even newer is accommodating resistance equipment, which automatically adjusts the resistance throughout an action to give just the amount you need at every stage, providing greater intensity of work.

Gym staff should always instruct you on how to use the machines.

Aerobic activity machines

Gymnasium bicycles, rowing and jogging machines provide the aerobic activity necessary to a training plan. They're all adjustable to suit different levels of fitness. Indoor jogging machines vary from simple rollers and treadmills to digital read-out electronic run-on-the-spot weight-sensitive pads. Newly developed is a type of mini-trampoline, which gives the benefits of jogging without the sting of the pavement. Again, gym staff will advise on how to use them.

Machines at home

Multi-gyms and their individual units are probably too bulky and too costly for home use; in any case, barbells and dumb-bells are sufficient for building stamina and strength to a reasonable level.

Exercise bicycles and rowing machines are not expensive, take up little room in use and can be stored away in a cupboard. Use the former to tackle heart-lung fitness or overweight – cycling is less fatiguing than the multi-muscle group action of a rowing machine so it's easier to keep up a steady rhythm for long periods, which is what counts in aerobics. Avoid bikes with rowing-action handlebars – they're confusing, uncomfortable and don't add much benefit to the exercise.

Rowing machines are suitable for those whose arms and back, rather than circulation, need strengthening. The action encourages short, sharp bursts of activity to build momentum, so get a version with adjustable resistance so you can warm up and cool down gently. On all machines, keep to your safe pulse rate (see pages 23–24).

1 Leg press machine
To strengthen the leg and lower back muscles. Lie on your back and with your legs raise and lower the board fixed to the weighted bar. It enables the standard squat (see also exercise 7, page 55) to be done in greater safety and with larger weights.

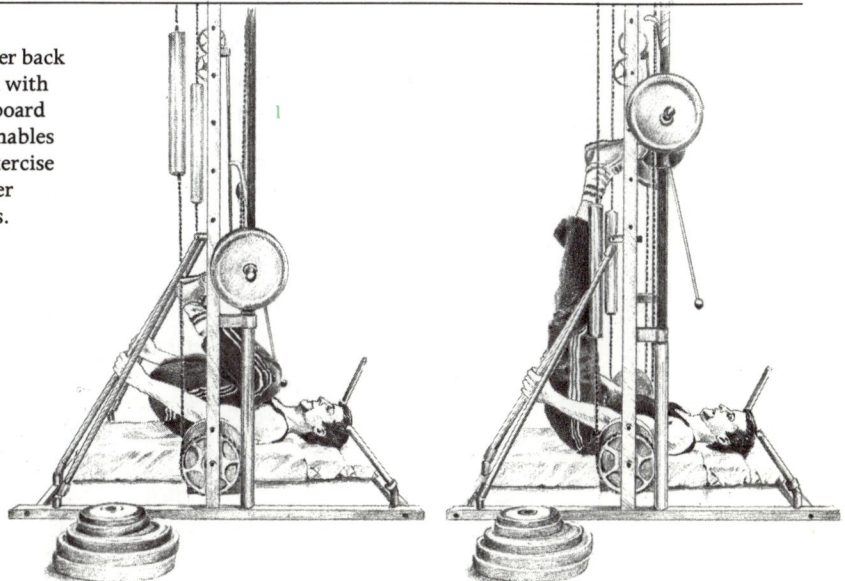

Exercise machines

The starting position is shown in pale green.

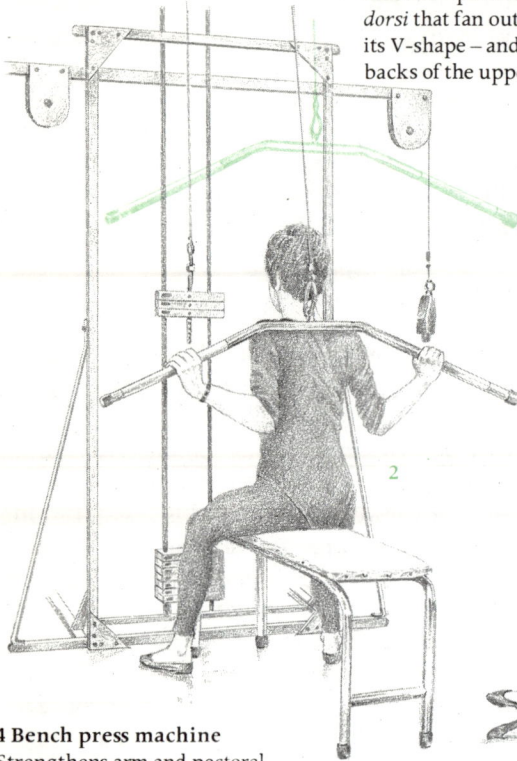

2 Lat machine
Strengthens and shapes the back muscles – particularly the *latissimus dorsi* that fan out to give the body its V-shape – and the muscles at the backs of the upper arms. The bar, on a cable attached via a pulley to weights, is grasped and pulled down. Use a wide grip to shape and tone the outer back area, and a narrow grip to work on the muscles of the inner back area.

3 Cable machine
The cable, ending in a leather cuff, is pulled against weights. It can be used standing, kneeling, sitting or lying. The exercise illustrated strengthens the inner thigh muscles: start with your right foot in the cuff, and right leg raised. Lower it to touch the left leg, keeping both legs straight. Raise it again. Repeat with the other leg.

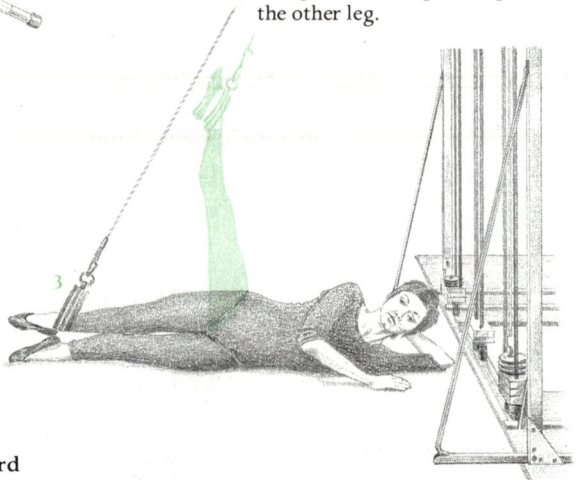

4 Bench press machine
Strengthens arm and pectoral muscles. The handles are grasped and pushed against the machine's resistance. It's a safer method of doing exercise 6 on page 55, since you can't be pinned down by the weight.

5 Twist board
Comes in single or double models, strengthens waist and leg muscles and is good pre-ski training. Standing on the disc, push against the fixed T-bar to right then left. Keep feet stationary on the disc as it swivels from side to side.

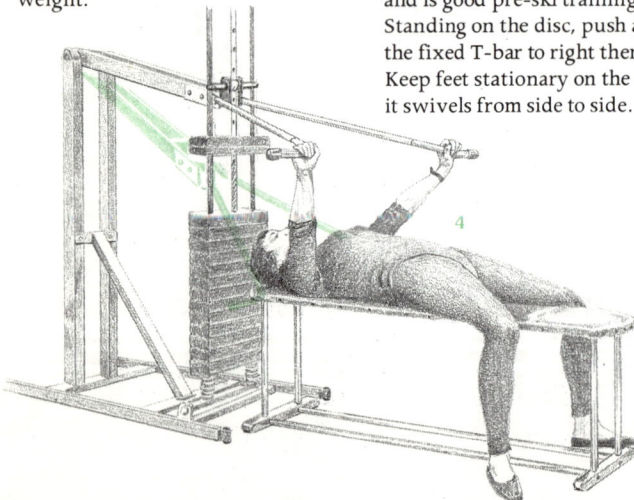

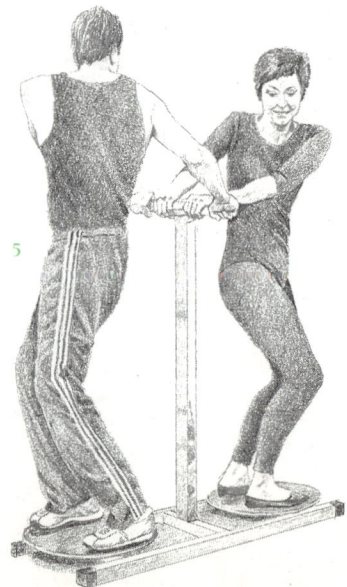

7 Exercise bicycle
Improves heart-lung fitness and strengthens leg muscles. Resistance, provided by a braking force on the wheel or pedals, can be increased as you get stronger. Usually calibrated so that effort can easily be measured. May include a heart-rate monitor and even a calorie read-out to show energy expended.

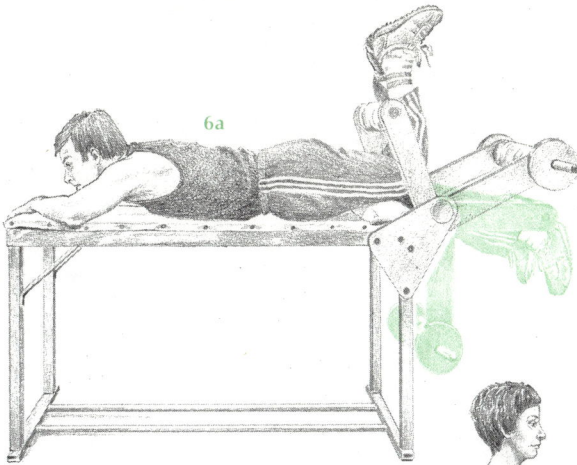

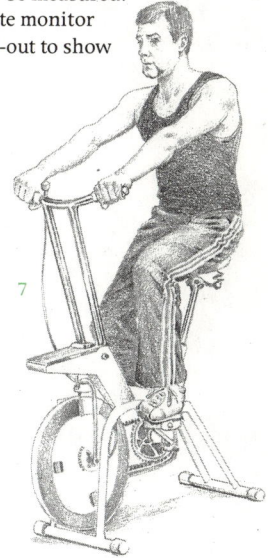

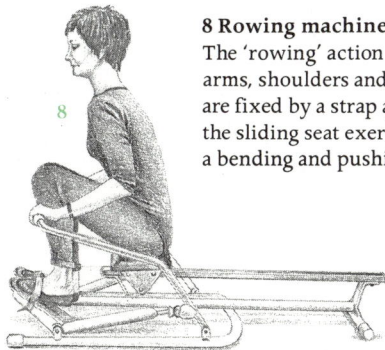

6 Leg curl and leg extension bench
The leg curl movement (a) strengthens the back thigh muscles. Lifting the upper bar raises the weighted bar below. Lie on your front and hook your heels under the upper bar. Hold the edge of the bench and keep your thighs and torso flat on the bench. Moving your lower legs only, pull the bar towards your buttocks; then lower it.

Leg extensions (b) strengthen front thigh muscles. Sit upright on the bench, shins against the weighted bar. Keep your back straight and grasp the bench sides. Smoothly push the bar up until your legs are straight. Lower them.

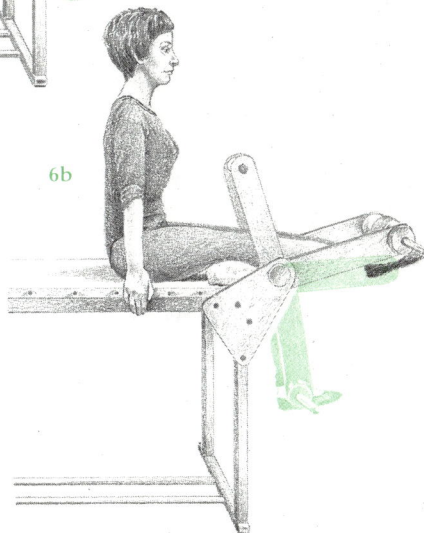

8 Rowing machine
The 'rowing' action strengthens arms, shoulders and back. The feet are fixed by a strap at the front, so the sliding seat exercises the legs in a bending and pushing movement.

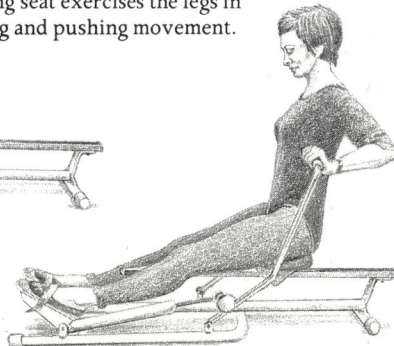

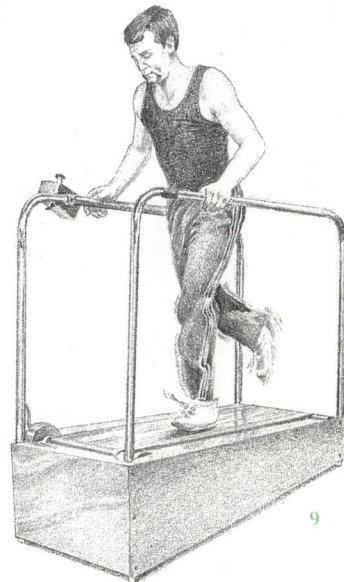

9 Jogging machine
For heart-lung fitness. Often takes the form of a motorized treadmill, with rails to hold on to; can be adjusted to run at various speeds for different levels of fitness.

59

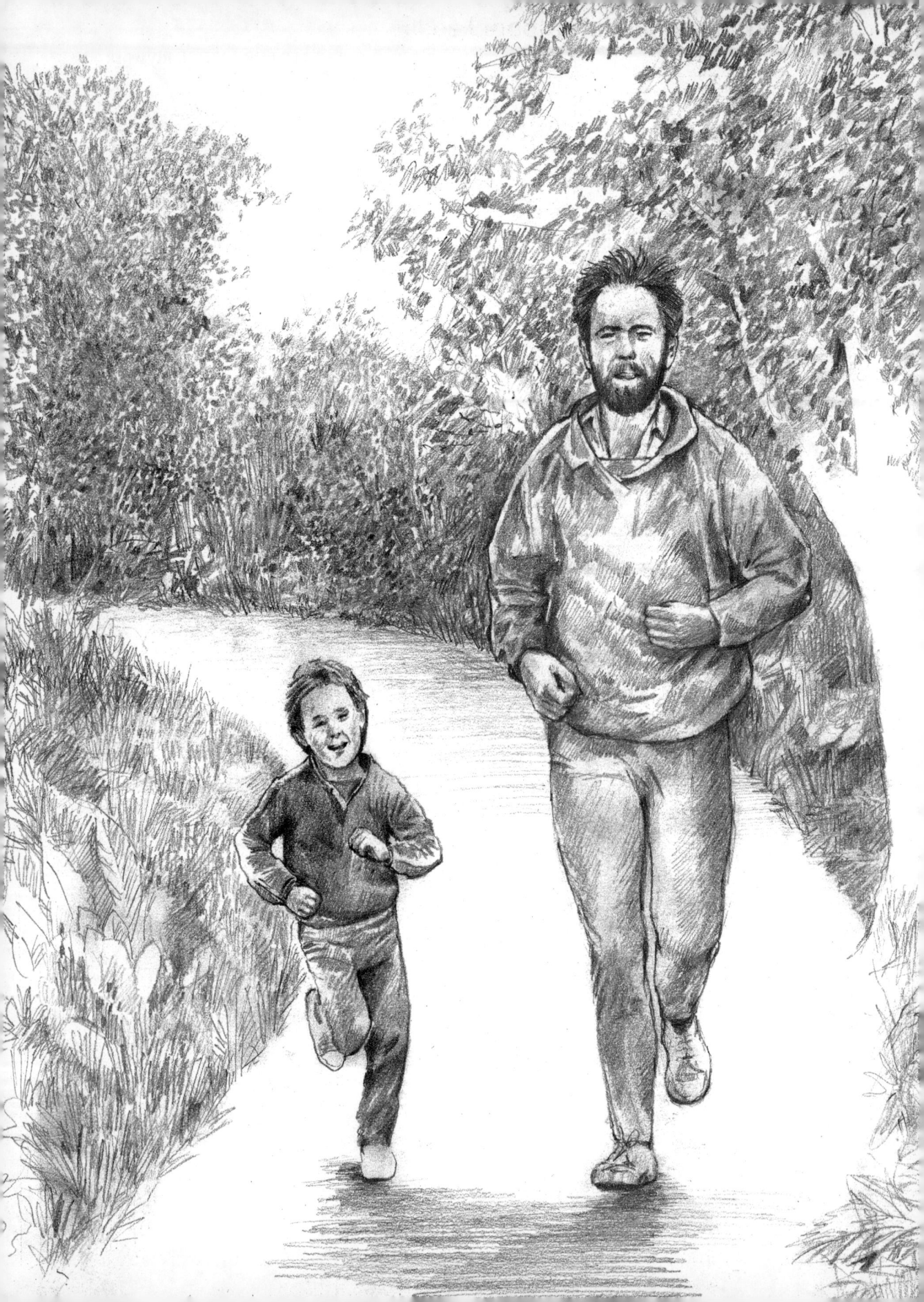

CHOOSE YOUR SPORT

Sport is an integral part of many people's lives. It's an acceptable way to release energy and aggression, it can be a means of starting or deepening friendships, and it offers a constructive escape from the pressures of the everyday world. In fact, you can change your life if you take up – and keep up – an activity suited to your character, abilities and lifestyle.

Sports for women

There's no sport that cannot be tackled by women *and* men. In fact, there is increasing evidence that women – with their lighter weight and greater stores of fuel in the form of body fat – may be better-equipped for some endurance events, for instance, long-distance running. Women often have quicker reflexes than men, making them good at fast-reaction, skill or intuition sports, including squash, racketball and target games such as archery.

Women are not necessarily more fragile than men, but it's worth bearing in mind that the development of women's protective equipment – even of something as essential as an efficient, comfortable sports bra – has lagged far behind that for men.

Family exercise

The favourite aerobic sports (see pages 67–75) – brisk or uphill walking, jogging, running, cycling and swimming – have much in common. They're available all year round, anywhere, at virtually any time, need the minimum of equipment, special facilities and instruction, and suit almost everyone. They are activities that the whole family can take part in together, and since they can be enjoyed non-competitively, all age-groups can participate. Other enjoyable family sports include roller-skating, ice-skating and skiing.

As a parent or grandparent, encourage children by exercising alongside them, not cheering them on from the sidelines and, as can happen, urging them to extend themselves too far, too soon. Don't set goals for children – they may feel they have to push themselves too hard to achieve them. If *you're* exercising with the children, you'll have a keener appreciation of when it's time to stop. Besides, there's the hope that they'll do the same for their own children some day. Don't drive the family everywhere by car. Encourage them to walk or cycle – and set them an example by doing the same yourself.

The earlier children start a balanced pattern of exercise the better. The spectacular success of athletes from developing countries at international sports competitions shows the standards that can be reached by those with a background of hard physical activity daily. Children accustomed to regular physical training will gain greater self-confidence, and the physical and mental well-being that is induced will help them to make the most of their education and to develop into well-rounded human beings – doers, not life-spectators hooked on hours of television each day. Indeed, this was one of the fundamental beliefs behind John F. Kennedy's bid to re-establish the physical tone of the United States with the foundation of the President's Council on Physical Fitness and Sports.

61

Children will experience competitive sports and regimented exercise at school; parents should balance this by re-emphasizing unforced, play-like activity. Most children don't lack flexibility, so early games should involve much aerobic exercise to lay a foundation of heart-lung fitness and should concentrate on stimulating the imagination. When they get into the teens, suggest some flexibility sessions so that they don't begin to lose range of movement; this is also a good time to help them develop their strength and muscularity. Leave team spirit to be instilled at school: introduce as many different games and sports as possible, and stress that the real competition comes from within the individual. Show children the possibilities for enjoyment rather than achievement.

Somatotyping

In the 1940s an American doctor, William Sheldon, developed somatotyping (see opposite). He categorized bodies according to three basic types, which he graded on a scale of one to seven. Thus an average body with equal parts of endomorph, ectomorph and mesomorph characteristics rates four-four-four, while the extreme endomorph, for instance, is rated seven-one-one since he has only minute shares of the attributes of the other two types.

Most people are a blend of types, but knowing which one you lean towards can help you to choose the sports to which you're physically best suited and in which you can maximize your potential, since some types are better suited to particular sports than others. This is especially helpful when you start out and are not used to regular, vigorous exercise: you can get basically fit by doing a sport you're well suited to before trying other sports.

For instance, if you know you're always going to be a bulky endomorph, you'll probably never be happy jogging – flesh wobbling, feet, ankles and knees taking a battering as your hefty body weight hits the ground with every step. So instead, try a sport where your bulk is less of a disadvantage – swimming or cycling are ideal because your weight is supported. You'll take the strain off your heart and lessen the risk of leg injuries.

Extensive somatotyping at an early age is thought to be one reason why Eastern block countries produce so many world-class sportspeople. But don't take it too far; the right body in the right sport is next to useless without enthusiasm and enjoyment.

Picking the right sport

Time is often the deciding factor in choosing a sport; not just the time it takes to exercise, but the time taken to prepare for it, to recover from it, to travel there and back, with the whole problem of fitting it in between work, meals, social engagements and sleep. If this is your main concern, choose an activity – such as jogging or cycling – that involves the minimum of extra time and bother. Whatever your sport, it's important to warm up beforehand and cool down afterwards, to prepare your body for the effort ahead and make you less liable to injury and post-exercise stiffness (see pages 69–71).

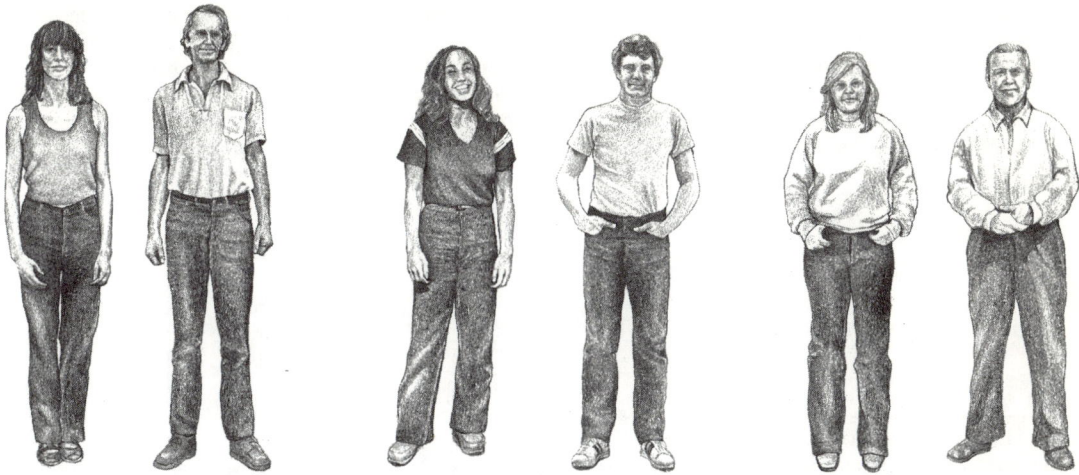

Ectomorphs may be tall and slender, or in extreme cases painfully thin. They put on fat with difficulty, which can be a plus, but also find it hard to pack on muscle, which makes their power-to-weight ratio low, although they are usually stronger than they look. They can excel in sports – such as long-distance running – where muscle-power is not too important, but heart-lung fitness is. Basketball players and climbers are often examples of this type.

Tarzan was a mesomorph – the key word here is muscle. Mesomorphs are naturally strong, well-built yet agile, and thus well suited to most sports. However, they can run to seed without regular work-outs. Look for this type in short-distance running events, body-building contests, or in aggressive body-contact sports such as the martial arts and all types of football.

Endomorphs are rounded. Well-covered all over they tend to run to fat yet are often weak relative to their size. The advantage in size and bulk makes them good weight-lifters, wrestlers and shot-putters, but they may need to work extra hard to build muscle and stay in shape. They can also be successful at bowling and archery. Long-distance swimmers, who tend to exaggerate their capacity to store fat in order to withstand long hours in cold water, are usually endomorphs.

If you're strong physically, but know that your staying power is limited – if you prefer activity in short, sharp bursts – find a sport that makes use of your strength, and will improve your heart-lung fitness. If you're competitive by nature, try a team activity – although this won't help you to relax if normally you're tense and anxious. Many people find that the camaraderie of a team encourages them to keep up their activity and even to train more frequently. They are motivated by being part of a group with a single aim, and often benefit from the feeling of support that this brings.

It's more important to do anything regularly than to hover indecisively between enthusiasms. You should spend at least three sessions a week on some form of exercise to have a minimum effect. If you pick something you enjoy, and that fits your requirements, you're more likely to stick to it.

The activity chart on the following pages lists just a few of the possibilities. All of them offer some fitness benefit: each is awarded ratings in different areas so that you can pinpoint the sports that capitalize on your strengths or will improve the areas in which you're aware that you're weakest.

63

Which sport?

These ratings are given as a guide to participation, and do not rate individual sports against one another. They indicate the effects of a sport if carried out at a reasonable level; they don't cover the requirements of a top-class performer.

The principal areas affected are: heart and lungs, muscle endurance, muscle strength, coordination, flexibility and relaxation.

The gradings, into low, medium and high, follow the system in *Maximum Performance* (see bibliography). Particoloured figures indicate an intermediate rating such as low-medium.

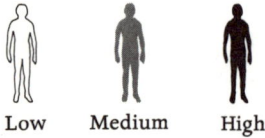

Low   Medium   High

Columns: Archery, Badminton, Baseball, Basketball, Bowling/Bowls, Boxing, Canoeing, Cricket, Cycling, Dancing (energetic), Fencing, Football (American), Football (Soccer), Golf, Gymnastics, Handball (court), Hockey

Heart-lung-circulation fitness
Commonly called endurance fitness.

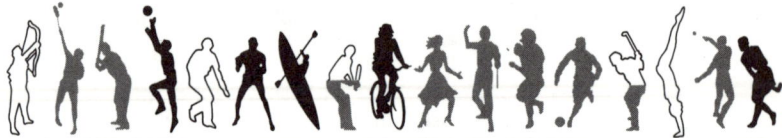

Muscle endurance, or ability of muscles to perform a set task over and over again.

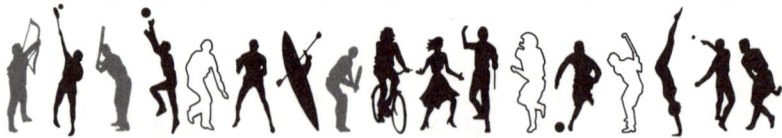

Muscle strength, or power of individual muscle groups.

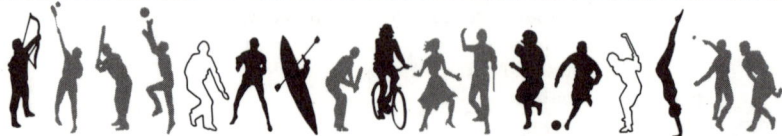

Coordination, or skill, including balance. High rating indicates tuition may be necessary, but don't be put off – 'poor' coordination is easily remedied with practice.

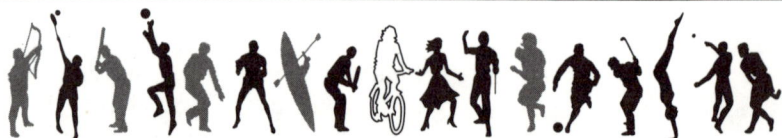

Flexibility, or ability to move freely in all directions.

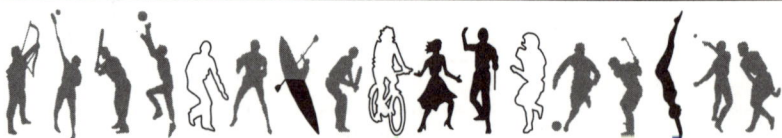

Relaxation, or whether the sport promotes freedom from tension and anxiety. Low rating indicates sport is likely to be competitive and may increase tension.

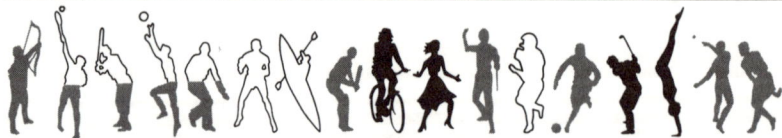

Access, or availability. High rating indicates sport is available to anyone, anywhere, any time, with minimum of necessary equipment or facilities.

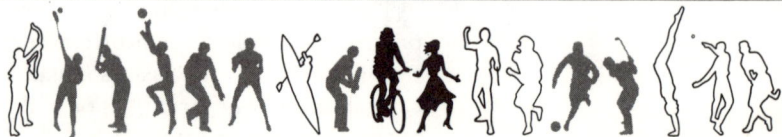

64

Horse-riding
Ice-skating
Jogging
Judo
Karate
Mountain climbing
Orienteering
Roller-skating
Rowing
Rugby
Running
Sailing
Scuba-diving
Skiing (cross-country)
Skiing (downhill)
Skipping
Squash/Racketball
Swimming
Table-tennis
T'ai chi ch'uan
Tennis
Volleyball
Walking
Water-skiing
Weight-training

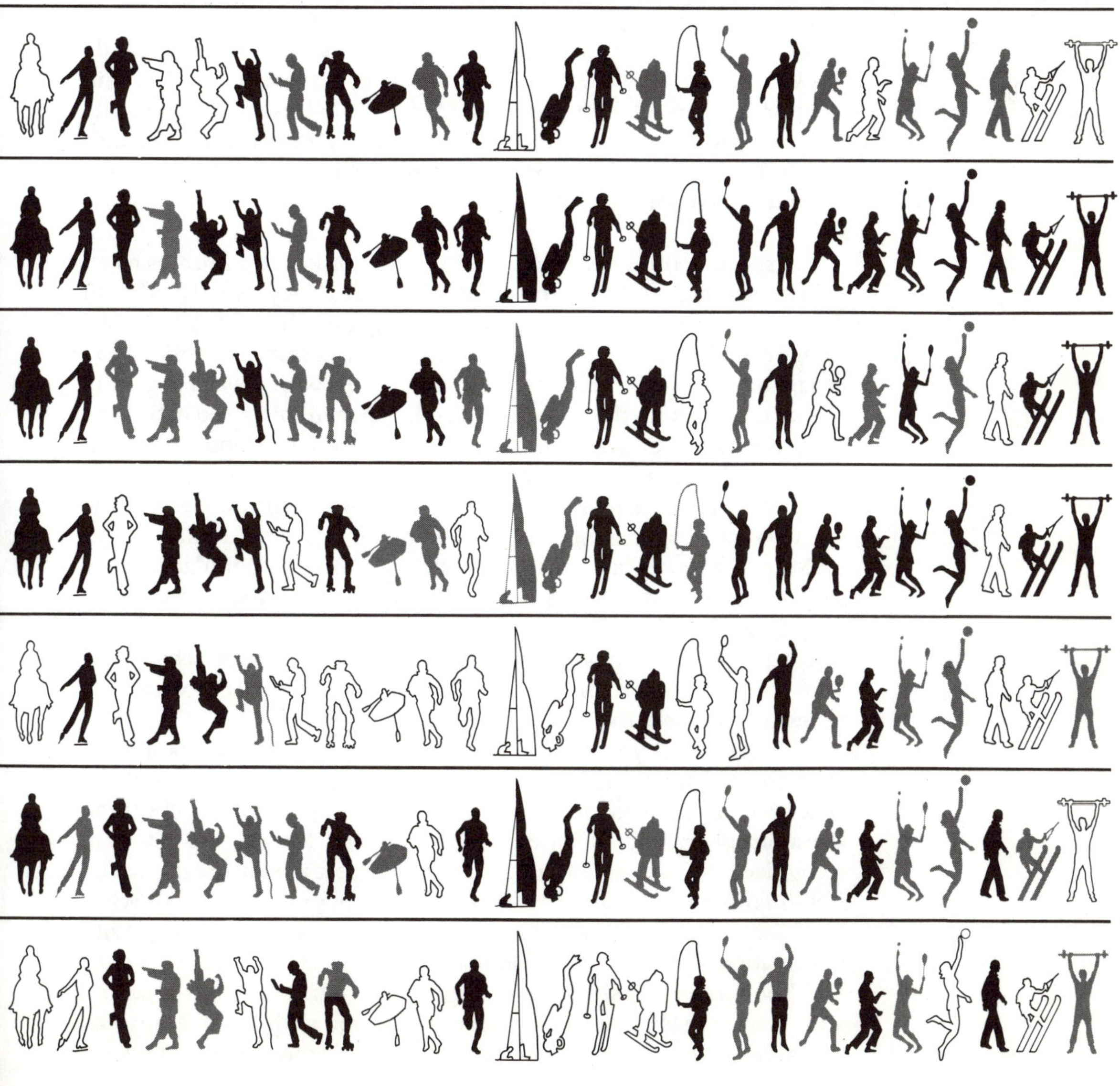

65

Where to go   If you want to exercise, there are hundreds of gyms, clubs and sports centres – varying from the primitive to the luxurious – to help you. Try to find one near your home or workplace: if it's convenient, you'll be more willing to continue going there. Always check that it's qualified and equipped to deal with novices and that there are first-aid or medical facilities. Rooms for indoor activities should have plenty of ventilation, and be well-lit and spacious enough for you to exercise in comfort.

The private gyms and health clubs that don't specialize in a particular exercise regime tend to centre on weight-training, circuit training, and keep-fit classes; they may also have jogging, swimming and weight-losing facilities. There are usually full-time health professionals on the staff: if you specifically request it they will prescribe you an individual exercise schedule. In this case they must first check your pulse rate and set you a gentle fitness test (if they don't do this you should view the club with suspicion). Subsequently they will monitor and control your progress. Membership fees are usually quite high, so you'll have to use the club regularly to get your money's worth. The accent tends to be on comfort, with perhaps a bar, restaurant and lounge. Many clubs cater for men and women separately, on alternate days.

The sports centres owned by communities or local authorities often provide the best facilities for the lowest price. They usually offer all the indoor sports, and many include jogging clubs that welcome beginners. The staff will be professionals but personal attention may be lacking. However, most centres remedy this with specialist tuition classes that back up the daily free-for-all of dozens of varied activities. They are excellent places to try out different sports and to get the whole family involved. The many YMCAs, to be found the world over, offer a similarly wide range of sporting facilities. Despite the organization's name, you need not be young, male or Christian to join a YMCA – anyone can become a member, although popular Ys may have a waiting list. They have good social facilities too – some even including a bar.

In some areas the sports halls and equipment at local schools are open to the public in the evenings and at weekends, and a variety of fitness classes held there.

Whatever sport you choose, there will be a specialist club or association for it. The public library will have the name and address of the club secretary of your local branch. It's then up to you to check on the atmosphere and facilities. Make sure that the club coaches are recognized by national organizations. One great advantage of joining a club is that you'll never have trouble finding people to play with. Established sports all have national organizations that can help with information and advice. They should have detailed calendars of events, will know of demonstrations or beginners' courses in your area and will provide lists of clubs or coaches registered with them. Many can also arrange discounts on equipment and insurance for members.

Aerobics

The word 'aerobic', popularized by Dr. Kenneth Cooper, the American fitness expert, means 'with oxygen'. Aerobic activities are endurance exercises that increase the body's ability to deliver blood – bearing the oxygen and nourishment used to produce energy – to muscles and organs. The most aerobically valuable sports are those that produce a high heart rate and a demand for large amounts of oxygen, and sustain it for long periods. This results in the improved functioning of the heart, blood vessels and lungs known as the 'training effect'.

The high heart rate required is 75 per cent of your maximum, in other words your safe pulse rate – see pages 23–24 for how to calculate this. The longer you maintain this rate the better, but an absolute minimum for a positive effect is 15 minutes.

The sports that achieve this include brisk or uphill walking, jogging, running, swimming, cycling, skipping and cross-country skiing. An activity like golf fails to produce a high enough heart rate to have a training effect, while sports like squash, football or sprinting stress the heart too much over too short periods, and are usually 'anaerobic' or 'without oxygen' – a sprinter may even hold his breath.

Aerobic exercise is 'isotonic', or dynamic, which means that it needs movement. Unlike isometric activity (such as weight-lifting), which involves static muscle contraction, it doesn't raise blood pressure without the release of movement; so it doesn't boost up pressure and strain the heart.

The training effect

This is the body's way of over-compensating for the stress of aerobic activity so that it will be ready for it next time. It adapts to the increased demand for oxygen-carrying blood in several ways.

The most obvious effect is on the heart. An aerobic sport should raise the pulse from its normal resting rate (average for men 70–85 beats per minute, for women 75–90) to well over 100 beats.

Aerobic exercise makes the major muscle groups work harder and blood is forced into them to such an extent that new avenues of supply, new capillaries, are opened up. Existing arteries and veins become more elastic, and free from blockages. In the event of an obstruction, the heart and muscles of a trained person can still get oxygen – and so keep him alive – through by-passing the blockage along what are called 'collateral' blood vessels.

The huge demand for air created during aerobic exercise means that breathing improves. Muscles of the chest and abdomen dormant from years of shallow breathing come alive; oxygen reaches more of the lungs than is normally used, improving the capacity to process oxygen and to clear out carbon dioxide and other toxic waste products.

Aerobic activity depends on the biggest and strongest muscle groups of the body to move body weight against gravity in pursuit of the training effect. The muscles that you use most every day are strengthened and shaped by loss of local stores of body fat; they also gain endurance fitness – the capacity to keep on working. In the upright sports like jogging and cycling, it's mainly the leg muscles

67

that benefit, but the muscles of the back and waist also are firmed by having to support the body weight. In swimming, skipping and running, the arm muscles are strengthened, with the bonus for women that the arm action works the pectoral muscles and helps to give the breasts firm support.

Further benefits

Metabolism and the production of energy are stimulated by aerobic exercise. The cells themselves develop greater efficiency in triggering the chemical activities that produce movement.

Research involving some 15,000 people at Ken Cooper's Aerobics Institute in Dallas, Texas, has shown that people who take regular aerobic exercise generally have lower blood pressure, lower levels of fats in the blood, lower body fat and fewer heartbeat irregularities than the average. In some cases of hypertension, aerobic sports have been used to lower blood pressure – although exercise for this purpose should always be prescribed by a health professional.

Dr. Cooper devised aerobics when he was developing a fitness system for the U.S. Air Force. He has consistently promoted aerobics as a way of life – rather than a part-time sport – and millions of Americans are reaping the benefits. There are now an estimated 27 million runners in the U.S.A., and the country has sustained a dramatic *decrease* in the rate of heart attacks in the last ten years. Although other factors, such as diet and cutting back smoking, are involved, it's been shown that regular aerobic exercise has played no mean part in achieving this reduction.

In Dr. Cooper's view aerobic sports can actually slow down the the aging process. All cells need oxygen; deprived of it, they die. Aerobic exercise force-feeds every part of the body with oxygen.

A chance to live a longer life is a doubtful advantage if it's not a happy one; but aerobic fitness improves the quality of that life. You'll look slimmer – and thanks to the 'high' it gives you, based on the extra production of hormone-like catecholamines, including adrenalin and noradrenalin – you'll feel happier and more alert. Keep a training diary, and you'll be able to *see* your fitness improving. Self-confidence is boosted when you realize that you can reach whatever goals you set.

Menstruation and pregnancy

Menstruation won't affect athletic performance. Aerobic exercise can lift pre-menstrual tension, relieve cramps and reduce fluid retention.

Pregnancy will slow performance, but need not stop it. The foetus is well-protected by the mother's muscles and pelvis, and by a wall of amniotic fluid. It's essential to consult a doctor, but as long as she's not experiencing any complications, a woman should keep training during pregnancy: the fitter she is, the easier the birth will be and the quicker she'll get back into shape afterwards. Athletic training seems to help both men and women deal with pain better, which means that labour will be less stressful. A woman should start training again as soon after the birth as feels good, generally about six weeks.

Warming up and cooling down

A warming up routine is particularly vital before aerobic activity because the heart, if launched into sudden action, reacts with abnormal rhythms which can kill an untrained person. As you warm up, your body temperature rises and the increasing need for oxygen in the newly exerting muscles stimulates a rise in the heart rate so that oxygen-laden blood can be pumped more quickly to the muscles.

Muscles also work better and faster when relaxed. In any activity you exert one set of muscles violently 'against' others: thus their range of movement is limited by the tightness of the antagonistic muscles. If you exercise without having warmed and relaxed them, you can sprain or tear the muscles, the tendons attaching muscles to bones, or the ligaments that wrap joints and help to keep them stable. They need to be loosened by 'static' or smooth stretches against their own resistance so that they won't crack up when asked to perform beyond their accustomed range of motion. Major joints are cushioned by cartilages; these thicken (by absorbing fluid) as you limber up, so that they fit better between the bones, giving a stronger joint.

A warm-up makes exercise much easier. As blood surges into the ends of the muscles, forcing open new capillaries and raising body temperature, nerve endings are prepared for fast reaction, while the loosened joints and muscles expand their range of movement. Stride length, for instance, increases – a flexible body needs less energy to move. On a day when you feel like dodging exercise, do your warm-up and then see how you feel. Going through an established routine may change your mind; if not, you've still done something positive for your health. The next day pick up your aerobic plan where you left off; if you interrupt it through illness, resume it by repeating your last day's exercise.

The cool-down, after strenuous exercise, is just as necessary. Don't stop suddenly: slacken your effort gradually. Again the aim is to take strain off the heart. During movement the other muscles help to pump blood back to the heart once it has delivered oxygen. After exercise their aid is especially important, since blood has been forced into areas it never normally reaches. If you come to an abrupt halt, the blood 'pools' in the extremities; as the muscles stop pumping, the lack of oxygen-bearing blood in the brain makes the heart, already beating fast to cope with demand, pump even harder. As a result you may faint.

A cool-down routine also helps to avoid post-exercise stiffness. During vigorous exercise two things happen that can cause problems later on. Firstly, the muscle fibres sustain microscopic tears. As these heal, inflexible scar tissue forms. If it's left to its own devices, you'll stiffen up as it heals, but if you stretch it with exercise as it forms, you'll keep the muscles flexible and efficient. Secondly, the body in action generates waste products: mainly lactic acid from the chemical reaction that triggers working muscles, and broken muscle tissue. As the blood recedes from the unaccustomed areas, the waste is left behind. If it remains, you'll be sore, but if you keep the heart and circulation exerting for a few minutes, they'll pump it away.

1 To relax the whole body. With arms loose by your sides, waggle your hands as if they were out of control. Work up to the elbows (a), then the shoulders, shaking the tension out. Now do each leg: shake the foot, then the leg below the knee and finally shake the whole leg around (b).

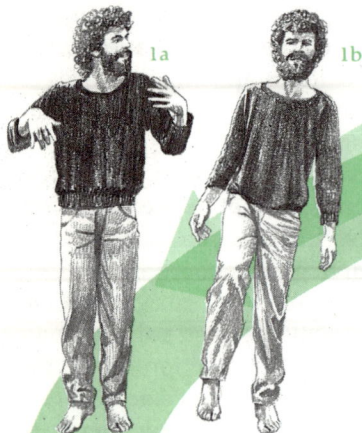

2 To loosen the shoulders. Stand with feet together. Raise both arms and rotate them forwards in large circles (a, b). Then rotate them backwards in the same way.

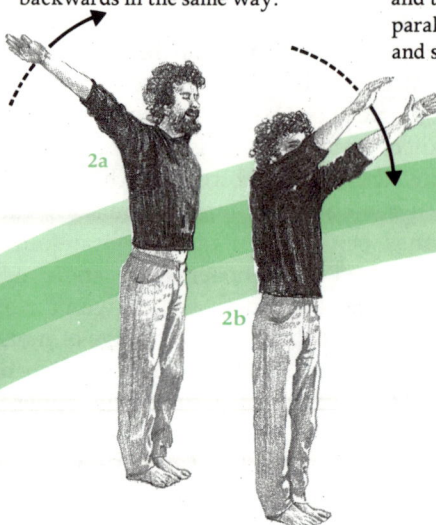

3 To relax the hip joints. Stand on tiptoe, supporting yourself with one hand, the other hanging loose. Swing your outside leg forwards and then back in a relaxed way, parallel to your support. Turn round and swing the other leg.

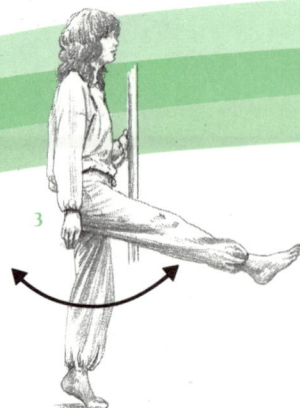

WARMING UP

COOLING DOWN

Warming up

Wear what you'll be exercising in, plus a loose oversuit, and begin with a good stretch, standing on tiptoe and reaching for the sky. Don't let your warm-up take more than 10–15 minutes, or you'll run out of breath and start to feel heavy. Do the stretching exercises smoothly and slowly: don't bounce, jerk or otherwise try to force a joint or muscle beyond its limits. Repeat each one until you feel loose.

Follow the exercises by relaxed practice of the activity you're about to do. For swimming, get into the pool, float, test your legstrokes: play around in the water.

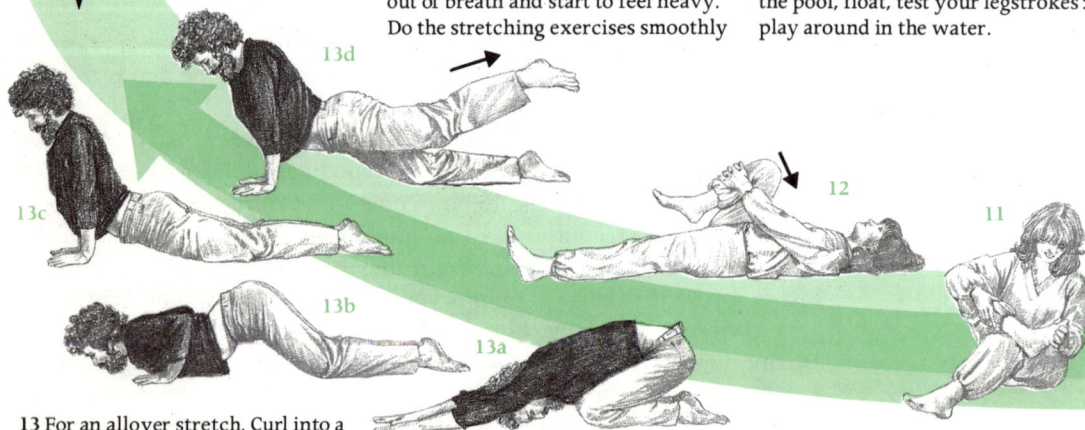

13 For an allover stretch. Curl into a ball, hugging yourself in. Keeping head and chest close to the ground, stretch your arms forwards (a) and hollow your back (b). Without moving your hands again, raise your head and chest (c). Carefully extend the left leg behind you and stretch it (d). Extend and stretch right leg.

12 To help relax abdomen, lower back and hamstrings. Lie on the ground, lift one knee into your chest and hug it there with both arms. Repeat with the other knee. Keep your head and trunk on the ground, but lift them if you feel strain.

11 This helps to prevent ankle injuries. Sit resting one ankle on the other knee, which should be slightly raised. Grasp the lower leg with one hand, and the sole with the other, and gently push the foot as far as it will go in all directions. Repeat with the other foot.

4 Let your head hang loose. Describe a vertical, clockwise circle with the point of your chin. Do the same anti-clockwise (a, b). Repeat this until all the tension in the neck has gone.

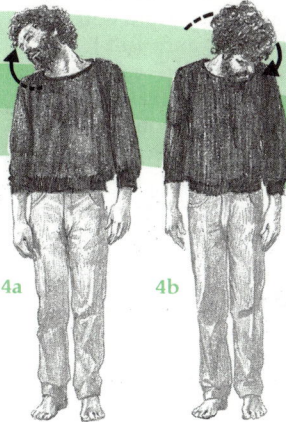

5 This stretches the muscles at the waist. Stand with legs apart. Keeping trunk straight and bottom tucked under, bend to the right from the waist. As you bend, lift your left arm up above your ear. Grasp your left hand with your right and pull down gently. Hold for 20 seconds; repeat to the left.

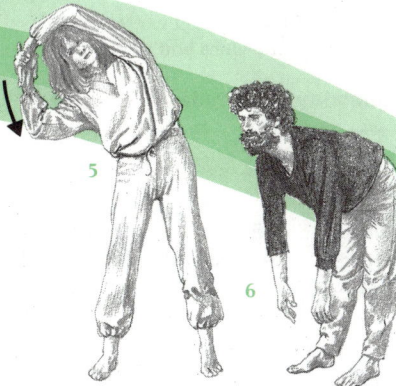

6 To stretch the muscles and tendons at the backs of the thighs. With feet apart and legs straight, bend over, keeping head up and back straight and letting the arms flop loose. Don't bend to touch your toes, just hang and feel the muscles at the backs of the legs take the weight. Hold for 20 seconds. Repeat until you feel loose.

7 To loosen your feet and ankles: squat with feet together, knees apart, heels off the ground and hands by the sides of your feet. Stand up smoothly and slowly, rising on to tiptoe. Repeat five times.

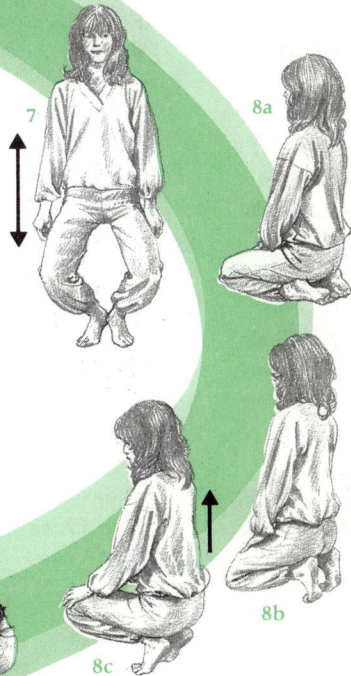

Cooling down

To cool down, do the warm-up routine in reverse order. First, continue your aerobic sport for 10–15 minutes at a slower pace, so blood circulates and clears out waste products. Breathe deeply and relax, while maintaining position and style. Don't pile on thick clothing if you're very hot, but slip into your oversuit as soon as your temperature cools. If possible change into warm, dry clothes before beginning the cool-down exercises. Now, when the muscles are warmed and relaxed, is the best time to work at mobility: any aches show you where you need it most.

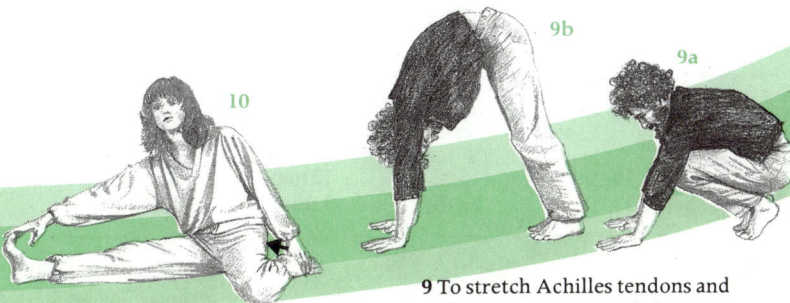

10 For hip and leg mobility. Sit with your right leg straight out in front, the foot flexed upwards. Double the left leg under you, as if hurdling; pull it back with your left hand. Reach towards your right foot with your right hand. Stretch for as long as comfortable. Repeat with your left leg in front.

9 To stretch Achilles tendons and calf muscles. Squat with feet together, knees apart and raised heels. Place your hands in front of your knees and put your weight on them (a), gently lowering your heels. Tuck in your chin and raise your bottom; keep heels down and hands flat or take your weight on the fingertips (b). Hold for 30 seconds; lift your heels if you feel strain.

8 This stretches the thigh muscles and helps ankle mobility. Kneel with feet together and knees a little apart. Gently lower your weight until you're sitting back on your heels, first with the tops of your feet flat on the floor (a), then with your toes supporting your weight (b). Get up, keeping a straight back, without using your hands to push yourself up (c).

71

Jogging

The only essential equipment is a pair of special running shoes, to protect your feet and cushion your whole body from the jolts of repeated impact. Don't run on your toes: lower the heels first, rocking forwards on them as in walking.

Never just rush out and jog. Go at a fast walk *interspersed* with brief jogs. In the progressive jogging plan beneath, the upper figure each day is the number of minutes you should spend exercising, the lower figure the length of each individual jog. Check your pulse after each one and stick to your safe pulse rate (see pages 23–24): it governs the number of times you can jog in a session. This will increase as you become fitter until you're jogging almost the whole time. Don't worry about your speed – it's the time spent exercising that's important. Once you've worked through the seven-week plan, aim to exercise for 15 minutes three days, and 30 minutes two days, a week.

Don't be afraid to take a day off if you're tired. If your pulse is ten beats per minute higher than usual first thing, don't jog, just walk.

If you're very unfit *walk* for the first week: 15 minutes continuous walking Monday to Friday; 30 minutes on Saturday and Sunday.

Week	Monday	Tuesday	Wednesday	Thursday	Friday	Saturday	Sunday
1	15min 15sec	15min 30sec	30min 30sec	15min 45sec	15min 45sec	15min 45sec	30min 45sec
2	15min 45sec	15min 1min	30min 45sec	15min 45sec	15min 45sec	15min 45sec	30min 1min
3	15min 45sec	15min 1min	30min 1min	15min 45sec	15min 1min	15min 45sec	30min 1min 15sec
4	15min 45sec	15min 1min 15sec	30min 1min	15min 1min	15min 1min	15min 1min	30min 1min 30sec
5	15min 45sec	15min 1min 30sec	30min 1min 15sec	15min 1min	15min 1min	15min 1min	30min 2min
6	15min 1min	15min 1min 30sec	30min 1min 30sec	15min 1min 30sec	15min 1min 30sec	15min 1min 30sec	30min 2min 30sec
7	15min 1min	15min 2min	30min 2min	15min 1min 30sec	15min 2min	15min 1min 30sec	30min 3min

Cycling

Cycling fits easily into the daily routine: start cycling to work, or follow this progressive plan showing the number of minutes you should cycle each day. The eventual aim is to cycle 30 minutes five days, and 45–60 minutes two days, a week.

Since the body weight is supported, cycling is excellent if you're very overweight or have problems with your joints; but as it's such an efficient method of propulsion you have to do it longer than other aerobic sports for it to have effect. Concentrate on the time spent exercising, not the speed, and keep the pace steady. Check your pulse rate regularly (see pages 23–24).

Any bike will do (including a stationary one, see page 59), but it must be the right size, so you can maintain good posture (see pages 12–15). Well-pumped tyres give an easier ride. So do flattish, hard shoes – running shoes tend to bend when you press the pedals. Push down with the ball of the foot, not the arch.

Week	Monday	Tuesday	Wednesday	Thursday	Friday	Saturday	Sunday
1	5	5	10	5	10	5	15
2	5	10	15	5	15	10	20
3	10	15	20	15	20	15	25
4	15	20	25	15	25	20	30
5	20	30	30	20	30	25	35
6	25	30	35	25	30	30	40
7	30	30	40	30	30	30	45

73

Skipping

The ground or floor should be level and free of snags, and there must be enough space overhead. Wear loose clothes – as few as possible – and running shoes if skipping on a hard surface. Make your own rope or buy a training rope at a sports store. It should be heavy enough to give a good action, and preferably be bearing-mounted to the handles so that it doesn't twist.

In the plan shown beneath, the upper figure each day is the total amount of time you should spend skipping. To begin with, this is built up in short periods of sustained skipping: the lower figure is the length of each period. Keep checking your pulse and stick to your safe pulse rate (see pages 23–24). As you get fitter cut down rests between the periods, until you're skipping continuously. The eventual aim is to skip for 15 minutes every day

with an extra 15 minutes on Wednesdays and Sundays.

Push off with your toes and land lightly on the balls of your feet. Start with the basic running step: one foot at a time over the rope, alternate feet leading. Progress to jumping the rope with both feet together. Only when you're well-advanced should you hop over: taking off and landing on the same foot, alternate legs.

Week	Monday	Tuesday	Wednesday	Thursday	Friday	Saturday	Sunday
1	5 min **30 sec**	5 min **30 sec**	7½ min **45 sec**	5 min **30 sec**	5 min **30 sec**	5 min **30 sec**	7½ min **45 sec**
2	5 min **30 sec**	7½ min **45 sec**	10 min **1 min**	5 min **30 sec**	7½ min **45 sec**	5 min **30 sec**	10 min **1 min**
3	5 min **30 sec**	7½ min **45 sec**	10 min **1 min**	7½ min **45 sec**	5 min **30 sec**	5 min **30 sec**	12½ min **1 min 15 sec**
4	5 min **30 sec**	10 min **1 min**	7½ min **45 sec**	7½ min **45 sec**	7½ min **45 sec**	5 min **30 sec**	15 min **1 min 30 sec**
5	5 min **30 sec**	12½ min **1 min 15 sec**	15 min **1 min 30 sec**	12½ min **1 min 15 sec**	12½ min **1 min 15 sec**	7½ min **45 sec**	15 min **1 min 30 sec**
6	7½ min **45 sec**	15 min **1 min 30 sec**	15 min **1 min 30 sec**	15 min **1 min 30 sec**	15 min **1 min 30 sec**	12½ min **1 min 15 sec**	15 min **1 min 30 sec**
7	10 min **1 min**	15 min **1 min 30 sec**	2 sessions of 15 min **1 min 30 sec**	15 min **1 min 30 sec**	15 min **1 min 30 sec**	15 min **1 min 30 sec**	2 sessions of 15 min **1 min 30 sec**

Swimming

Swimming is gentle, whole-body exercise with high aerobic value. Since the body weight is supported, it's good for those who are overweight or have back or joint troubles.

The plan beneath involves swimming either three or five times a week. The number of minutes to swim for each day is shown: the three-day plan in black, the five-day one in green. The eventual aim is a minimum total of 90 minutes swimming a week.

To begin with you may not be able to swim for the whole period: a five-minute session could mean swimming one width, then a walk back to your starting point before doing another width. Judge roughly by your pulse rate and by the ease of your breathing whether you need to add walks back to your session.

Float until you feel at home in the water, then try backstroke – leg-kicking only. Progress to sidestroke, breaststroke, and, for the young and fit, the crawl. Keep the pace steady and slow at first.

For walking to and from the poolside you'll need plastic or rubber slippers – available at sports stores and some pools; you may also want anti-chlorine goggles. While in the pool, try some of the water exercises on pages 76–79.

Week	Monday	Tuesday	Wednesday	Thursday	Friday	Saturday	Sunday
1	3	5	3	3	3	3	3 / 5
2	3	5	3	3 / 5	3	3	8 / 10
3	5	10	5	10	5	5	15 / 15
4	7	15	7	15	7	7	20 / 20
5	10	20	10	20	10	10	25 / 25
6	12	25	12	25	12	12	30 / 30
7	20	30	20	30	20	20	30 / 30

75

Exercising in water

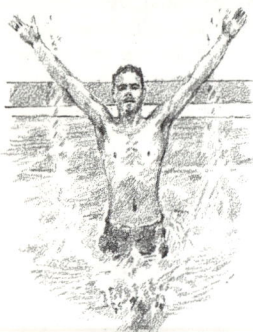

To warm up, jump vigorously, stretching in all directions.

Water is an ideal medium for exercise: its resistance helps to build strength while at the same time its buoyancy supports the weight of the body. This relieves the pressure of gravity on the spine and allows the muscles at the back of the body and legs, which usually keep the body erect, to relax. As movements in the water involve less tension, this helps to prevent the build-up of the waste products in the bloodstream that make the muscles feel stiff and leaden. Exercising in water is particularly useful for those with back, knee, hip or ankle problems, as it's possible to do many weight-bearing exercises without the jarring effect of exercising on land.

These exercises are suitable for non-swimmers as well as swimmers, as most of them are practised in chest-deep water with the help of a hand-rail. For non-swimmers they help to build confidence in the water. They are also a good way for parents to stay warm and active while keeping an eye on children. Some people do, however, find it hard to float – this is determined by weight distribution and body shape – and so they will find some of these exercises more difficult.

Try not to rest too long between exercises, as this lowers the temperature of the body and prevents proper relaxation. At first you may feel slightly stiff the next day because the resistance of the water is greater than it seems. However, this will wear off within the next few days – one of the best ways of relieving it is to exercise again. As the muscles firm up, the exercises become easier.

1a

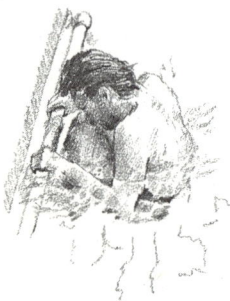

1 Strengthens hand muscles and biceps and stretches Achilles tendons, calf muscles (often shortened in women who wear high heels), and hamstrings, thus helping to prevent a common football injury. Face the rail, holding it with both hands, and crouch up close to it, with your head relaxed on your knees (a). Straighten your arms and legs, pushing away from the edge and pressing your heels on the wall (b). Repeat 12 times.

1b

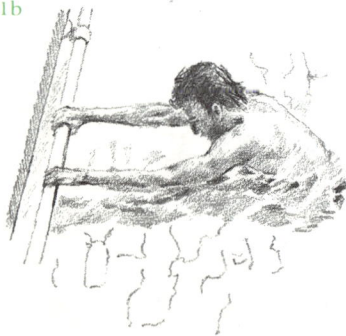

2 This increases the mobility of the neck and lower spine, slims the waist and strengthens the arms. Stand close to the pool edge, facing sideways; hold the rail with your left hand (a). Turn your head to the right and stretch your right arm out (b). Lean right out from the rail, straightening your left arm but keeping your feet by the pool edge. Stretch your right hand up and arch your body over to the left (c). Repeat eight times to each side.

2a

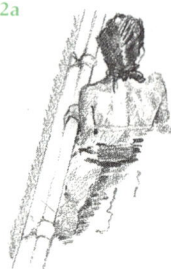

2b

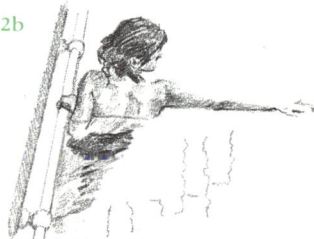

2c

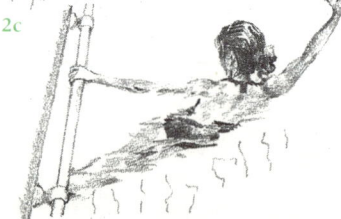

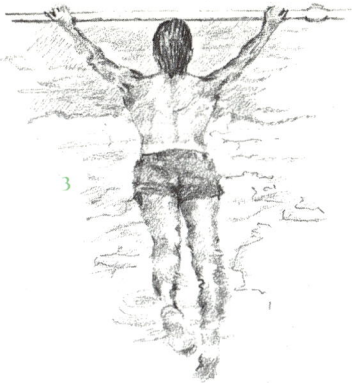

3 This exercise allows the spine to stretch out. The water's resistance helps to slim the thighs; its buoyancy relaxes the ankles – thus helping to prevent ankle injuries – and reduces articular tension and pain common in arthritic conditions. You may not be able to do this exercise if you don't float easily. With your hands on the rail, lie prone in the water. Kick your legs, keeping your knees straight and relaxing your ankles. Don't kick too hard; a movement of about 30 cm [12 in] is sufficient. Do about 16 kicks in all. You can also do this exercise lying on your back.

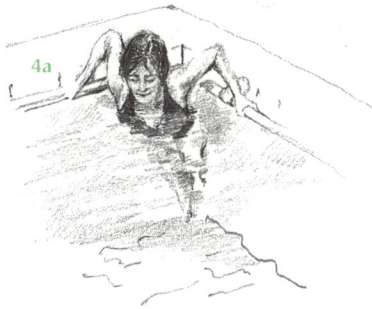

4 Good for upper arm flab. The water's buoyancy means that even those with weak arms can do it. It's best done at the deep end as it strengthens the arms more if you can't push with the feet. With your back to the edge, hold the rail fairly close to your body (a). Straighten your arms to lift your weight upwards (b). Hold for a second before going down. Repeat eight times.

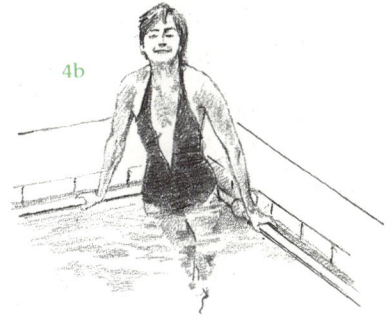

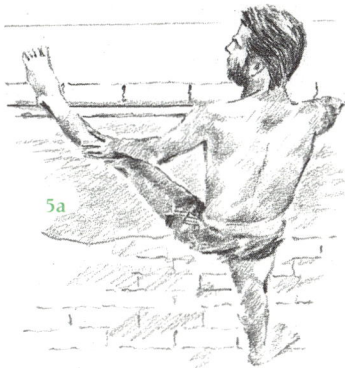

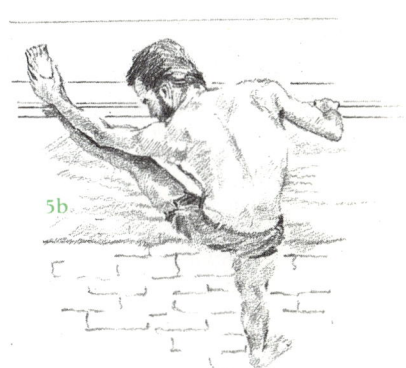

5 To stretch the inside thigh and hamstring muscles, and so prevent muscle tears in sports players. Face the edge and lift your left leg to place the heel on the rail. Holding the rail with your right hand, rest the left hand on your left knee (a). Stretch out the left hand to clasp the left foot, keeping the right leg straight (b). Hold for five seconds, relaxing and feeling your spine stretch. Return to (a). Repeat six times to each side.

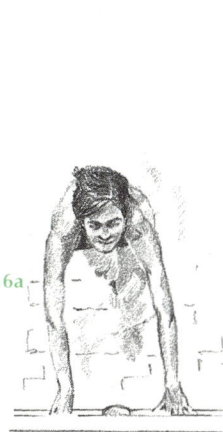

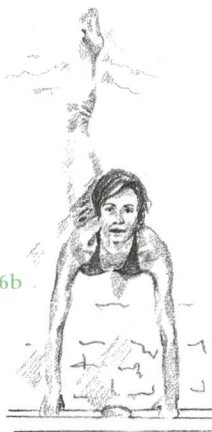

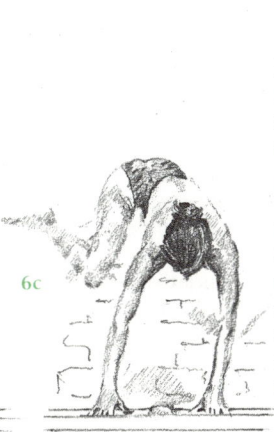

6 This slims the buttocks and thighs and stretches the muscles at the inside of the thighs. Stand facing the pool side and hold the rail with both hands (a). Swing your right leg back behind (b). Bring it forwards as if jumping a hurdle, bending the knee, but keeping the thigh parallel to the ground (c). Circle the leg back down to the starting position (a) again. Repeat eight times to one side and eight to the other.

77

▷

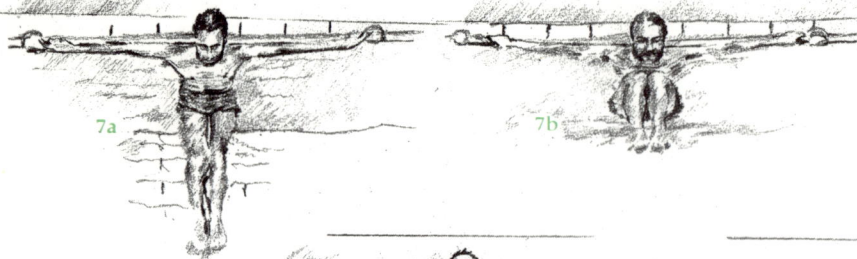
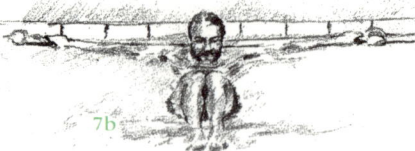
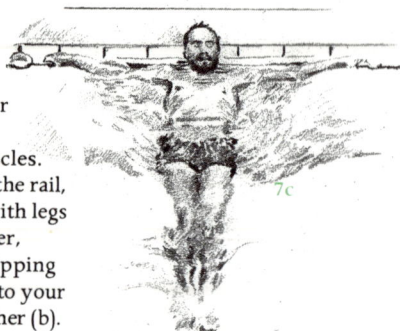
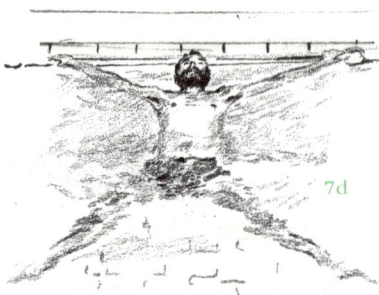

7 This is particularly good for slimming the thighs. It also exercises the abdominal muscles. Stretch your arms out along the rail, your back to the pool side, with legs outstretched and feet together, resting on the bottom (a). Gripping the rail, bend your knees up to your chest, keeping the legs together (b). Straighten your legs out again, allowing them to float (c). Stretch out as far as possible, so your shoulders move away from the side of the pool, and spread your legs apart (d). Return to the starting position (a) without bending your knees. Repeat five times.

8 Stretches inside thigh and hamstring muscles. The arm movement strengthens and firms the pectoral muscles, while the head movement reduces a double chin. Face the rail and hold it with both hands. Hook both feet up under it and stretch them wide apart. Pull yourself into the side without bending your knees (a). Straighten your arms, pushing away from the edge and stretching your head back (b). Hold for three seconds, then straighten up. Repeat eight times.

9 To slim the outside of the thighs and the waist; also to exercise the arms gently, open up the chest, and reduce a double chin. Stand on your right leg. Lift your left leg straight up to the side, so it's parallel with the water surface. Stretch your arms right out to the sides to help your balance, and turn your head to the left to tone up the muscles in your neck. Hold for three seconds. Repeat four times to each side.

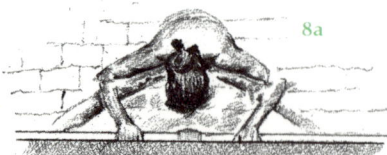
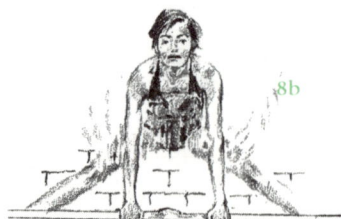

10 This slims the waist, stretches the hamstrings, and helps to strengthen thigh muscles. Face the rail and hold on with both hands. Lift your legs to tuck the toes under the rail, keeping them straight and stretching the feet as far apart as possible (a).

Still holding the knees straight, touch your right foot with your left hand (b); switch to left side. Repeat ten times.

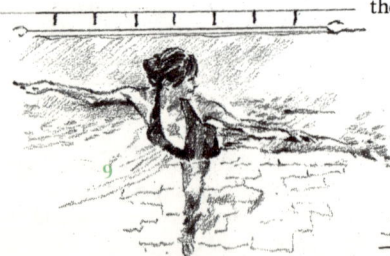
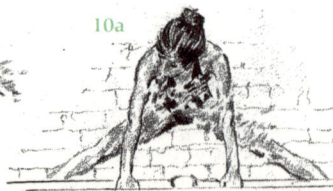
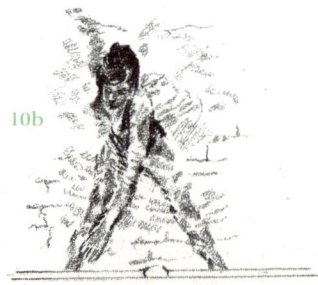

11 This tones and strengthens the muscles of upper arms, shoulders and chest, and those down the front of the legs. It also helps to relieve fibrositis of the shoulders. Lie on your back on the surface of the water at right angles to the pool side, feet tucked under the rail and arms at your sides (a). Make yourself as tall as possible to lengthen the spine. Raise your arms above your head (b). Turn your hands, so the palms face outwards, and pull against the water (c) to bring them back to the sides of the body. Repeat ten times.

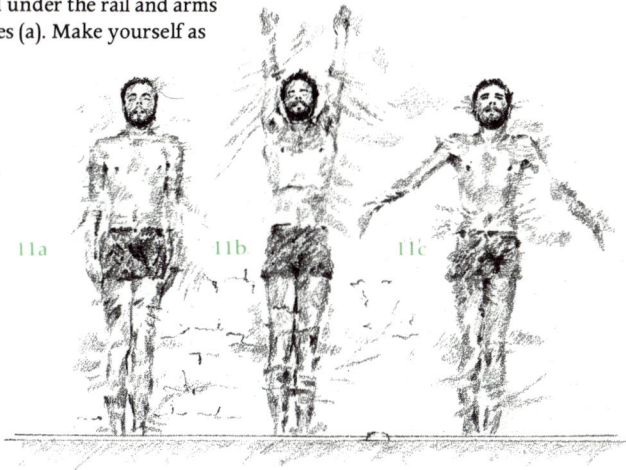

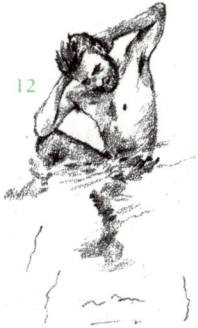

11a 11b 11c

12

12 This strengthens and slims the abdominal muscles and thighs, and mobilizes the spine. Stand away from the side of the pool and clasp your hands behind your head. Lift your left knee up and bring the right elbow down to meet it. Repeat with right knee and left elbow. Do ten times, alternating sides.

13 You'll need a partner for this exercise. It stretches and strengthens the abdominal, chest, arm and thigh muscles, and helps to counteract bad posture. Stand back to back with your arms stretched above your head and hands clasped (a). One partner now bends forwards from the waist, stretching out the arms as far as possible and extending the spine at the same time so that the other partner is stretched backwards with his or her feet off the pool floor (b). Hold for five seconds, before returning to central position. Repeat with partners changing roles, six times to each side.

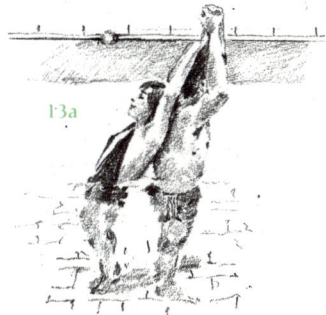

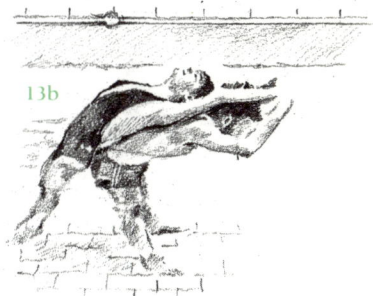

13a 13b

14 Another exercise for two people. It slims the waist and improves breathing by opening the ribcage. Stand with feet apart, holding nearest hands. Your arms should be stretched out to the sides as far as possible (a). Keeping your arms straight, stretch over to touch outer hands and form a diamond shape with the arms (b). Don't allow your feet to move. Hold for two seconds. Repeat ten times.

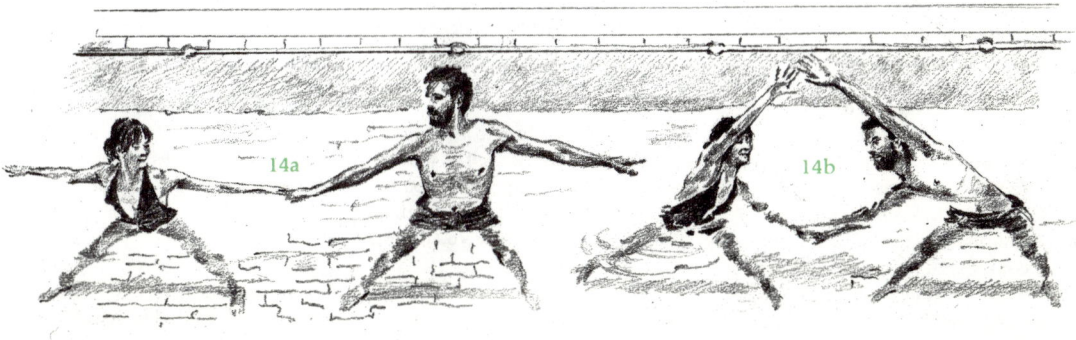

14a 14b

SPECIAL NEEDS: Fit for childbirth

Pregnancy is a good time to start making your body more flexible and to create new habits of regular exercise, correct posture, relaxation and good breathing. This is because the ligaments and joints of the body loosen so that room can be made in the pelvis for the baby.

Carrying the baby

While you are carrying the baby, your abdominal muscles, spine and pelvic floor have to be strong enough to support the growing weight. Strong leg muscles encourage good circulation, and this helps prevent tiredness, cramp and varicose veins. Because so much extra weight is concentrated in one part of your body, posture is also important; above all, try to ensure your pelvis is tilted correctly (see page 12).

In late pregnancy it may be hard to find a comfortable position for resting and sleeping. Try lying on your side with your top leg bent and placing a cushion under the knee. The extra support stops the top leg pulling on the lower back.

Having the baby

Supple hip joints, legs and feet help you to move into useful positions for labour and birth. Practise squatting with your heels on the floor to strengthen the lower back, hips, knees and ankles. The abdominal muscles should be strong to help with delivery and the pelvic floor in good shape so it can cope with stretching as the baby passes through it. If you can breathe well and relax (see pages 208–09) you will be able to keep control and be as comfortable as possible during labour.

After the baby

The body undergoes many changes and much hard work during pregnancy, delivery and immediately after the birth, and restoring it through exercise is essential to avoid later problems, particularly with the pelvic floor. The ability to relax and breathe well is helpful in coping with the strains of parenthood and the hard work involved in looking after a baby. The fitter you are, the less likely you are to tire easily. Babies spend a lot of time on the floor, so if you can squat and sit on the floor in comfort, you will both enjoy playing more.

Strengthening the pelvic floor
While you are pregnant and after the birth, strengthen the pelvic floor muscles with this exercise. Breathing normally, lift, tighten and squeeze the pelvic floor to a count of four, and then release. Try this lying down at first, but it can be done in any position, preferably as often as possible; it can also be combined with pelvic tilts (see exercise 8, page 33). It helps to keep the pelvic area strong and healthy, which encourages full enjoyment of sex, and will prevent problems such as incontinence later on.

Exercise tips
Don't strain or overdo any of the exercises. It's best to practise a little, regularly. Once you've overcome any initial stiffness, the exercises should be pleasant and should make you feel better.

Don't hold your breath; relax, release and breathe well as you exercise. This will prepare you for breathing during labour. Take a deep breath before and after you do each exercise.

Do each exercise four times only.

Turn on to your side first as you sit up or lie down.

Don't lie on your back and try to lift both legs up in the air. It's quite unnecessary and much too strenuous. Instead do this routine of gentle but effective exercises.

Don't do exercises that make you overarch and squeeze the small of your back.

In late pregnancy you may find lying on your back uncomfortable. If so, lie on your side instead.

Ante-natal exercises

Make this gentle routine part of your daily relaxation time. Where appropriate, try the exercises lying on your back to begin with so that the trunk is supported. A cushion placed under your head may make you more comfortable. Progress to doing the exercises sitting, first with your back supported and then without, but go cautiously. Always be gentle with yourself.

If the ante-natal routine isn't enough, you may safely add any of the post-natal exercises, but don't strain or hold your breath.

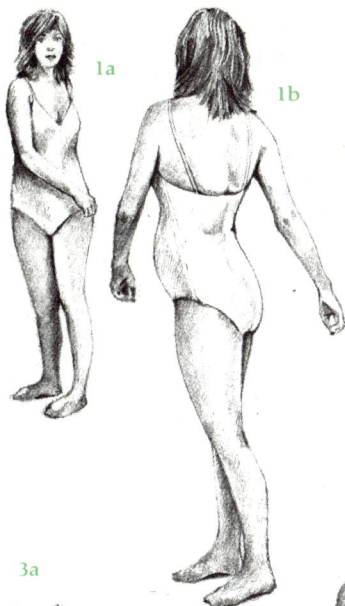

1 For spine and abdomen. Stand with good posture (see page 12), feet a little apart and arms by your sides. Keeping your feet firm, twist gently to the left (a) and to the right (b). Check your posture again. Don't do this exercise if you find that it hurts your lower back.

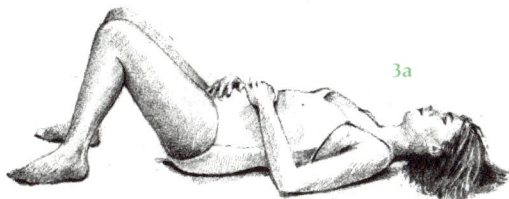

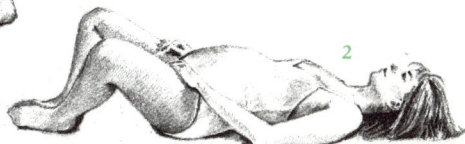

2 For supple hips, knees and feet. Lie on your back and bend your legs up. Bring the soles of your feet together and let your knees fall outwards. Hold for a while and practise the pelvic floor exercise opposite; otherwise, pull in the abdominal muscles or stretch your arms up. This exercise can also be done sitting, with your back supported if necessary.

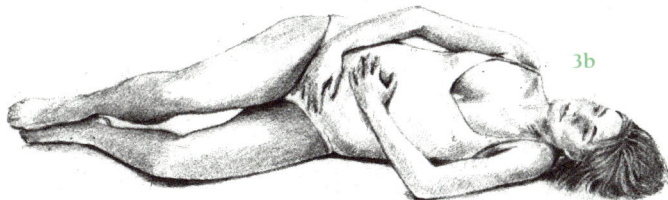

3 To keep the abdomen in shape. Lie on your back (a) or side (b), with your knees bent and your hands on your abdomen. Breathe in; breathing out, pull your abdomen in gently. Hold for a while, breathing normally. Practise this whenever you think of it, in any position.

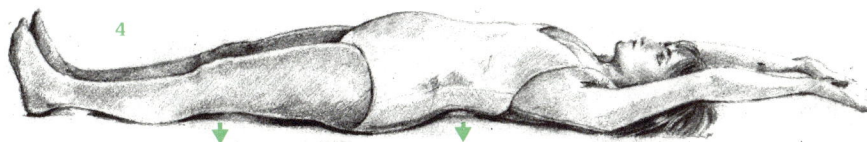

4 Good for posture. Lie on your back, with your arms stretched over your head; breathe in and really stretch, pressing your lower back and knees into the floor. Breathe out and stop stretching. If your lower back feels uncomfortable, put a cushion under your thighs. If you're still not comfortable, bend your legs up, keeping your feet flat on the floor, and stretch your arms and trunk only. This exercise can also be practised sitting cross-legged with your back against a wall.

5 For spine, hips, knees and feet. Sit with your legs crossed, on a cushion if it's more comfortable. Breathing in, straighten your spine and lift the front ribs. Hold for a while, breathing normally. If you find this difficult at first, rest your back against a wall for support. Stand up slowly after the exercise. Try to sit cross-legged often, even on a sofa.

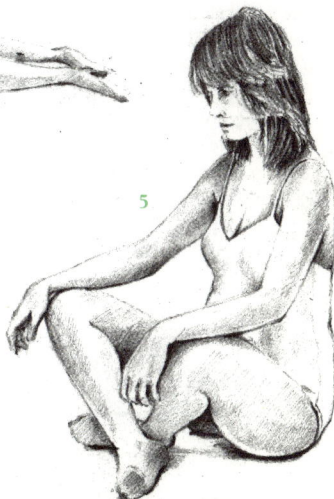

81

Fit for childbirth

Post-natal exercises

1 To improve posture and shorten and tighten the abdominal muscles. Stand with your feet apart, knees slightly bent. Put one hand on your abdomen with the fingertips on the pubic bone, the other on your lower back, fingers pointing down (a). Breathe in; breathe out and tilt the pelvis, pulling the abdominal muscles in and lifting the pubic bone forwards and up so your bottom is tucked down and in (b). Hold for a while, breathing normally.

This can also be done sitting or lying. Try tightening abdomen, buttocks and pelvic floor at the same time.

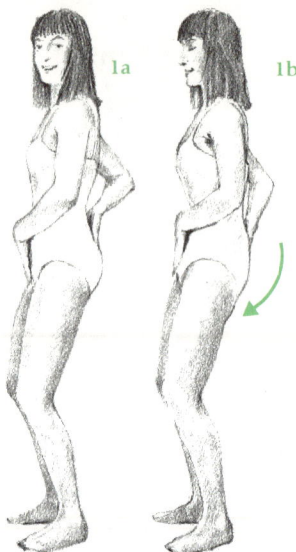

1a *1b*

Exercises 1–4 on pages 38–39 can be included in the ante- and post-natal exercise routines. No. 5 on page 40 is beneficial after the birth.

2 Works diagonal abdominal muscles and mobilizes pelvis and spine. Lie facing upwards, legs bent up to your chest, hands clasped behind your head and breathe in (a). Breathing out, roll your legs to the right, keeping the knees together and turning your head to the left (b). Breathe in and lift your knees back to the centre. Repeat to the other side (c), breathing out as you roll your legs over, and in as you lift them back to the centre.

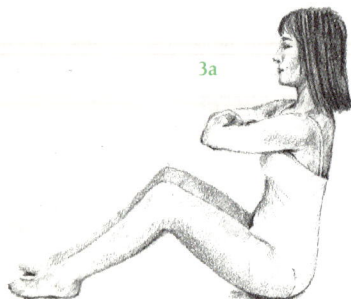

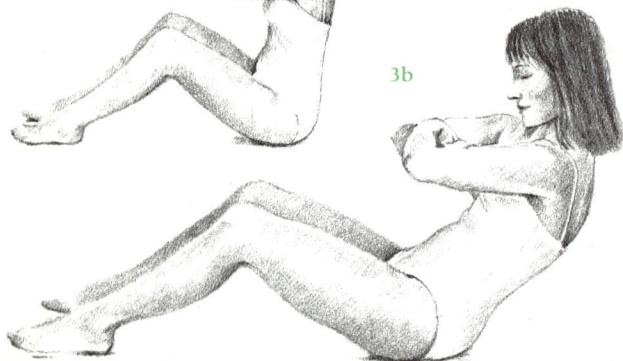

3a

3b

2a

2b

2c

3 For the vertical muscles of the abdomen. Sit up tall, legs bent, arms folded but held away from the body with elbows up and breathe in (a). Breathing out, do a pelvic tilt, as in exercise 1, and lean back until the abdominal muscles begin to tighten (b). Breathing normally, hold for a while; breathe in and sit up.

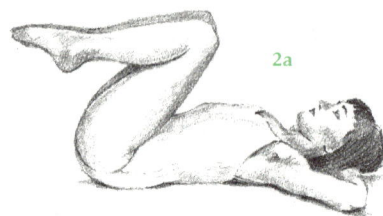

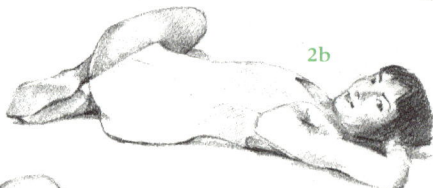

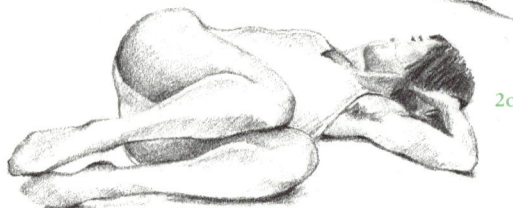

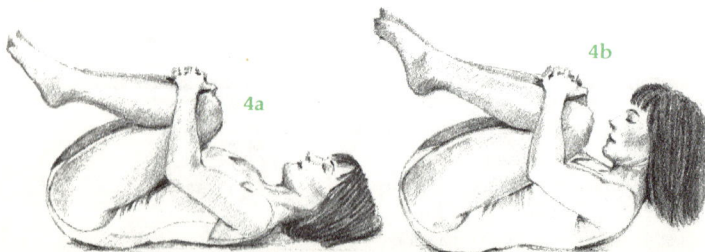

4 For abdomen and spine. Lie on your back with your legs bent up to your chest and hands clasped round your knees. Breathe in; breathing out, suck your abdomen in, trying to pull the navel to the spine, and press your knees against your chest (a). Breathe in and release. For an extra stretch try this with your head lifted up to your knees (b).

4a

4b

Relieving aches and pains

Many everyday aches and pains can be healed, or at least eased, by movement, if it's done at the right time and in moderate amounts.

First check with your doctor or practitioner that your condition will benefit from exercise and describe the exercises you plan to do. He may recommend complete rest at first.

Always work gently, never force or overdo movement. Little and often is the rule. Do each exercise up to five times, performing it rhythmically and smoothly. To progress, repeat your set of exercises at intervals up to three times a day, providing you don't get tired; always work within your own capacity. As you do them, bear in mind that done quickly they give mobility, and done slowly they strengthen, so vary the pace as you go. You're bound to feel some stiffness at first: this is normal and will wear off as you exercise regularly.

If commonplace problems go on for longer than a few days, or recur frequently, consult your doctor.

Ankles: *swollen*
Often a result of standing or sitting for too long, these can occur when circulation in legs, ankles and feet is bad. Placing the legs at three successive levels will restore their circulation, reduce swelling and make them feel rested.

Lie on your back, arms by your sides, with your legs up at a comfortable angle against a wall, or placed on a chair or similar surface so that they're more than 60 cm [2 ft] above your heart (a). Rest in this position for two minutes. Then lie flat for two minutes (b). Finally, sit on a chair or sofa with your legs down for two minutes (c).

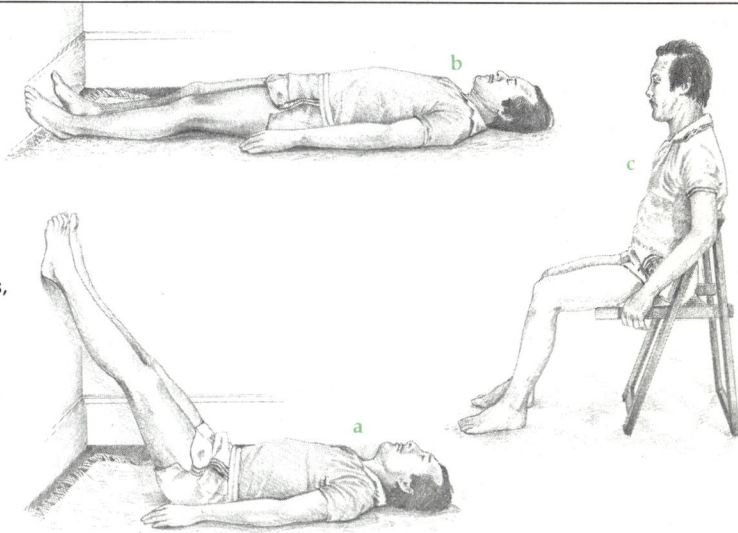

Arms and hands: *pain or tingling*
May be caused either by tension or by carrying heavy objects that pull down the arms and overstretch the nerves. Do exercise 5, page 29, and those on pages 36–37. If exercise does not relieve the problem, see your doctor. These exercises also help chilblains and poor circulation in the hands.

Arthritis: *see* OSTEOARTHRITIS

Asthma
A respiratory condition. Teach yourself to breathe *out* as an attack comes on, since this collapses the lungs and so allows you to breathe in. Having an item to blow may help you to practise this: blow a crumpled tissue off a surface or puff out candles. It can be very frightening when you keep trying to breathe in but find that you can't draw air into your lungs. Fright may make you hang on tightly to something, but this fixes the chest and ribs and further prevents breathing. Relaxing your shoulders, arms and hands (see pages 208–10) as you blow out will help you not to do this. Learn the routine – don't panic, think, breathe out, relax – until it's second nature.

Asthma can be much relieved by sprays given on prescription and by carefully graded exercise. Avoid anything that's too strenuous and makes you out of breath.

Try to increase the mobility of the chest: exercises 4 and 5 on page 32 will help. So will good posture (see pages 12–15) and all chest-opening exercises (see pages 34–35). Yoga (see pages 214–20) helps to teach breathing control; see also Breathing, page 211. These exercises also help bronchitis sufferers.

83
▷

Back pain

In most cases this can be prevented and remedied by good posture (see pages 12–15) and by exercise. Check that nothing – a sagging bed or a badly adjusted chair – is aggravating the problem (see pages 18–21).

During severe attacks of back pain in which the muscles are in spasm, rest and warmth are essential. Lie on your back with a pillow under your knees and a soft hot-water bottle in the painful area. For immediate relief tilt the pelvis forwards (exercise 2a, page 39) as often as you can: do it very gently, lying down at first.

As soon as a spasm has gone, practise the pelvic tilting routine (exercise 8, page 33), gently and calmly. Finish on a forward tilt. Move the pelvis in all directions a few times each day with exercises 3, page 28, and 7, page 33. Try 5, page 32; 12, page 41, or 4, page 82; 5, page 28, or 9, page 33. As soon as is comfortable, do the whole Daily minimum. Exercising in water also helps (see page 76).

1 Learn to release the lower back by squatting – against a wall for balance if necessary. If you can't get your heels flat on the floor at first, put a book beneath them for support.

Weight-bearing exercises strengthen the back but mustn't be done until the pain is *completely* gone: doing them then will help prevent it happening again. Start with exercise 5, page 40; when that has become easy, go on to exercise 4, page 43.

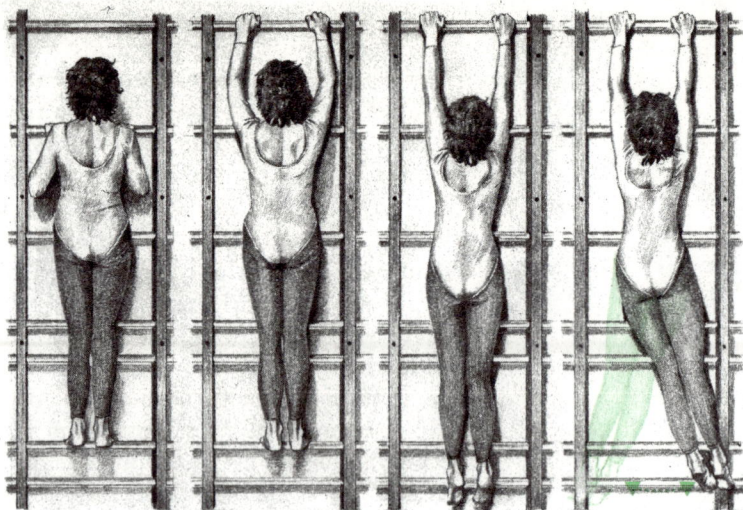

2a   2b   2c   3

Hanging gives marvellous relief to back sufferers since gravity and the weight of the hips and legs lengthen and release the lower back. Wall-bars are ideal, but at home you can install an exercise bar: have a partner on hand so that you can stand on a book or box beneath

the bar, grasp the bar, then ask your partner to remove the support gently, and to replace it when you've finished, so you won't jar the spine by jumping up or down.

2 Stand on a low bar (or a support) (a). Raise your arms and grasp the bar above you (b). Slowly take your feet off the lower bar (or ask your partner to remove the support) (c). Hang there: less than a minute may be enough at first. Work up to three or four minutes. Replace your feet as in (b) and slowly step down.

3 While hanging, lift the legs together to one side then the other. This is particularly good for those with one leg longer than the other (see LEGS, page 86). In such a case do twice as many lifts on the *short*-leg side.

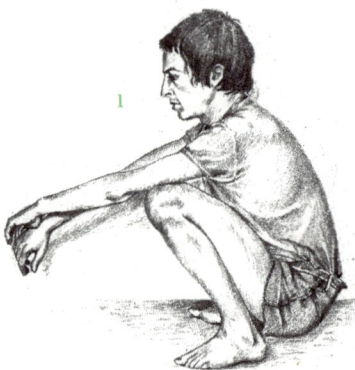

Bronchitis: *see* ASTHMA

Chilblains: *see* ARMS AND HANDS and FEET

Constipation

First make sure there is enough fibre in your diet (see pages 109–11). Lack of exercise can cause constipation, as can being in a hurry. Once again relaxation helps, and adopting a

squatting position with heels flat on the floor (see BACK PAIN exercise 1) can release the muscles of the rectum. Abdominal exercises may help; see pages 38–41 and 81–82; also pose 3, page 215.

Cramp

May be caused by constriction of circulation, or by lack of calcium. It tends to happen if muscles are out

of condition or cold; the rule is to stretch them gently away from the position in which they have contracted. To relieve cramp in the front of the thigh, see exercise 5, page 45.

For cramp in the calves and under the feet: sit down, hold your toes and pull them towards you. Or get someone else to do it for you (exercise 3, page 27).

Eyes: *aching*
Often the result of tiredness or tension – a common symptom of tension is to fix the face and eyes, and stare. Practise relaxation exercises, see pages 208–10. Get into the habit of blinking to relieve the eyes every few moments. Looking down helps, too. Try screwing up the eyes tightly, then opening them wide. Moving the eyes up, down and side to side is also beneficial.

Face: *stiff*
Try face exercises if sitting in a draught has made parts of your face stiff. They are good for circulation and a youthful appearance. Try to use the facial muscles as much as you can, to avoid the face taking on a dead-pan expression.

1 Purse your lips slightly and push your mouth towards your right ear (a), then towards the left (b). Men who shave needn't do this exercise, since shaving usually involves these movements.

2 Open the mouth as though you're screaming loudly (a), and stick your tongue right out (b) to release the throat. This exercise will also relieve tension.

Fill your cheeks with air, purse the lips and blow out slowly – this is particularly good for asthma and bronchitis sufferers.

3 Brace the muscles at the front of the throat by pushing the chin down strongly and pulling back the sides of the mouth.

Feet
Always try to wear good shoes in which the feet are not cramped and can bend freely. Go barefoot as much as possible and encourage children to do the same.

High heels – more than 25 mm [1 in] – worn regularly ruin the feet and often the spine (see pages 12–13). They can cause deformed toes, enlarged big toe joints, fallen arches, soreness in the balls of the feet, tightness behind the ankles and up the back of the calves, and exacerbate varicose veins. If you insist on wearing them you should do the exercises below, and those on pages 44–45, to compensate.

Chilblains, cold or aching feet, poor circulation
Improve circulation by doing the exercise for ANKLES (see page 83). All exercises on pages 44–45 will help. Stimulate circulation by dipping your feet into bowls of hot and cold water alternately. Massage the feet (see page 229). Move and wriggle the toes as much as possible. Yoga standing postures strengthen the feet and help to improve poor circulation (see pages 214–20).

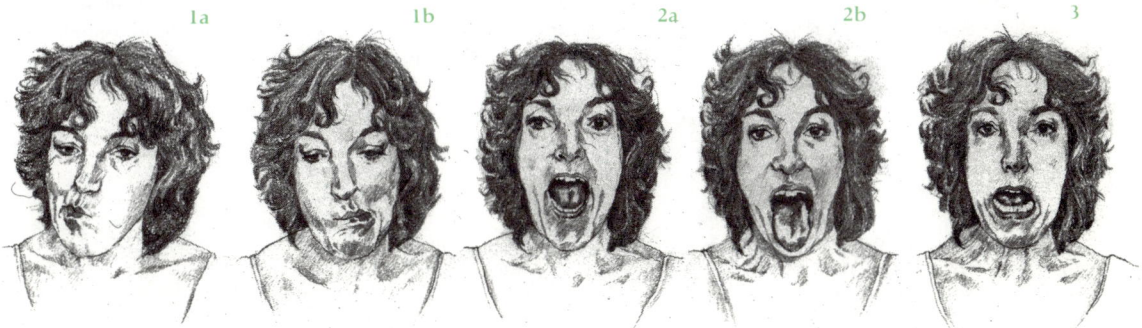

1 Massage the feet and restore circulation by rolling a ball in circular movements under one foot. Repeat with other foot.

Enlarged big toe joints (bunions)
These can be hereditary but are usually the result of wearing bad shoes. Rubber pads worn between the big toe and second toe will help. Do exercise 8, page 45, and 2, below.

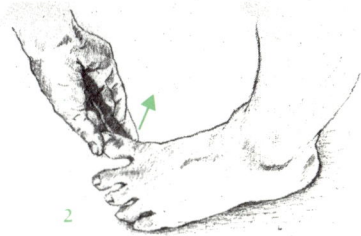

2 Pull the big toe away out from the other toes. Do as often as you can.

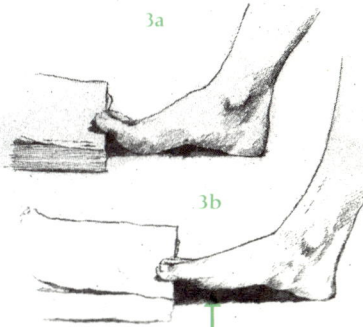

Fallen arches
3 To improve fallen arches. Place the tips of your toes on a book or similar support, resting the ball of the foot on the floor (a). Lift the ball of the foot (b), and lower it again. Repeat with other foot. Eventually you'll be able to contract the arch under your foot without supporting the toes (exercise 9, page 45); providing you're wearing comfortable shoes, you'll be able to do this at any time.

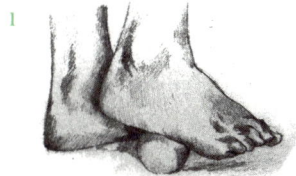

Relieving aches and pains

Headache and **Migraine**
Often the result of anxiety, tension and tiredness. The first priorities are to learn to relax, see pages 208–09, and to maintain good posture (see pages 12–15).

Migraine is an extremely severe type of headache, which takes many forms and can have many stages from disturbance of vision to bilious sickness and intolerable pain in various parts of the head. The exact causes are not known, but research has shown that certain foods can spark it off in some people (see page 133).

Try the following to get rid of a headache or to ease a migraine: massage, see pages 227–28 (always using a downward movement on the back of the neck); relaxation exercises, pages 208–10; the SHOULDERS exercises on page 88. Or try the following technique:

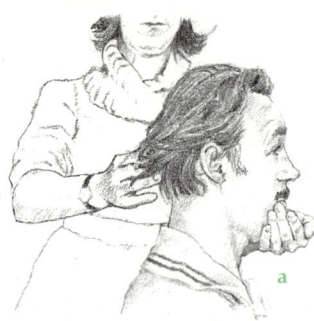

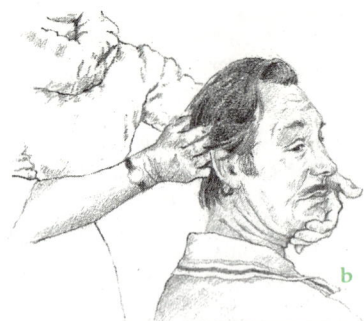

Place the middle finger of each hand at the base of your skull, on either side of the spine. Push them upwards on to the two large knobs just above the hairline – the occiput bones. Place a finger on each knob and press firmly. Hold a few seconds then remove your hands. Slowly turn your head from side to side. Massage the back of your neck in superficial circular downward movements.

It's even better if you can persuade someone else to do this for you. Your partner should support your chin with one hand, while pressing your occiput bones with the thumb and forefinger of the other one (a). He or she should next turn your head to one side and then to the other (b), before gently massaging the back of your neck in circular downward movements.

Incontinence
In women, incontinence may be caused by weak pelvic floor muscles, so contract the pelvic floor as often as you think of it (see page 80). Yoga poses 9, page 217, and 18, page 219, are very helpful because when you are inverted, gravity pulls the pelvic floor into your body.

Exercise cannot usually help incontinence in men.

Knees: *painful*
Discuss the possibility of osteo-arthritis with your doctor. Painful knees can also result from sports injuries or overweight. Always use a pad when kneeling to avoid pressure on the knees. For all these problems the answer is to strengthen the muscles at the fronts of the thighs: do OSTEOARTHRITIS exercise 1.

Legs: *one longer than the other*
Don't let your spine suffer as a result of this unevenness.

To help this condition, do the hanging exercises, BACK PAIN 2 and 3 on page 84, regularly, and exercise 7 on page 33, doing twice as many lifts

on the short-leg side, since normally this hip will be pulled down to meet the longer leg. Don't do any forward-bend standing exercises unless the short leg is supported on something, so that both hips are even; otherwise by stretching unevenly, you'll do more harm than good. Nor should you do forward-bends sitting; instead bend one leg out when you stretch forwards to the other (see pose 12, page 218).

Neck: *painful, stiff*
Often the result of tension or of sitting in a draught, this can be eased by rest, heat, gentle exercise and massage (see pages 227–28). Try the exercises on page 210, and if stiffness also affects the shoulders, those for the SHOULDERS on page 88. Should the condition persist, see

your doctor, particularly if you have had any kind of jolt, because something may be out of place.

First turn your head from side to side to test what movement is possible. Place one hand at the back of your neck and pick up the skin firmly, lifting it away as though picking up a kitten by the scruff of the neck. If the skin slips out of your hand during the exercise, stop and pick it up again. Holding the skin, nod your head up and down (a). Shake your head from side to side (b). Inscribe vertical circles with your nose, five times clockwise, and five anti-clockwise (c). Take the hand away from the back of your neck and turn your head from side to side again as at the start. It should feel much easier.

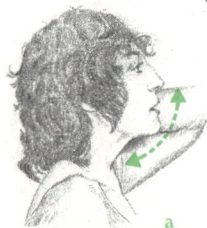

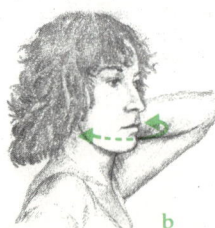

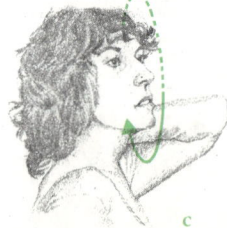

Osteoarthritis

Rheumatoid arthritis is a medical condition – patients must be under professional care.

Osteoarthritis is a wearing-away of certain joints in the body, most commonly the knees, hips and those in the hands. Overweight exacerbates it. The quadriceps – the long muscles that run down the front of the thighs and enclose the knee-caps – must be kept strong enough to support the knees, otherwise the knee joints may wear away. Since women have weaker thigh muscles than men, overweight women who spend much time standing are extra liable to get arthritis in the knees.

The rule is to keep moving. Try to exercise in warm water, as warmth and the elimination of gravity make movement easier. In any case, exercise when you're warm, with movements that don't require you to use your body weight but simply to work the relevant muscles. Try exercising on your bed in the mornings and evenings. To prevent the hips from stiffening, sit on the floor as much as possible. See page 27 for useful floor exercises.

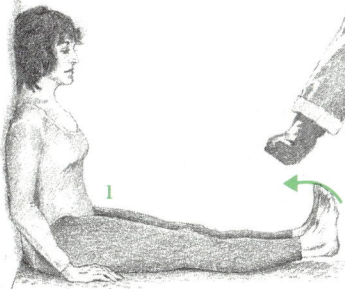

1 To strengthen the knees by tightening the quadriceps. Sit with your legs straight out in front, with your back supported for comfort. Draw your toes strongly towards you. Don't worry if your heels don't come off the floor at first – they will do so, as the muscles become stronger. You can also do this exercise lying on your back, or sitting in an easy chair with your legs straight out in front of you on a footrest.

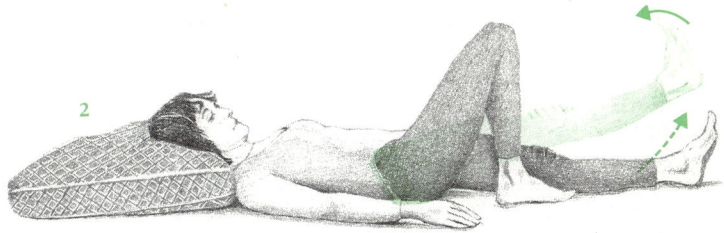

2 To strengthen the hips and knees. This can be done lying in bed with your head supported. Bend the right leg up along the bed. Straighten it a little above the bed, then draw the toes towards your nose. Lower the leg to the bed. Repeat with your left leg.

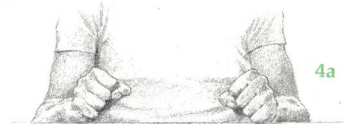

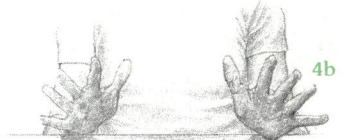

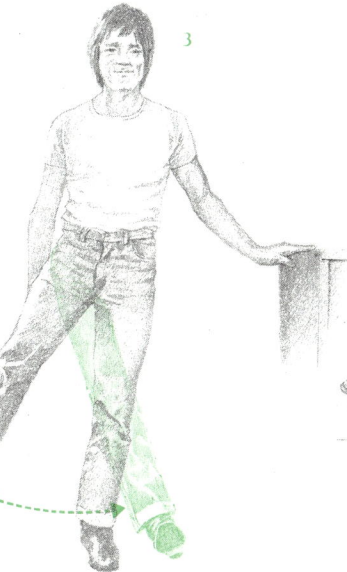

3 For hip joint mobility. Stand sideways on to a wall or bar, and hold it for balance. Stand on the leg nearer the wall, and gently and rhythmically swing your outer leg forwards and back. Also try gently swinging the outer leg across your body and then out (as shown). Repeat with other leg.

4 To improve mobility, strength and circulation in hands and wrists. Support your wrists on your thighs or on a table. Clench your fingers and thumbs strongly together (a).

Then stretch your fingers and thumbs out wide, making space between each finger (b). Continue supporting your wrists. Keeping your fingers together throughout, lift your hands and turn them in as far as you can (c); brush them across your thighs or the table and turn them as far out as possible (d).

Pre-menstrual tension and Period pain

Movement often helps the congestion and makes you feel better and less tense. Any exercise is recommended providing it's not too vigorous and doesn't tire you too much. Try the relaxation exercises on pages 208–09; some yoga poses, such as 7, page 217, also help.

Sciatica

Inflammation of the sciatic nerve, running from the low spine through the buttocks and down the backs of the legs. Apply warmth to the sore spot, and rest, lying with a cushion under the small of the back. Your doctor may advise a painkiller when inflammation is severe. When the pain has gone, exercise will help to ward off further attacks. Women may feel sciatica during pregnancy – particularly if they're unfit – owing to the extra weight.

Hanging, see BACK PAIN exercises 2 and 3 on page 84, is recommended as a first, gentle step. Then go on to the strengthening exercises, 5 on page 40, followed by 4 on page 43. Do these carefully. Later, sitting on the floor will help mobility.

In late pregnancy women should avoid back exercises lying on their front, or hanging. Instead do OSTEOARTHRITIS exercise 3 on page 87, and the following: sitting in a chair, press your thighs well down into it, which will make your bottom rise. Squeeze your buttocks together a moment. Once mastered, this can be done lying or standing.

Shoulders and upper back:
'frozen', immobile after a stroke, painful, tension knots (fibrositis)
Massage (see pages 227–28), relaxation (see pages 208–10) and yoga (see pages 214–20) help to ease shoulder problems. Also try the following two sequences.

1 Turn your head from side to side and shrug your shoulders up and down to see how stiff they feel. Place your right hand between your left shoulder and neck, and pick up the flesh. Hold it firmly. Let your left arm hang passively at your side throughout the exercise (a). Shrug your left shoulder up and down twice. Make circles with the shoulder (b), two back, two forwards and two back again. Shrug up and down twice more. Release your right hand. Turn your head and shrug as you did before starting – the side you've worked should feel looser. Repeat on the other side.

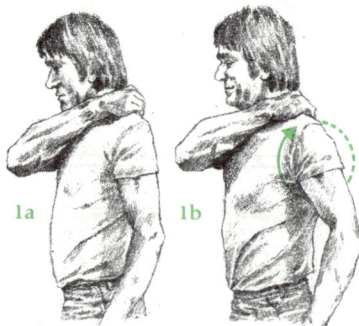

2 In the second sequence the shoulder is fixed down with the opposite hand and it's the arm that works, within the shoulder joint. Place your left hand inside your right shoulder, pressing firmly down to keep the shoulder still. Place your right fingertips on your right shoulder (a). Lift the right arm up as far as it will go, then lower it (b), repeating this five times. Lift the arm forwards (c) and back (d) gently and rhythmically. Then circle the arm forwards and back. Finally remove your left arm; take your right arm across your body, hugging it in with your left arm (e), then take the right arm out again. Repeat the sequence to the other side.

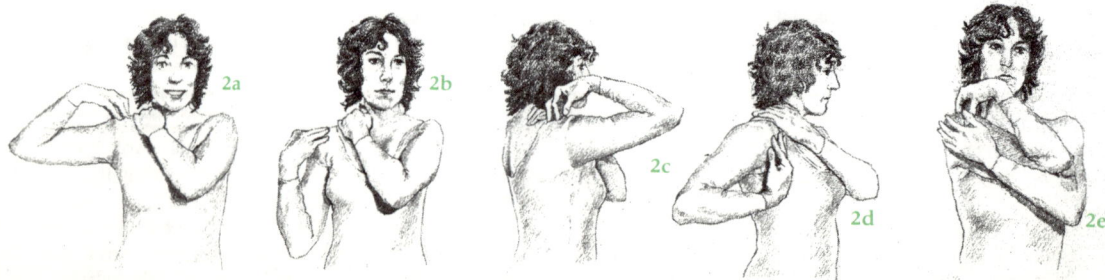

3 Particularly helpful after a stroke or for 'frozen shoulder'. Stand facing, but a little way from, a wall, with feet together. Place your lower arms on the wall (a) and gradually creep your fingertips and arms up the surface (b).

Varicose veins

Distended veins, due to sluggish circulation, common in pregnancy. Diet is important, particularly fibre (see pages 109–11). Varicose veins usually appear in the legs and can be greatly helped by movement. Circulation is the key, so do the ANKLES exercise on page 83. Try the exercises on pages 44–45, particularly 4; exercise 3, page 27; and the positions in exercise 1, page 38. Walking is helpful; see page 13 on how to do this correctly.

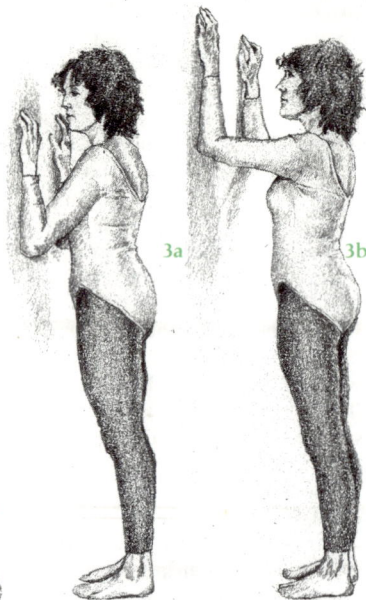

EATING
FOR
LIFE

Eat well, stay healthy

Just as ill-health can make life a misery, good health is the key to enjoying life to the full. It means having a strong body, able to recover from or fight off disease. It means having the zest to get the most out of what every waking moment has to offer. And the first step towards good health is one everybody can take. One of the simplest and most effective ways to keep healthy is to eat properly – and that means eating the right foods in the right amounts.

A good diet is what everyone needs to be aiming for – but alas there is no magic formula for this. It simply isn't possible to draw up a list of foods divided into those that are 'good' for you and those that are 'bad' for you; how much you eat of a food compared with how much you need (or can get away with) are highly individual matters. People vary, in what they need, in what they like, and in the risks they run of harming their health.

Most of us have at least a vague idea of the link-up between what we eat and how we feel. We suspect, when we tuck into a sugary pudding covered with lashings of cream, that we're probably not doing ourselves much good. But we go on because we like it. We know what we *like* but we don't always know what we *need*.

Some people know that they put on weight easily and that they ought to watch what they eat. Other people feel a bit under the weather and suspect that an improvement in diet might help them feel fitter. However, it's not uncommon to feel fit despite having a serious disorder like high blood pressure or atherosclerosis. A spreading waistline or a regular check-up for high blood pressure can give some indication of the kind of shape we are in physically, but they don't tell the whole story. For one thing, we can't take a look at the inside of our arteries to see how healthy they are. By the time we do find out that something is wrong, the disease has often reached such an advanced stage that matters can't be put right in a few weeks, months, or even years. This is why preventing disease is so important.

The fact that you're reading this chapter at all probably indicates that you already know something about the importance of preventing disease, but you may not have got as far as actually doing anything about it. It may stiffen your resolve to know something more about what you're eating and why it's good or bad for you. That is the purpose of this chapter. It looks at why a balanced diet is important and what can go wrong if you eat an unbalanced one. There are plenty of practical hints on how to make eating wisely easier and pleasanter. We'll also be looking at some of the food fads and fancies that seem to get a grip on people, often for no apparent reason, other than that they're fashionable. Some fads are harmless enough, and some are positively helpful – but others can be dangerous if taken to extremes.

Diet and disease

If you'd been living in Europe or North America 80 or so years ago instead of today, the most serious threats to your life would have been infectious diseases like diphtheria, influenza or tuberculosis. Around the year 1900 more than a quarter of boys died from infectious disease before the age of 15. And four out of every ten boys who survived into adult life died from infectious disease before reaching 65.

In the last 80 years the picture has changed dramatically so far as youngsters are concerned. Today only 2 per cent of boys fail to reach the age of 15. But life expectancy hasn't improved so much among adults. Despite modern drugs and vaccines to protect people against diseases like tuberculosis and influenza, one out of every four working men still can't expect to reach the retirement age of 65. The biggest killer of men in this age group is heart disease; the second biggest, cancer. Where women are concerned, more die of breast cancer between the ages of 35 and 54 than from any other disease. With both heart disease and cancer, experts are becoming increasingly convinced that what people eat has a lot to do with how likely they are to be among the disease's victims. Of course, with heart disease things like smoking, lack of exercise, high blood pressure and a history of heart disease in the family are also important, but few experts now doubt that the diet typical in most affluent parts of the world is also partly to blame. Defining the role of diet in causing cancer is more controversial – but evidence is mounting that eating too much fat can increase the risk of developing certain cancers (see pages 94–95).

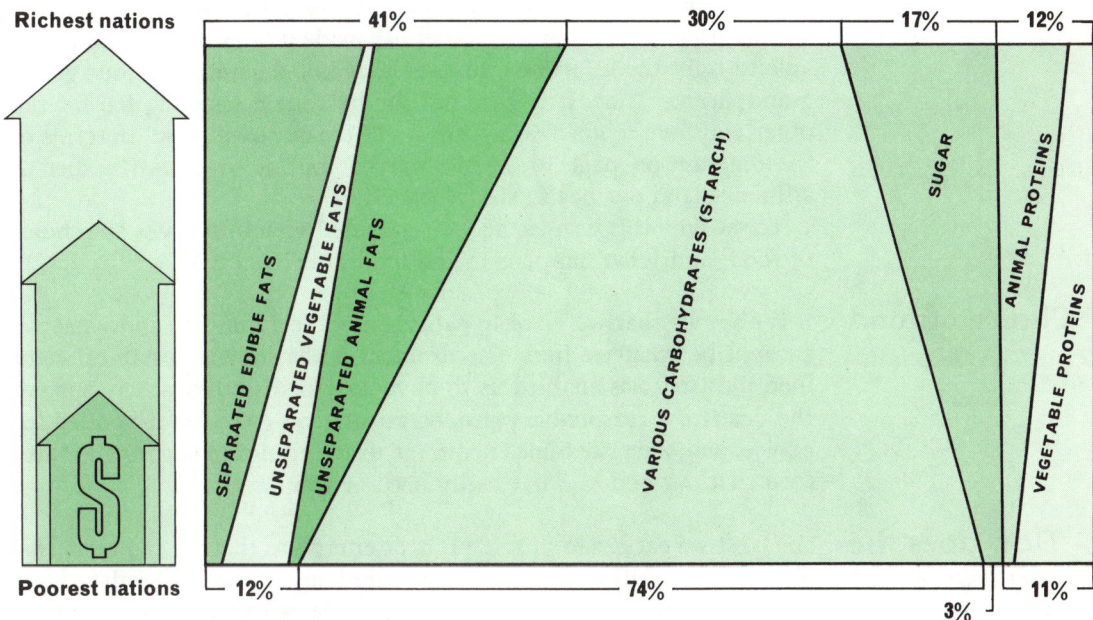

Richest nations — 41% — 30% — 17% — 12%

SEPARATED EDIBLE FATS / UNSEPARATED VEGETABLE FATS / UNSEPARATED ANIMAL FATS / VARIOUS CARBOHYDRATES (STARCH) / SUGAR / ANIMAL PROTEINS / VEGETABLE PROTEINS

Poorest nations — 12% — 74% — 3% — 11%

This diagram, based on World Health Organization data, shows the percentage of energy provided by various nutrients for people in rich and poor countries. The richest get very much more energy from fats (both separated, or visible, and unseparated, or hidden) and sugar, and less than half as much from starch as people in the poorest areas.

The interplay between diet and health shows up in the pattern of diseases that prevail at the extremes of diet illustrated above. In very poor regions the diet is too dilute in nutrients for many young children, who tend to die from disease and malnutrition. In the wealthiest areas, overnutrition is one of the major causes of the 'diseases of affluence', such as heart disease.

91

But it's not just heart disease and cancer that have a link with diet. One of the scourges of modern times is obesity – itself a contributory cause of heart disease. Surprisingly, the total amount of food eaten these days is actually less than it was a generation ago, yet obesity is more of a problem. Why? Part of the reason is that people are less active than they were then, and so are burning up less energy. As a result appetites are smaller. But instead of eating less of the foods that produce a lot of energy – like fats, sugar and alcohol – we've cut down on bulky foods like bread and potatoes. On the plate it may look as though we're eating less, but appearances are deceptive. In fact, there's more energy – more calories – on the plate than we need, so we get fatter. Apart from the diseases mentioned, our present diet also encourages illnesses like gallstones, diabetes and strokes (which we'll be looking at in more detail on pages 94–99). Less dramatic than these, other diet-linked conditions such as migraine, allergies, low resistance to illness and a general feeling of being below par can take much of the fun out of life.

It would be foolish, however, to blame all our modern ills on food. In fact, comparing what we eat now with what our great-grandparents probably ate 100 years ago, we now do very well indeed, and our health shows it. In developed countries these days we rarely see diseases caused by nutritional deficiency, or people starving to death, as they used to. Our improved diet has made us all stronger and better able to fight the infectious diseases that killed so many in our great-grandparents' time. It is just that the balance has swung too far the other way: we're now eating too 'well' for our own good. In terms of the diagram on page 91, we've moved too far towards the diet of affluence, and our health shows the effects.

To see why this is so we need to consider what influences our choice of food, and what happens to the food after we eat it.

Choice of food

It is obvious that we want to eat when we feel hungry, and what we eat will be what we like. The problem is that nowadays an efficient food industry has enabled us to have any food we like at any time of the year for a reasonable price. So far as food goes, we're spoiled for choice, and our taste buds encourage us to indulge in sugary and fatty food that our bodies don't really need or want.

How does the body use food?

The food we eat has to provide fuel or energy so that we can carry out our daily activities. Energy is measured in calories (scientists have recently taken to talking of joules; 1 joule is roughly equivalent to 4 calories). The average man needs 2,900 calories a day, the average woman slightly fewer – 2,200 a day. Two-thirds of this energy the body needs simply to stay alive – to maintain the heartbeat, to keep the lungs breathing, and the rest of the body ticking over. The remaining third is used for growth and movement.

The work of keeping the body ticking over is called the resting metabolism. Babies and young children have faster metabolic rates

One gram of fat PROVIDES →	C + C + C + C + C + C + C + C + C
One gram of alcohol PROVIDES →	C + C + C + C + C + C + C
One gram of protein PROVIDES →	C + C + C + C
One gram of carbo-hydrate PROVIDES →	C + C + C + C

Analysis of the energy, or calorie, content of the pure nutrients shows that fat and alcohol are the richest sources, and so the most fattening. Fatty foods provide more than twice as many calories as starchy ones.

Note that foods (and drinks) are a mixture of the nutrients analysed here: wine, for example, contains water, some carbohydrate and other solids as well as ethyl alcohol (the main nutrient).

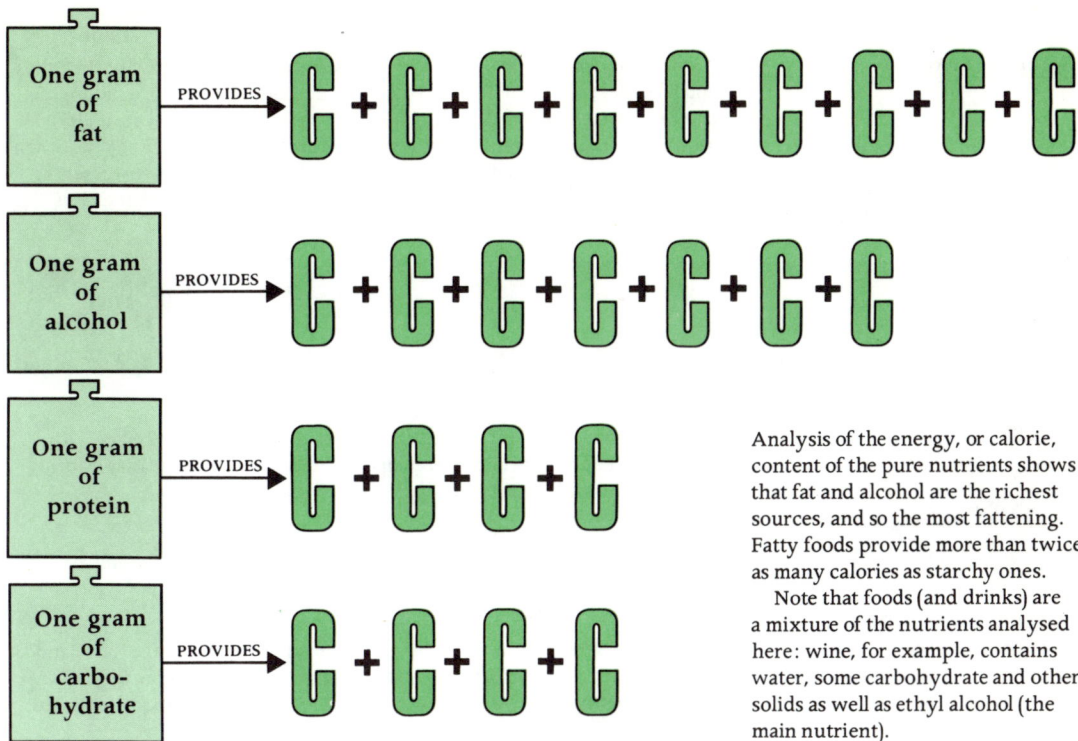

than adults and so they need proportionately more energy just to stay alive. Very fat people, on the other hand, become much more efficient at using as little energy as possible and they have a slower metabolic rate (this may return to normal after they have lost weight).

Apart from providing energy, food also provides the body with protein, vitamins and minerals (like calcium and iron), which together supply the bits and pieces that in different combinations make bone, flesh, and blood. If the body can't get enough energy either from food or from its stores of body fat, then it converts protein into energy (it can convert protein in the diet, or protein already stored in the form of lean body tissue). Conversely, if we eat more than we need, the surplus – whether it's protein, fat or carbohydrate – is either burnt off as heat or converted into fat and stored.

The amount of energy or fuel provided by nutrients varies greatly; as you can see from the illustration, weight for weight, fat provides more than twice as many calories as either carbohydrate or protein. Water, vitamins, minerals and roughage (fibre) provide no calories.

Most people connect calories only with dieting, but we'll return to this subject later in the chapter, after taking a look at some of the diseases that have been linked with our affluent diet.

Note Following standard practice the fat, carbohydrate, protein and fibre content of foods is given in grams only (28.3 g = 1 oz).

93

Illness: the link with diet

NAME	WHAT IS IT?
ATHEROSCLEROSIS	A thickening of the walls of arteries that reduces their diameter (see below) and impedes the flow of blood to the heart muscle. The result can be angina or a heart attack. Blood clots can block a narrowed artery and cause a heart attack (coronary thrombosis) or, if the clot forms in the brain, a stroke. Much of the slowing down that goes with old age is in fact the effect of worsening atherosclerosis. Until women reach the menopause, they seem much less prone to atherosclerosis than men.

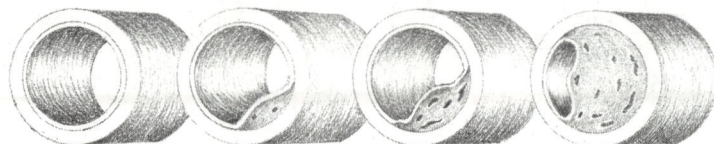

CANCER

Not one disease but many, involving abnormal, uncontrolled cell growth. One in five people dies of cancer in one or other of its 200 identifiable forms (one in three develops it).

Cancer of the breast

This type of cancer is the major killer of women between the ages of 35 and 54. One woman in 17 in Britain gets the disease; one in 30 dies of it. In the U.S.A. something like 90,000 new cases of breast cancer are expected each year.

Women over the age of 20 should examine their own breasts for lumps at least once a month, and consult a doctor if they find anything that worries them. Four out of five lumps turn out to be quite harmless, but those that aren't need treatment as soon as possible.

Cancer of the colon/rectum

This type of cancer kills more people in the U.S.A. than any other type, and it ranks second only to lung cancer as a killer in Britain. Even so, in the U.S.A. over 40 per cent of people with cancer of the colon are still alive five years after the condition is diagnosed and (as with all cancers) the earlier it's treated the better the prospects of survival.

In Africa and Asia this type of cancer is much less common than it is in Western countries, where its toll is still rising year by year.

LINK WITH DIET

The arteries get furred up as a result of the build-up of a fatty substance that includes cholesterol. Although some cholesterol comes from foods that contain it (see Group 2), the body makes most of its cholesterol out of fats in the foods you eat (especially saturated fats).

Very little is known about the causes of cancer, but it has been suspected for many years that diet plays an important part where some types of cancer are concerned. Different dietary factors are linked with different forms of cancer.

This type of cancer is also linked with overnutrition, particularly a high intake of fat. Girls who because of their good diet grow fast and start menstruating early have a slightly greater chance of developing breast cancer later on. Changes in the balance of hormones (caused by too much fat or too much total energy in the diet) may create the predisposition to develop this disease. Of course, other factors are important too: there is a lower rate of breast cancer among women who have their first child by the age of 25, for example.

This disease seems to be related to the typical high fat, low fibre diet of developed countries. The explanation may be that bacteria in the waste matter passing through the colon produce a substance that causes cancer. If so, then concentrated, slow-moving waste (typical of people on a low fibre diet) may produce more concentrated carcinogens, which remain in contact with the lining of the rectum and colon for a long time. It's also possible that a high energy intake increases the sensitivity of tissues to cancer-causing chemicals.

WHAT TO DO

Cut back on the fatty foods listed in Group 1. Although cholesterol is found only in animal fats, it's safer to cut down on all fats. Some *less* fatty foods are high in cholesterol too (see Group 2); if you think you are prone to heart trouble, don't eat these often.

A woman who stays near the ideal weight for her height (see page 152) and starts her family by her mid-twenties stands less chance of getting breast cancer.

Cut back on the fatty foods listed in Group 1. Increase the amount of fibre in your diet by eating more of the foods in Group 4.

1 FOODS HIGH IN FAT
Visible fats: Butter; cream; dripping; fat on meat; lard; margarine; oil; suet; top of milk.
Hidden fats: Bacon; cakes; cheese; chips [fries]; chocolate; crisps [potato chips]; eggs; fried foods; ice cream; meat, especially pork and lamb; nuts; oily fish; pastries and biscuits [cookies]; processed meat products like sausages, salami, pâté and meat pies.

2 FOODS HIGH IN CHOLESTEROL
Brains; butter; eggs; heart; kidney; liver; shellfish.

3 FOODS HIGH IN SALT
Bacon; canned vegetables; corned beef; cornflakes; ham; hard cheese; margarine; salami; salted butter; sausages; savoury biscuits [crackers]; shellfish; smoked fish; some bread; tomato juice; tomato ketchup; Worcester sauce; yeast extract. Any food to which salt has been added.

4 FOODS HIGH IN FIBRE
Brown rice; fruit (especially dried fruit such as dates and raisins); nuts; vegetables (especially peas, beans, lentils); wholegrain cereals; wholemeal [wholewheat] bread, pasta and crispbread.

NAME	WHAT IS IT?
Cancer of the liver/stomach	Liver cancer is a rare disease, but cancer of the stomach still kills over 13,000 people a year in Britain. Worldwide, stomach cancer is on the decline, even in Japan where this condition is 20 times as common as it is in the U.S.A. or Canada.

DIABETES

Inability to control the amount of glucose in the blood by normal metabolic means. This may happen either because the body isn't providing enough insulin (the principal hormone that controls the amount of glucose sugar in the blood) or because it's unable to use effectively the insulin it produces. By and large, those who develop diabetes under the age of 40 are unable to make enough insulin and so must be treated with drugs. Those who develop diabetes in later life, however, are usually unable to use the insulin they make. Both types of diabetes are linked with increased rates of heart disease. Four out of five diabetics die early from this cause.

At present about 2 per cent of people in Europe have diabetes, and in the U.S.A. this figure may be as high as 5 per cent. In the future the number of diabetics is likely to rise. For one thing those affected are no longer dying young, and so more genes that predispose towards diabetes are being added to the gene pool. For another, those with a predisposition towards the disease have a greater chance of getting it in a society where 'middle age spread' is considered the norm. Those who develop diabetes in later life are generally overweight.

DIVERTICULAR DISEASE

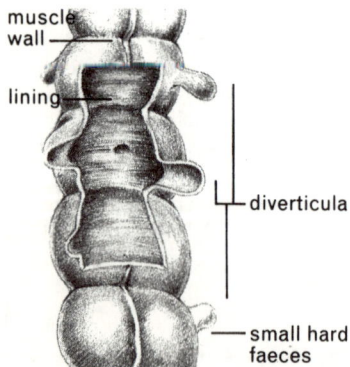

muscle wall
lining
diverticula
small hard faeces

When pressure inside the colon is high (as it is when the tube is full of hard waste matter), parts of the walls of the colon may be unable to take the strain and may give way in places to form diverticula, little pocket-like protrusions from the colon itself (see left). This condition is known as diverticulosis. Among the symptoms it can produce are pain or discomfort in the stomach, nausea and a feeling of being bloated. Should the neck of one of the diverticula become blocked, things get more serious. The diverticulum may become inflamed (diverticulitis), and eventually the waste matter trapped inside it may become infected.

The disease becomes more common as people get older: by the age of 80, between 50 and 70 per cent of people suffer from it. It's only in the past 70 or 80 years that diverticular disease has become rife among the middle-aged and elderly (the first death from the condition was recorded only in 1923), and it's virtually confined to the affluent West. In Africa and Asia, the disease is almost unknown.

LINK WITH DIET

There is a strong suspicion that toxins present in some kinds of mouldy food may be carcinogenic. Mouldy peanuts, for instance, contain aflatoxin, which is a known carcinogen. The development of cancer of the liver or stomach is thought to be related to having eaten food contaminated by these toxins. The drop in deaths from these types of cancer probably reflects improvements in food preservation over the past few decades.

Before the discovery of insulin the only way of treating diabetes was by severely restricting the intake of carbohydrates (starch and sugar) so that only a little glucose was released into the bloodstream. But although this may once have been an effective treatment, too much carbohydrate in the diet is not necessarily the *cause* of diabetes. In fact carbohydrate intake probably has no influence on the development of this condition. For the person who develops diabetes in middle life, too much food is the root problem. This leads to obesity, which in turn seems to stop the body using effectively the insulin it makes. Once the excess weight is shed, things often go back to normal again.

When the diet is low in fibre, the waste material passing through the colon tends to be solid and dense rather than bulky, and the colon itself tends to be narrow. This can lead to the build-up of abnormally high pressure when the colon contracts to move the waste along. The greater pressure (over many years of eating a low fibre diet) increases the risk of damage to the walls of the colon and the formation of diverticula.

WHAT TO DO

Play safe by throwing away any food that has begun to go mouldy – you can't tell just by looking which moulds are the dangerous sort. If you eat a lot of whole grains and health foods, check that you're getting them from a reputable supplier with a rapid turnover.

Stay near the ideal weight for your height (see page 152). Slim by cutting back on fats (Group 1) not on starchy food. For guidance on how to lose weight, see pages 158–62.

People who already have diverticular disease tend to improve on a high fibre diet (although existing diverticula won't disappear). As a safeguard against the condition developing, eat more of the foods in Group 4.

1 FOODS HIGH IN FAT
Visible fats: Butter; cream; dripping; fat on meat; lard; margarine; oil; suet; top of milk.
Hidden fats: Bacon; cakes; cheese; chips [fries]; chocolate; crisps [potato chips]; eggs; fried foods; ice cream; meat, especially pork and lamb; nuts; oily fish; pastries and biscuits [cookies]; processed meat products like sausages, salami, pâté and meat pies.

2 FOODS HIGH IN CHOLESTEROL
Brains; butter; eggs; heart; kidney; liver; shellfish.

3 FOODS HIGH IN SALT
Bacon; canned vegetables; corned beef; cornflakes; ham; hard cheese; margarine; salami; salted butter; sausages; savoury biscuits [crackers]; shellfish; smoked fish; some bread; tomato juice; tomato ketchup; Worcester sauce; yeast extract. Any food to which salt has been added.

4 FOODS HIGH IN FIBRE
Brown rice; fruit (especially dried fruit such as dates and raisins); nuts; vegetables (especially peas, beans, lentils); wholegrain cereals; wholemeal [wholewheat] bread, pasta and crispbread.

NAME	WHAT IS IT?

GALLSTONES

One of the jobs of the liver is to produce bile, a fluid needed to help digest fats. Until it is called for, the bile is stored in a little sac near the liver, known as the gall bladder. The hard deposits of calcium salts and cholesterol that may form within the gall bladder are called gallstones.

Most gallstones cause no trouble at all, provided they remain within the gall bladder. Those that are a problem are the ones that try to get out of the gall bladder into the bile duct (the route along which the bile flows to the duodenum). This happens with around a third of all gallstones, and it can be a very painful process.

Gallstones are one of the commonest diseases of developed countries, and they are becoming increasingly rife. Women are the main victims. Once upon a time the typical patient used to be 'fat, forty and fertile'; now she's more likely to be young, taking oral contraceptives and dieting. Female sex hormones seem to favour gallstones, and treatment with oestrogen, even in the small doses used in some contraceptive pills, doubles the risks. The Pill also tends to make women put on weight, by preventing ovulation and the surge of metabolism that follows it, so taking the Pill often goes with periods of dieting.

HEART (OR CORONARY ARTERY) DISEASE (ISCHAEMIC HEART DISEASE)

The tiny vessels feeding blood to the heart muscle to enable it to go on pumping become furred up and narrow. This can hamper blood supply to the heart muscle so that in periods of exertion or excitement (when the heart is pumping rapidly) the sufferer feels an acute pain in the chest (angina). A blockage may form in one of the blood vessels, starving part of the heart of oxygen so that some of the muscle dies (myocardial infarction). This can cause acute pain and other typical symptoms of a heart attack. The heart itself may stop beating.

Heart disease is the major cause of death among men of working age. Women are less prone to it (although its incidence is increasing among younger women) until they reach the menopause, after which male and female rates of heart disease converge.

HIGH BLOOD PRESSURE (HYPERTENSION)

We can measure how hard the heart has to pump to push the blood around the body. Normal systolic blood pressure (when the heart is pumping) should be around 120 mm of mercury when measured at the upper arm; normal diastolic blood pressure (when the heart is resting) is around 80 mm. This is written as 120/80. The second figure is really the one to worry about. If diastolic blood pressure goes much above 90, there is a much greater risk that the patient will die from kidney failure or a disease like atherosclerosis than if his blood pressure were lower. (The systolic pressure is not so significant, because it can rise as a result of exertion or emotion.)

The most troublesome thing about high blood pressure is that you may not know you have it: people don't necessarily feel unwell when their blood pressure is high. The tendency towards high blood pressure is partly inherited, so if your family are known to have it, the chances are much greater that you may too, which makes it worth having a regular check to find out what your blood pressure is. Although it's considered normal in Europe and North America for blood pressure to rise with age, in many developing countries this is far less common. A different diet or lifestyle may be the key to this discrepancy.

LINK WITH DIET

Girls who are dieting often go in for periods of fasting, and they cut out carbohydrate foods like bread and potatoes. Fasting tends to raise the cholesterol saturation of the bile, and cutting out starchy food means cutting fibre intake. This leads to lower production of bile salts (needed to wash out the surplus cholesterol) and greater risk of gallstones.

WHAT TO DO

Cutting back on foods in Group 2 will do no good. Try instead to stick near the right weight for your height (see page 152) and eat plenty of wholegrain cereals and foods high on fibre (see Group 4). If overweight, diet sensibly (see pages 158–62), not by fasting.

1 FOODS HIGH IN FAT
Visible fats: Butter; cream; dripping; fat on meat; lard; margarine; oil; suet; top of milk.
Hidden fats: Bacon; cakes; cheese; chips [fries]; chocolate; crisps [potato chips]; eggs; fried foods; ice cream; meat, especially pork and lamb; nuts; oily fish; pastries and biscuits [cookies]; processed meat products like sausages, salami, pâté and meat pies.

2 FOODS HIGH IN CHOLESTEROL
Brains; butter; eggs; heart; kidney; liver; shellfish.

The clogging of the arteries is thought to be caused by the build-up of a fatty substance (that includes cholesterol) on the inner walls of the arteries. Too much fat in the diet encourages this process – saturated fat (see pages 100–03) is particularly suspect.

Cut right back on the amount of fat you eat (Group 1). Consider the case for switching from saturated to poly-unsaturated fats where possible (see pages 102–03).

3 FOODS HIGH IN SALT
Bacon; canned vegetables; corned beef; cornflakes; ham; hard cheese; margarine; salami; salted butter; sausages; savoury biscuits [crackers]; shellfish; smoked fish; some bread; tomato juice; tomato ketchup; Worcester sauce; yeast extract. Any food to which salt has been added.

Restricting the amount of sodium (and hence of salt) in the diet helps patients already suffering from high blood pressure, and taking a great deal of salt is thought to encourage high blood pressure to develop. An Australian study suggested that if people halved their salt intake (which is between 5 g and 18 g a day on average) the current epidemic of high blood pressure in Australia would be halted.

Cut back on Group 3 foods and add less salt in cooking and at table. See also page 123.

4 FOODS HIGH IN FIBRE
Brown rice; fruit (especially dried fruit such as dates and raisins); nuts; vegetables (especially peas, beans, lentils); wholegrain cereals; wholemeal [wholewheat] bread, pasta and crispbread.

The facts about fat

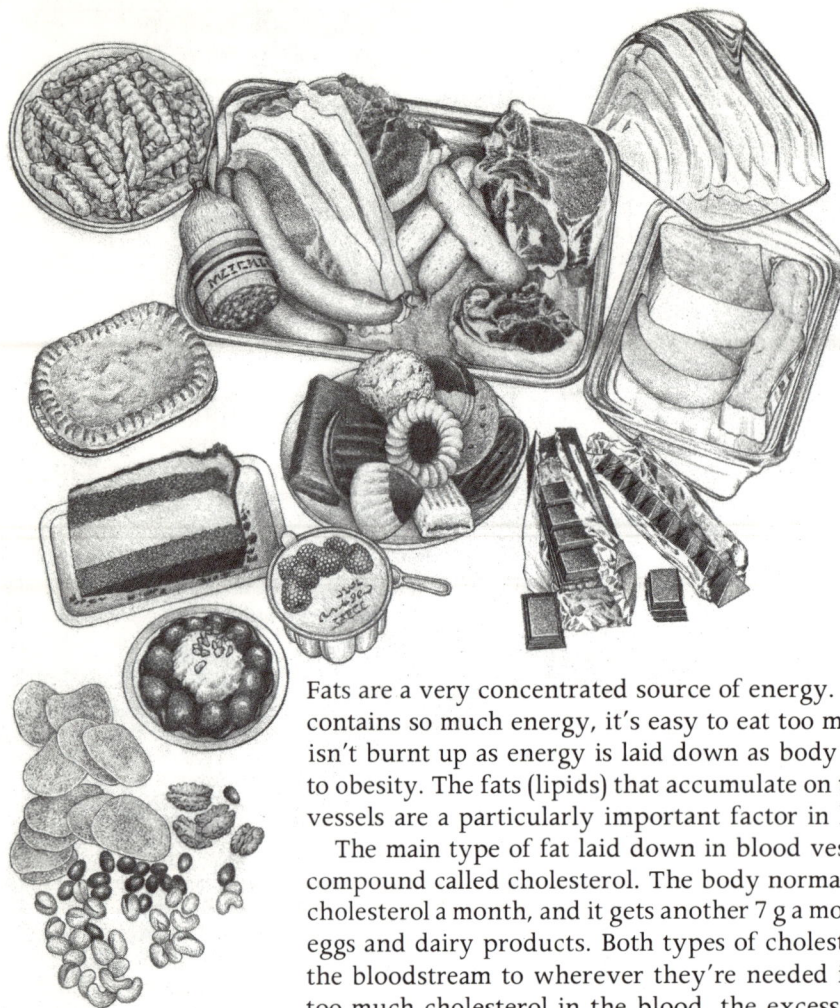

HIDDEN FAT
Bacon
Biscuits [cookies]
Cakes
Cheese
Chocolate
Crinkle cut chips [fries]
Crisps [potato chips]
Gammon [ham]
Ice cream
Meat, especially pork
    and lamb
Nuts
Pastries
Processed meat products
    such as meat pies,
    salami and sausages

Fats are a very concentrated source of energy. Because a little of them contains so much energy, it's easy to eat too much of them; and what isn't burnt up as energy is laid down as body fat, leading eventually to obesity. The fats (lipids) that accumulate on the inner walls of blood vessels are a particularly important factor in heart disease.

The main type of fat laid down in blood vessels is a fatty chemical compound called cholesterol. The body normally makes about 28 g of cholesterol a month, and it gets another 7 g a month directly from meat, eggs and dairy products. Both types of cholesterol are transported in the bloodstream to wherever they're needed in the body. If there is too much cholesterol in the blood, the excess is deposited along the inner walls of the blood vessels, where it can eventually lead to a narrowing of the arteries (atherosclerosis, see pages 94–95). If nothing happens – like a change of diet – to interfere with the gradual build-up of cholesterol deposits, the result can be a heart attack.

The villain of the piece is the cholesterol in the bloodstream, so what can be done about it? The first step towards a solution is to understand how the fat we eat is classified.

What kinds of fat are there?

About 80 per cent of the fats we eat are made up of fatty acids. There are a host of different kinds of fatty acids, with three different basic chemical structures. The carbon atoms in *saturated fatty acids* (like butyric acid) contain all the hydrogen they can hold; this makes them very stable. *Monounsaturated fatty acids* (such as oleic acid) can take a little more hydrogen, and *polyunsaturated fatty acids* (such as linoleic acid) can take a lot more. Results of many studies suggest that saturated fatty acids encourage high levels of cholesterol in the blood, while polyunsaturated ones may help to reduce blood cholesterol. Mono-unsaturated fatty acids seem to be neutral, neither raising nor lowering the level.

Saturated fatty acids are mainly found in animal products, and unsaturated ones in plant products (but there are exceptions). Saturated fats tend to be solid at room temperature – lard, butter and most margarine, for example. Unsaturated fats, like those in corn oil, tend to be liquid at room temperature. However, some plant fats, such as coconut oil and palm oil, are highly saturated, and some naturally unsaturated fats can be artificially saturated by forcing in extra hydrogen (hydrogenation) during food processing. Artificially hydrogenated fats end up with a different structure from naturally saturated fats, and it's quite possible that they add to the problems the body has to cope with. So an ordinary soft margarine may not necessarily be as polyunsaturated as a margarine that is actually labelled as such. Incidentally, polyunsaturated oils contain just as many calories as animal fats.

Is eating a lot of fats dangerous?

The most telling evidence for this comes from epidemiological studies that analyse differences in health of different human populations. In most developed countries coronary heart disease has shot up over the last 30 to 40 years. All social classes are now at risk. The rise in heart disease has been especially marked among the poorer socioeconomic groups, and among men aged 35 to 44. There is some evidence that the rates of death from heart disease are remaining stable (if high) in Britain, while in the U.S.A. and several other countries the rates are falling, especially among men. No one can say why for certain, but perhaps the campaign to get people to eat less fat, stop smoking and take more exercise is beginning to pay off, in some quarters at least.

One early epidemiological study showed that heart disease in Norway fell during the Second World War after the German invasion, but rose when the war was over. Much the same took place in England and Wales during the war, and the reason may be that people ate more frugally.

Another kind of study compares what happens to people when they leave their native country to live elsewhere. For example, people in Asia and Africa have little heart disease, probably because of their generally lower fat and lower calorie diet. But Asians and Africans who move to Europe or America, or adopt our lifestyles and diet, tend eventually to adopt our heart disease patterns too.

Some studies have tried to identify the link between diet and heart disease by following a group of men over many years, noting their eating habits and other health-related factors like exercise and smoking, to see if common links emerge between those who develop heart disease. One of the most famous studies is known as the Framingham Study, after the small town in Massachusetts where it took place. Beginning in 1949, it followed 5,000 men for many years. One finding was that men on a high fat diet were more at risk of heart disease.

101

The evidence points strongly to there being a firm link between heart disease and a high level of cholesterol in the blood – which, in turn, is linked with a diet rich in fats, especially saturated fats. (Cholesterol in *food* seems to be much less important.) Factors like smoking and genetic inheritance influence blood cholesterol, too, but in general the link between blood cholesterol and diet holds. In countries where the average saturated fat intake is just over 30 g a day, as in the Third World, heart disease is rare. Where it's 110 g a day, as in many developed countries, heart disease is rife.

How much do you need?

The aim is to cut the proportion of calories derived from fats from around 40 per cent to no more than 30 per cent. A maximum fat intake of 80 g a day is quite feasible, and already more than you need.

Saturated versus polyunsaturated

There has been a lot of argument recently about whether or not people should switch from a diet high in saturated fats to one high in poly-unsaturates. Organizations with a vested interest in the outcome of the controversy – the dairy industry on the one hand, the makers and sellers of polyunsaturated margarines and oils on the other – have thrown themselves into the debate. Here are some of the commonest arguments advanced by the dairy industry.

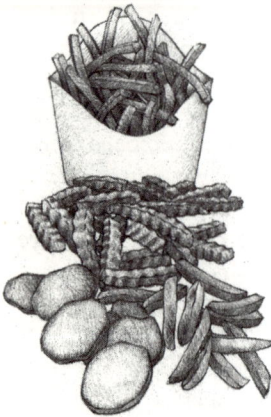

'**A high intake of polyunsaturates could be bad for you.**' Although there may be long-term side effects of eating polyunsaturated fats, none has been found that is as serious as heart disease. The suggestion that polyunsaturates might predispose people to develop cancer is now discounted. In fact there is some evidence that taking in more linoleic acid can be beneficial for health, by reducing the tendency to thrombosis. Anyway, no one suggests that you eat a lot of polyun-saturated fats – simply that you swop some saturated fats for them.

The way you prepare chips [fries] makes a difference to the amount of cooking fat they absorb, and hence the number of calories they contain. As the figures below for 120 g [4 oz] servings show, crinkle cut are the most fattening as their crinkled edges provide the greatest surface area for fat absorption:

crinkle cut	348 calories
thin cut	336 calories
average cut	264 calories
thick cut	156 calories

'**The studies that condemn saturated fats are poorly designed, and of only marginal significance.**' While this may be true in strictly scientific terms, the evidence examined is the best there's likely to be. Any controlled trial designed to prove the link conclus-ively could well be unethical. It would be necessary to find several thousand people willing to eat a diet high in saturated fats over many years, to see if more than the normal number among them died from heart disease. On current knowledge, the risk would be too high.

In fact something along these lines was done in the past, during a 12-year study of two mental hospitals in Helsinki. In one hospital, patients were given a diet with nearly one and a half times more poly-unsaturated fats than saturated fats. Over the next six years the levels of cholesterol in the blood of these patients fell, and they had fewer heart attacks than those in the neighbouring hospital who were on their usual diet rich in saturated fats. For the second six-year period the diets were switched over so that the patients who had previously had a diet rich in polyunsaturates had a diet high in saturated fats.

This time the first set of results was reversed, and the other group of patients had fewer heart attacks.

'A switch to polyunsaturates would spell disaster for the agricultural and food industries.' This claim seems implausible. Any change in eating patterns would take place gradually, and the food industry should have time to adapt. People have to eat *something*, and it will presumably have to be grown by farmers and processed by the food industry.

'Reducing blood cholesterol levels by drugs hasn't led to fewer heart attacks.' This is irrelevant. Drugs don't necessarily mimic a change in diet; and they have side effects, which distort the picture.

HOW TO CUT DOWN ON FAT

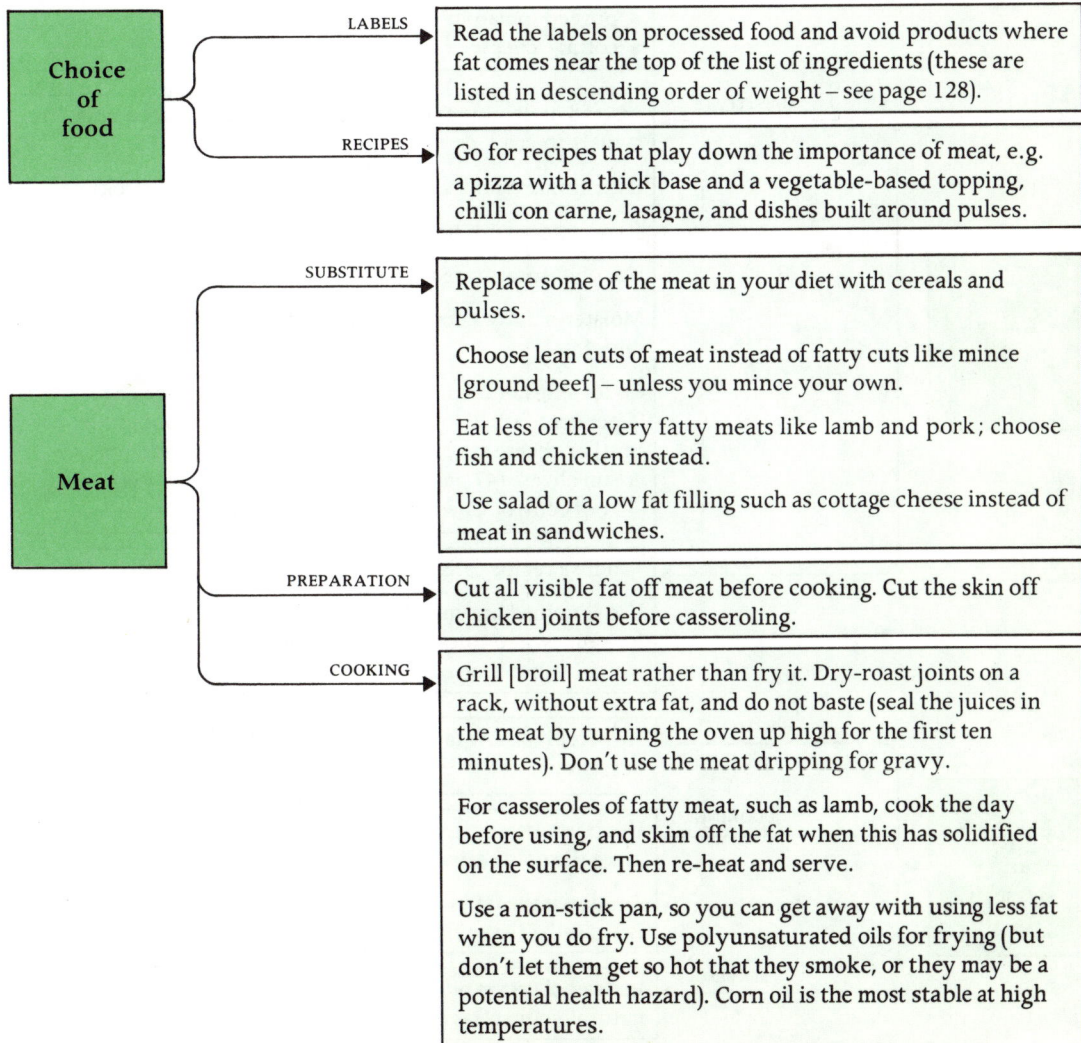

Choice of food	LABELS	Read the labels on processed food and avoid products where fat comes near the top of the list of ingredients (these are listed in descending order of weight – see page 128).
	RECIPES	Go for recipes that play down the importance of meat, e.g. a pizza with a thick base and a vegetable-based topping, chilli con carne, lasagne, and dishes built around pulses.
Meat	SUBSTITUTE	Replace some of the meat in your diet with cereals and pulses. Choose lean cuts of meat instead of fatty cuts like mince [ground beef] – unless you mince your own. Eat less of the very fatty meats like lamb and pork; choose fish and chicken instead. Use salad or a low fat filling such as cottage cheese instead of meat in sandwiches.
	PREPARATION	Cut all visible fat off meat before cooking. Cut the skin off chicken joints before casseroling.
	COOKING	Grill [broil] meat rather than fry it. Dry-roast joints on a rack, without extra fat, and do not baste (seal the juices in the meat by turning the oven up high for the first ten minutes). Don't use the meat dripping for gravy. For casseroles of fatty meat, such as lamb, cook the day before using, and skim off the fat when this has solidified on the surface. Then re-heat and serve. Use a non-stick pan, so you can get away with using less fat when you do fry. Use polyunsaturated oils for frying (but don't let them get so hot that they smoke, or they may be a potential health hazard). Corn oil is the most stable at high temperatures.

103

▷

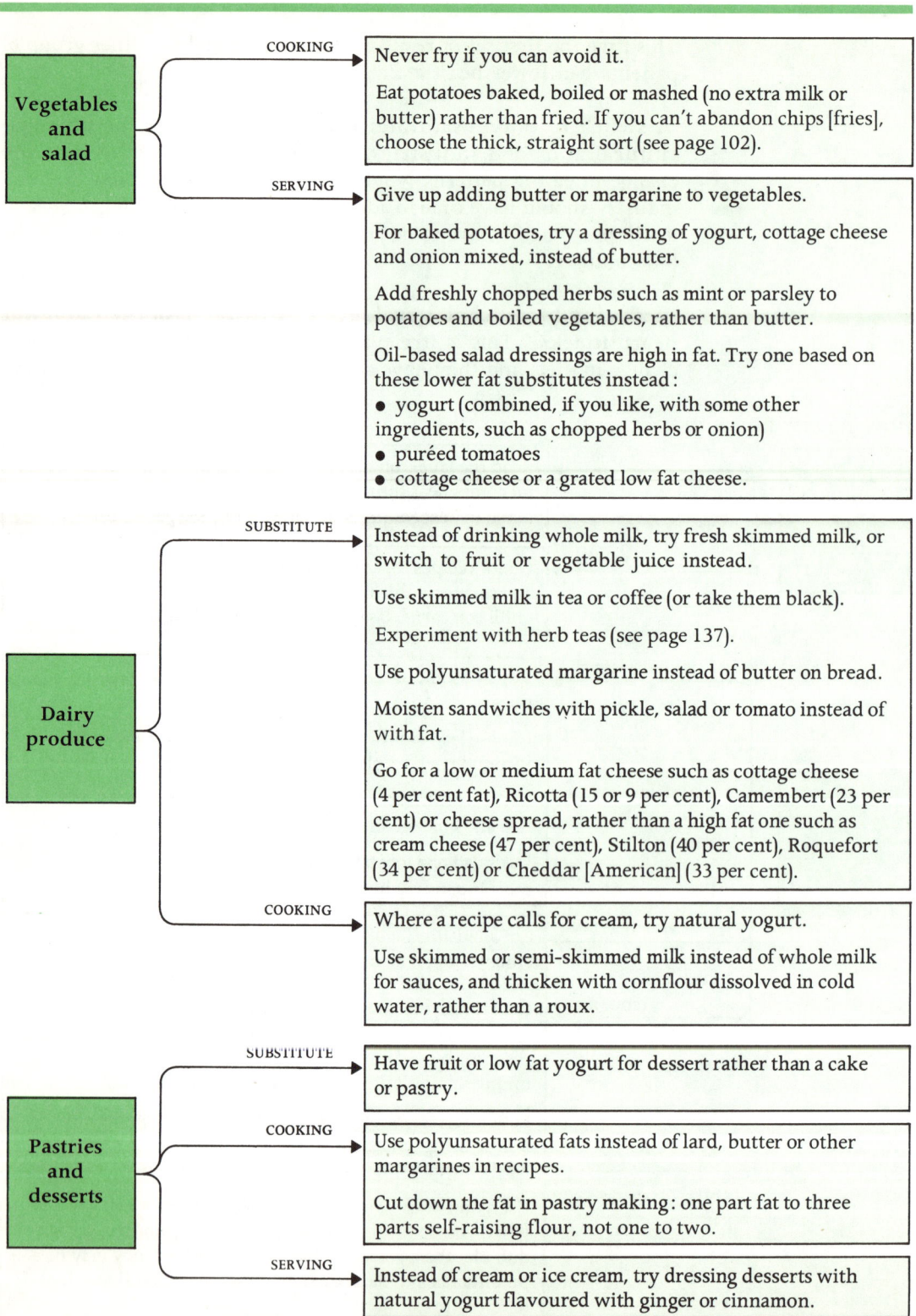

Vegetables and salad

COOKING

Never fry if you can avoid it.

Eat potatoes baked, boiled or mashed (no extra milk or butter) rather than fried. If you can't abandon chips [fries], choose the thick, straight sort (see page 102).

SERVING

Give up adding butter or margarine to vegetables.

For baked potatoes, try a dressing of yogurt, cottage cheese and onion mixed, instead of butter.

Add freshly chopped herbs such as mint or parsley to potatoes and boiled vegetables, rather than butter.

Oil-based salad dressings are high in fat. Try one based on these lower fat substitutes instead:
● yogurt (combined, if you like, with some other ingredients, such as chopped herbs or onion)
● puréed tomatoes
● cottage cheese or a grated low fat cheese.

Dairy produce

SUBSTITUTE

Instead of drinking whole milk, try fresh skimmed milk, or switch to fruit or vegetable juice instead.

Use skimmed milk in tea or coffee (or take them black).

Experiment with herb teas (see page 137).

Use polyunsaturated margarine instead of butter on bread.

Moisten sandwiches with pickle, salad or tomato instead of with fat.

Go for a low or medium fat cheese such as cottage cheese (4 per cent fat), Ricotta (15 or 9 per cent), Camembert (23 per cent) or cheese spread, rather than a high fat one such as cream cheese (47 per cent), Stilton (40 per cent), Roquefort (34 per cent) or Cheddar [American] (33 per cent).

COOKING

Where a recipe calls for cream, try natural yogurt.

Use skimmed or semi-skimmed milk instead of whole milk for sauces, and thicken with cornflour dissolved in cold water, rather than a roux.

Pastries and desserts

SUBSTITUTE

Have fruit or low fat yogurt for dessert rather than a cake or pastry.

COOKING

Use polyunsaturated fats instead of lard, butter or other margarines in recipes.

Cut down the fat in pastry making: one part fat to three parts self-raising flour, not one to two.

SERVING

Instead of cream or ice cream, try dressing desserts with natural yogurt flavoured with ginger or cinnamon.

Carbohydrates

Carbohydrates have a bad image. People tend to think of them as especially fattening, and try to give them up when they diet. In fact, as you can see by looking back at the illustration on page 93, dieters would do much better to cut out energy-rich fats.

Plants make carbohydrates out of water and carbon dioxide, using the energy provided by the sun. The cellulose that makes up the plant's rigid structure is one form of carbohydrate, but since the digestive system can't break this down, it passes through the body unchanged (see Fibre, pages 109–11). The two main kinds of carbohydrate that can be digested are starch and sugar.

Starch In developed countries, bread and other flour products and potatoes are the major sources of starch in the diet, but they're being eaten in far smaller quantities than they used to be. A century ago poor people in industrial countries ate half a loaf of bread at a meal, with maybe a little cheese or meat. Now sandwiches are made from bread so thin that the butter and cheese are thicker than the bread.

Weight for weight potatoes have only about a quarter the calories of beef steak and only a tenth as many calories as a similar weight of butter. So there is nothing intrinsically fattening about them. Of course, eating too much of any food will lead to excess weight, but carbohydrates are not particularly blameworthy in this respect.

Cereals, such as rice, oats and barley, play a fairly small role in the diet of affluent society today, but they are important foods for anyone who intends eating more carbohydrates. Rye bread and oatcakes make tasty and interesting alternatives to bread or biscuits made from

105

wheat. Rice contains high quality protein as well as carbohydrate, and so does oatmeal – slightly higher on oil. For how to eat more starch (and fibre) see pages 110–11.

Sugar

There are two types of sugar. The simpler type, monosaccharides, includes glucose (also called dextrose) and fructose. Disaccharides are more complicated structurally, and sucrose, the sugar most commonly used, falls into this category. From the nutritional point of view one type is just as good (or bad) as the other. To the body, sugar is sugar, whether it's brown, white, powdered, granulated or cubed, and whether it comes in the form of syrup, sweet wine or a mouthful of banana. Whatever form it's in originally, it will be broken down within the body and either used as a source of energy or stored as fat.

You could get along perfectly healthily if you never ate any sugar whatsoever. It provides calories but no other nutrients at all, and the body can use starch in just the same way as sugar. But – probably because people like the taste of sweet food – over the past 100 years or so sugar consumption has shot up, while that of starch has fallen.

It takes longer for the body to break down a complex structure like starch into glucose than it does to handle a relatively simple one like sugar. This may be what lies behind the common belief that taking a sweet drink or teaspoonful of sugar can give a person an immediate 'lift', which disappears within a few hours to leave a sensation of depression and irritation. In fact, the body is very efficient at keeping the level of sugar in the blood constant, so taking in sugar should not normally have much physiological impact. Mood swings like this are more likely to be caused by the fact that being hungry makes people feel cross. The crossness disappears quickly when the hunger is temporarily banished by eating sugar, but it reappears as soon as the hunger returns (which will be as soon as the liver has removed the sugar from the blood). A sandwich or meal, by contrast, leaves a reserve of food in the stomach to be absorbed gradually.

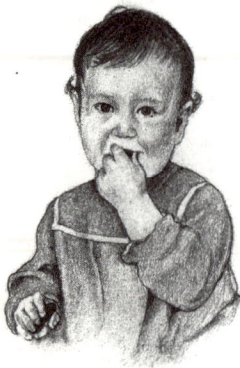

Don't encourage your children to develop a sweet tooth by giving them sweets [candies] as rewards or pacifiers early in life.

Is sugar bad for you?

There are two ways in which sugar certainly does no good. First, it tempts you to eat too much. Sweet foods crowd out more nourishing and less fattening items, and people who eat a lot of them can easily wind up fat. As you can see from pages 152–53, obesity is a real health hazard.

Second, sugar causes tooth decay. This may not put your life at risk but it's quite important enough to warrant a change of diet. Natural fluoride in water can help strengthen teeth, but not everyone has fluoride in their water; if you live in a low fluoride area, you could give your children fluoride tablets instead. Particularly for children, it's important to cut down both on the amount of sugar eaten and the frequency of eating it – a continual trickle of sugar in the mouth, while sucking a peppermint or lollipop, say, is extremely damaging. Restricting sweet-eating to after a meal would do a lot to prevent dental decay.

Is honey healthier? Honey is a form of fruit sugar or fructose. As a sweetener, it may have marginal advantages over sucrose (ordinary table sugar): it takes longer to absorb; less honey than sugar is needed to provide the same sweetness; it contains some trace elements; because of its water content, honey supplies just under 3 calories per g [85 per oz] as opposed to nearer 3.5 per g [110 per oz] for sugar – but if you eat more than a little honey, you'll still get a lot of surplus calories without a worthwhile amount of nutrients.

There's no scientific evidence to back honey's healer reputation, although some people swear by it on burns and ulcers, for constipation and throat problems.

The third and most controversial charge laid against sugar is that it is a factor in causing heart disease. Considering the length of time since this theory was first proposed, surprisingly few scientists support it. It has not been proved that heart attack patients have a particularly high intake of sugar, and some countries with relatively low rates of heart disease are high on sugar consumption. This supports the generally accepted view that sugar is not one of the major causes of heart disease, if it is a cause at all.

Artificial sweeteners An alternative to sweetening food and drinks with sugar is to use an artificial sweetener. These are widely used today, both by the general public and by the food industry. Most artificial sweeteners have no nutritive value, and hence don't encourage tooth decay or add calories to food. All they do is make the food taste sweet.

Saccharine is the best-known artificial sweetener; it's about 400 times as sweet as sugar, which makes it very economical to use (a little saccharine equals a lot of sweetness). The main drawback from the food industry's point of view is that saccharine is destroyed by heat, and so is useless in some forms of food processing.

A new sort of sweetener, cyclamate, was introduced in 1950 but in 1969 research on animals suggested that there could be a link between cyclamates and cancer, and cyclamates were banned. Since then saccharine has come under renewed scrutiny as a possible health hazard, but it is still available (and cancer does not seem to be any more frequent among diabetics – who consume large amounts of saccharine over years – than among the rest of the population).

Doubts about the safety of saccharine have nevertheless led to new interest in alternative artificial sweeteners and some promising ones have been found. However, none is ideal: some break down when heated, some cause stomach upsets if eaten in large quantities, and they are all expensive to make.

Using an artificial sweetener in place of sugar isn't going to cure anyone's sweet tooth. So taking saccharine rather than sugar in your tea or coffee is just dodging the issue. Cutting down on sweet foods is the only real solution; for tips on how to do this, see page 108.

107

HOW TO CUT DOWN ON SUGAR

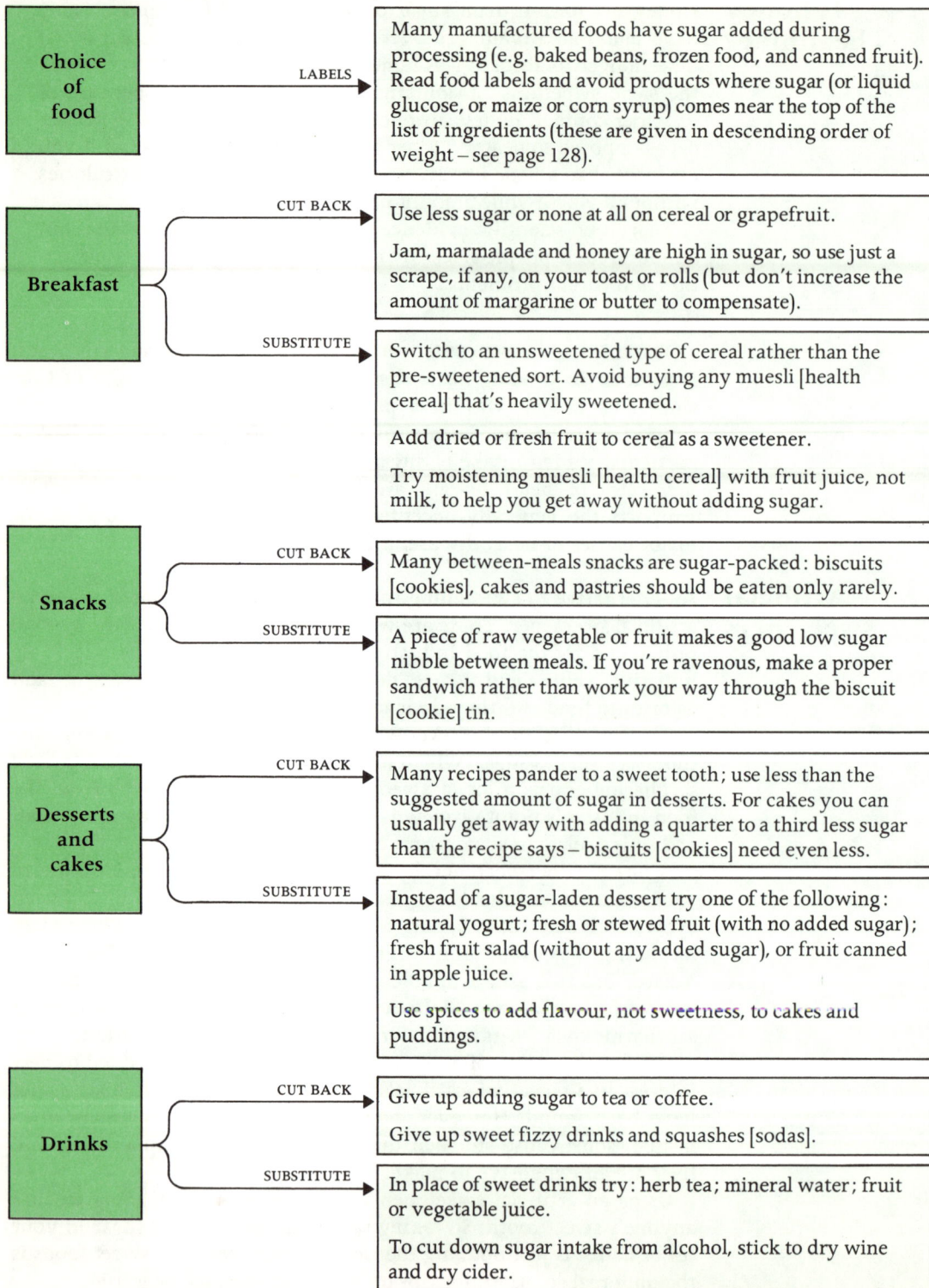

Choice of food	LABELS	Many manufactured foods have sugar added during processing (e.g. baked beans, frozen food, and canned fruit). Read food labels and avoid products where sugar (or liquid glucose, or maize or corn syrup) comes near the top of the list of ingredients (these are given in descending order of weight – see page 128).

Breakfast

CUT BACK → Use less sugar or none at all on cereal or grapefruit.

Jam, marmalade and honey are high in sugar, so use just a scrape, if any, on your toast or rolls (but don't increase the amount of margarine or butter to compensate).

SUBSTITUTE → Switch to an unsweetened type of cereal rather than the pre-sweetened sort. Avoid buying any muesli [health cereal] that's heavily sweetened.

Add dried or fresh fruit to cereal as a sweetener.

Try moistening muesli [health cereal] with fruit juice, not milk, to help you get away without adding sugar.

Snacks

CUT BACK → Many between-meals snacks are sugar-packed: biscuits [cookies], cakes and pastries should be eaten only rarely.

SUBSTITUTE → A piece of raw vegetable or fruit makes a good low sugar nibble between meals. If you're ravenous, make a proper sandwich rather than work your way through the biscuit [cookie] tin.

Desserts and cakes

CUT BACK → Many recipes pander to a sweet tooth; use less than the suggested amount of sugar in desserts. For cakes you can usually get away with adding a quarter to a third less sugar than the recipe says – biscuits [cookies] need even less.

SUBSTITUTE → Instead of a sugar-laden dessert try one of the following: natural yogurt; fresh or stewed fruit (with no added sugar); fresh fruit salad (without any added sugar), or fruit canned in apple juice.

Use spices to add flavour, not sweetness, to cakes and puddings.

Drinks

CUT BACK → Give up adding sugar to tea or coffee.

Give up sweet fizzy drinks and squashes [sodas].

SUBSTITUTE → In place of sweet drinks try: herb tea; mineral water; fruit or vegetable juice.

To cut down sugar intake from alcohol, stick to dry wine and dry cider.

Fibre

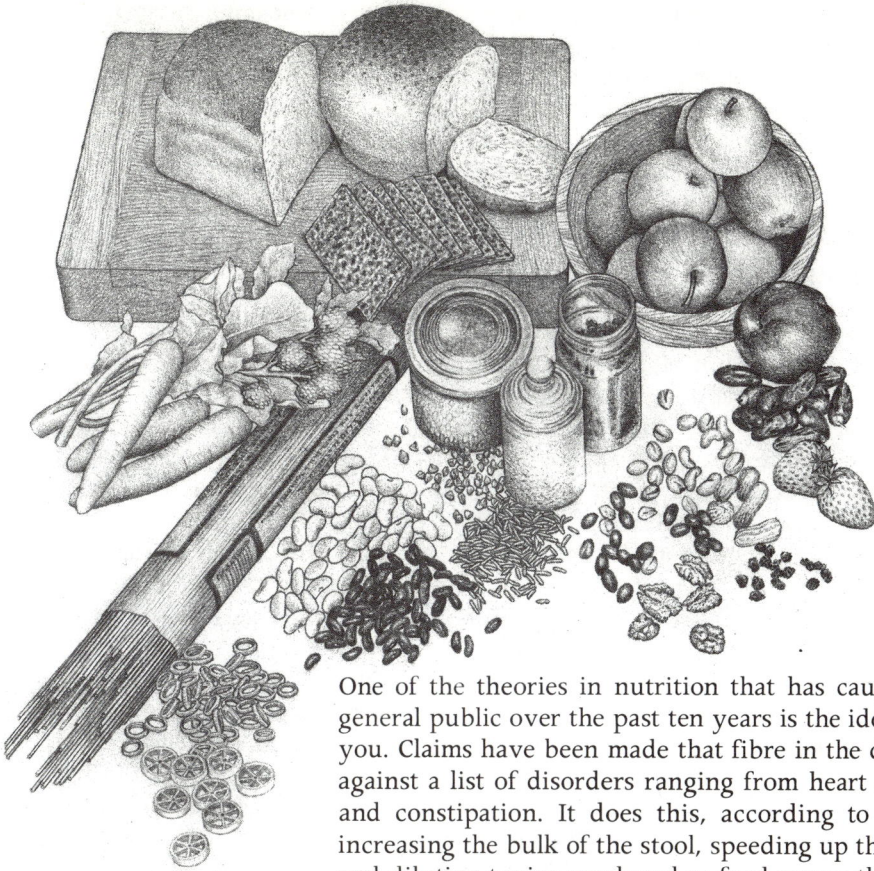

HIGH FIBRE
Brown rice
Fruit, especially dried
    fruit, such as dates and
    raisins, and berries
Nuts
Vegetables, especially
    beans, peas and lentils
Wholegrain cereals
Wholemeal [wholewheat]
    bread, crispbread and
    pasta

One of the theories in nutrition that has caught on fast among the general public over the past ten years is the idea that fibre is good for you. Claims have been made that fibre in the diet can help to protect against a list of disorders ranging from heart disease to appendicitis and constipation. It does this, according to different theories, by increasing the bulk of the stool, speeding up the transit time of waste, and diluting toxins produced as food passes through the body.

Recognition that removing fibre from foods (refining them) may not be improving them is by no means new. Hundreds – even thousands – of years ago, people were saying the same, albeit on less scientific grounds. The big change in recent years is not simply the popularity of fibre but the mounting evidence as to *why* fibre is important. A recent report by the Royal College of Physicians in Britain (where most of the research on this topic is being carried out) came to the conclusion that everyone should try to eat more fibre. Though there is, as yet, no official recommendation, around 30 g a day would be a sensible target. At the moment people in industrialized countries are eating, on average, 20 g a day, compared with over 60 g a day for the typical rural African or Asian.

What is fibre? Dietary fibre is a cover-all term for a large group of substances that make up the supporting structure in plant cell walls, plus substances intimately associated with them, such as the pith of fruit. These mostly pass unchanged through the digestive system, because the human alimentary canal lacks the enzymes to enable it to break them down. 'Fibre' is also used to include such things as gums – fruit pectin, for instance. Each kind of fibre has different effects on the body.

109

Sources of fibre

The best-known source of fibre is cereal grains. The outer covering, or husk, of the grain accounts for about 13 per cent of its total. One of the special properties of cells in this husk is their ability to take up and retain water – and this special feature may explain some of the beneficial effects of dietary fibre. In refined white flour, the husk is removed as part of the milling process; the discarded material makes up the bulk of what is known as bran. The precise fibre content of bran varies, but it is usually between 40 and 50 per cent depending on the milling process. This makes bran the richest source of fibre available (but not necessarily the ideal way to increase fibre intake – see below and opposite).

The amount of fibre bread contains depends on the type of flour used for the dough: about 8.5 per cent in wholemeal [wholewheat] bread, 4.5 to 5 per cent in 'wheatmeal' and 'brown', and 2.7 per cent in white. Brown rice, wholemeal pasta, and biscuits [cookies and crackers], cakes, pastry and breakfast cereals made from whole grains are also a good source of cereal fibre.

Fruit and vegetables contain less fibre than cereals, but because we eat a lot of them, they make an important contribution to total fibre intake. For details of fibre content of specific foods, turn to the tables on pages 241–49.

How much fibre do you eat?

As people get more affluent they tend to eat more meat and animal products and less of the staple starchy foods such as bread and potatoes. In Britain and the U.S.A., for instance, consumption of fibre from flour has fallen dramatically over the past 100 years, both because less bread and flour are being eaten, and because the flour people do eat has less fibre in it. This decrease in cereal fibre intake has been offset to some extent by a rise in the amount of fibre taken in from fruit and vegetable sources; and although the typical fibre intake of a North American or a European today is probably only fractionally less than it was a century ago, no one knows yet what the full effect of this switch in type of fibre may be.

Among European peoples, the British eat less fibre than the Yugoslavs, Germans, Swedes and Irish. They also eat less fibre than people in many African countries (less than half as much) and in India and North America. There are geographical variations within countries, too, and tremendous variations between different individuals.

How to eat more fibre and starch

Although it would be simple to increase fibre intake merely by sprinkling bran on your ordinary breakfast cereal, this isn't the best solution. Bran contains only one group of fibres; fruit and vegetables contain vitamins and minerals, too, and other whole foods contain starch as well. The best plan is to eat more fibre-rich foods rather than those to which bran has been added. A dramatic increase in fibre intake can lead to flatulence, so increase the fibre you eat little by little over two or three months, so that your system has a chance to adapt to it gradually.

FIBRE AT WORK

Mouth
Fibre in food makes it chewy, which stimulates saliva production. This helps neutralize acid formed on the teeth, reducing **dental decay.**

The extra chewing slows down food intake and so helps cut calories if less ends up being eaten.

Gall bladder
More fibre in the diet may reduce the cholesterol saturation of the bile and so make it less prone to form **gallstones** (see pages 98–99).

Small intestine
Digestion is slower and energy absorption, probably from fats, is lower on a high fibre diet: about 92.5 calories are absorbed per 100 eaten, compared with 98 on a low fibre diet. Over the long term, this could help weight loss. On a diet of around 2,500 calories a day, you could lose about ½ kilo [1 lb] a month.

Rectum
Too little waste material causes constipation, as the signal to the muscles to evacuate is weak. The softer, bulkier stools of a fibrous diet are easier to pass and help to prevent **haemorrhoids** (piles), **varicose veins,** and possibly **cancer of the rectum.**

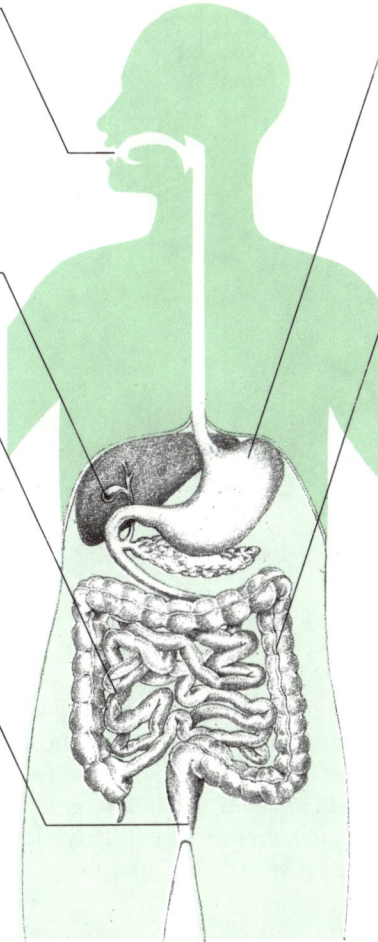

Stomach
The stomach feels fuller as the bulk in the stomach is greater after fibrous food has been eaten. This is partly due to extra saliva being swallowed and more gastric juices being produced. Fibre also holds and retains water. This full feeling helps you eat less.

Large intestine
On a low fibre diet, pressure inside the colon tends to be high, which can lead to **diverticular disease** (see pages 96–97).

Colitis, or 'irritable bowel syndrome', with its symptoms of distension, cramps, and alternate diarrhoea and constipation, generally improves on a high fibre diet. Bowel habits in general seem better regulated when the diet is high in fibre.

Fibre also seems to help protect against **cancer of the colon** (see pages 94–95).

Other links with health
There is some evidence that the type of **diabetes** common among overweight adults (see pages 96–97) is less often seen in people eating a high fibre diet.

Low fibre diets have been linked with **heart disease,** but the high fat content of this type of diet may be the real culprit (see pages 98–99).

- Eat breakfast – particularly wholegrain breakfast cereals (check the label), and wholemeal [wholewheat] toast. Make your own muesli [health cereal] from oats, fresh and/or dried fruit, nuts and wheatgerm (by doing this you'll get less sugar than from most commercial types).
- Eat brown rice and wholemeal [wholewheat] pasta, and leave the skin on potatoes (unless it's green).
- Eat wholemeal [wholewheat] bread and crispbreads.
- Don't throw away the outer leaves of vegetables – these are a richer source of fibre than the inner ones. Chop them up finely and add them to soups and stews.
- Eat more pulses (lentils, beans and peas) – add them to soups and to stews.
- Use wholemeal [wholewheat] or part wholemeal flour for cooking.

Proteins

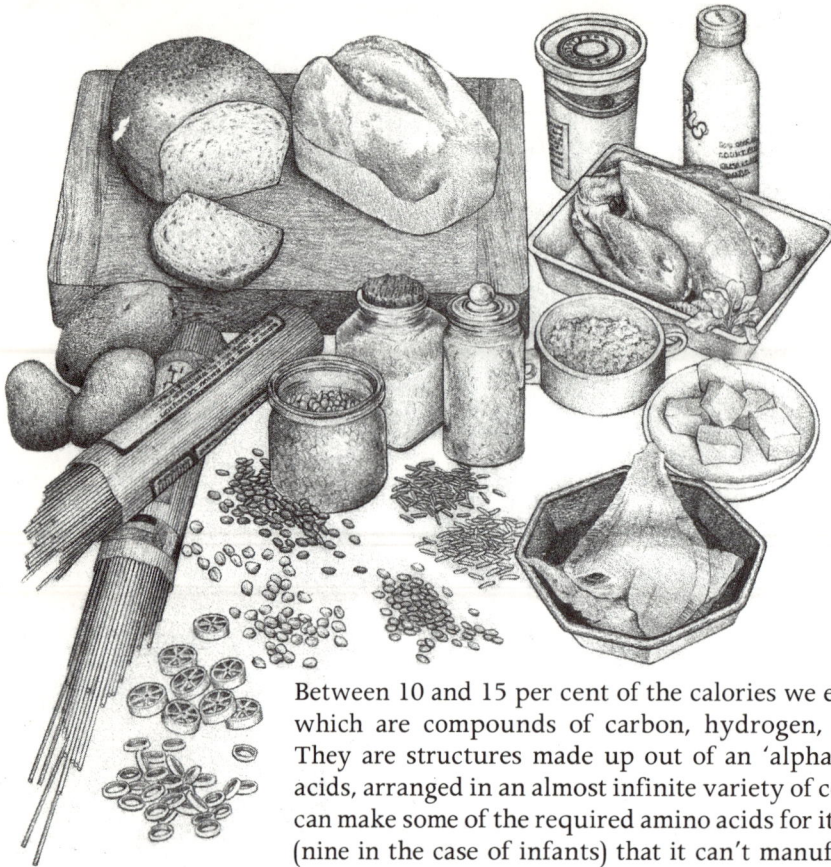

LOW FAT PROTEIN
Beans
Bread
Cottage cheese
Lentils
Low fat yogurt
Pasta
Potatoes
Poultry (skinless)
Rice and other grains
Skimmed milk
Tofu [soya bean curd]
White fish

Between 10 and 15 per cent of the calories we eat come from proteins, which are compounds of carbon, hydrogen, oxygen and nitrogen. They are structures made up out of an 'alphabet' of 20 or so amino acids, arranged in an almost infinite variety of combinations. The body can make some of the required amino acids for itself, but there are eight (nine in the case of infants) that it can't manufacture, and these have to be obtained from food. The essential amino acids are isoleucine, leucine, lysine, methionine, phenylalanine, threonine, tryptophan and valine (plus histidine for infants).

Why you need protein

Many of the body's cells consist of protein, and the body needs a steady supply of the essential amino acids to enable it to repair and replace these tissues. Different patterns of amino acids are needed for the protein in different body structures (skin, hair, nails and so forth).

The demand for protein is highest when the body is growing, during childhood and puberty, but adults need protein, too, for the continuous process of replacement of body tissue. Protein is also needed to manufacture digestive and other enzymes. If there is too little protein in the diet, or if total calorie intake is so low that the body has to burn protein to supply its need for energy, protein deficiency diseases can result; these are, however, rare outside developing countries.

There is no way the body can store amino acids, so if you take in more protein than you need, the surplus is converted into glucose in the liver, and either stored as body fat or simply burnt as a source of energy.

One of the popular myths about diet for generations has been the theory that an active man needs plenty of protein. Subscribing to this myth has often led a poor family to allocate too much protein to the working man in the household, while the mother and children go short. In fact things should be the other way round: growing children are the ones who need the protein most. What working adults need is energy, which can be provided by other foods, like carbohydrates and, in an even more concentrated form, by fats.

A new-born baby probably needs about five times the amount of protein, in relation to body weight, that an adult needs. As the child gets bigger, it grows more slowly and its need for protein drops – but children's protein requirements stay above those of an adult until they stop growing.

How much protein should you eat?

There is really no exact answer to this, but for an adult a protein intake of around 45 g a day is reckoned to be sufficient. Most people eat much more than this in a normal day. For instance, a handful of roasted peanuts, 25 g [roughly 1 oz] of cheese and a couple of slices of wholemeal [wholewheat] bread would supply ample protein to take an adult through one day.

For babies and children, protein requirements range from between 15 and 20 g a day under the age of one, to between 30 and 53 g a day at the age of seven or eight, peaking at puberty to 44 to 58 g a day for girls, 50 to 75 g for boys.

Protein intake in adults can vary quite a lot without seemingly affecting health greatly. Some people have remained perfectly healthy on a diet containing as little as 40 g of protein a day, for periods of up to a year. Some people, by contrast, eat as much as 300 g of protein daily all their lives, without seeming any the worse for it.

Is one sort of protein better than another?

Some proteins contain all the amino acids you need in roughly the right proportions: this is true mostly of animal protein (meat, fish, milk, cheese, eggs and so on). For this reason it used to be thought that vegetable proteins were not as good as animal ones, but this is not true in practice. Some vegetable proteins are virtually as good as meat, and indeed are used as substitutes for animal protein in modern food processes (see page 115). Many traditional dishes are based on good sources of vegetable protein (see the suggestions on page 114).

Different vegetable sources are low on different essential amino acids. Mix them suitably and you end up with just as nutritious a meal as one high on animal protein. Beans complement wheat in this way, since beans are high in lysine, which wheat is short of. This makes baked beans on toast, for instance, a good combination nutritionally. Nuts and seeds make good accompaniments to pulses (lentils, beans and peas) in this respect too.

A typical affluent diet takes about two-thirds of its protein from animal sources. This tends to be expensive, since far more land and energy are needed to produce meat and dairy produce than vegetable protein such as cereals or beans. The classic example of this is the disastrous experience of Germany during the First World War, when

113

German farmers were advised to concentrate on rearing large herds of cattle and sheep. No extra pastures were ploughed up, although cereals can yield up to six times more dietary energy per acre than cattle. When food in Central Europe became in short supply as a result of the Allied blockade, it was too late to increase cereal production effectively.

Expense is not the only drawback to meat-eating, however. Meat and animal products are high in fat, so if you eat a lot of them, your fat intake will end up too high to be healthy (see pages 100–03). And if you take in a high proportion of your calories in meat, then either you have to cut back on carbohydrates, which is considered undesirable, or you will probably take in too many calories overall and wind up overweight, which is a major health hazard (see pages 152–53). It makes sense to try to get as much as possible of your protein from low fat sources such as white fish, grains, pulses, low fat dairy foods, bread, preferably wholemeal [wholewheat], rice and potatoes.

VEGETABLE PROTEIN
Here are suggestions for sources of vegetable protein and ways of using them. Bear in mind that nuts are higher in fat than grains and pulses, so don't overdo them.

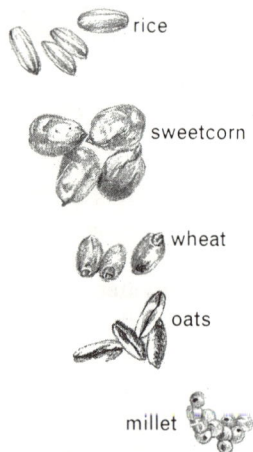

rice

sweetcorn

wheat

oats

millet

Grains
Barley stew, biscuits [cookies], bread, breakfast cereals, Chinese and Indian rice dishes pancakes, pasta pastry, pitta bread pizza, Scotch broth
Other uses:
for sprouting, in salads

Pulses
Baked beans, beanburgers
bean casserole
bean salads, beansprouts
chilli con carne
dhal (curried pulses)
humus, from chick peas [garbanzos]
lentil soup, minestrone
pease pudding
savoury loaf

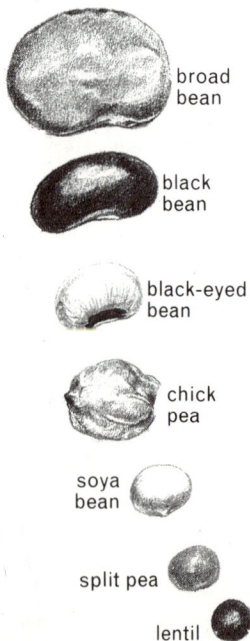

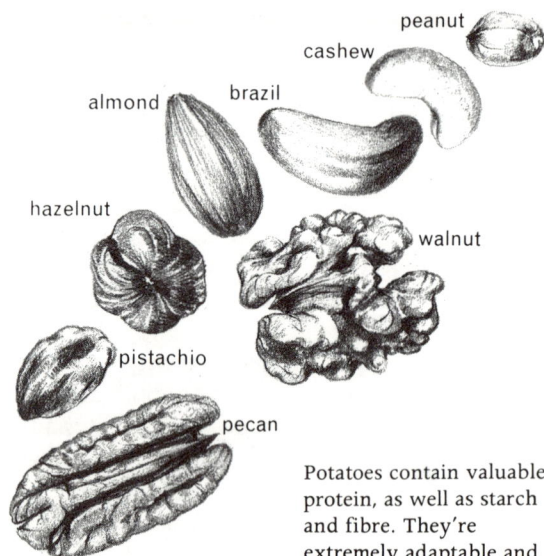

broad bean

black bean

black-eyed bean

chick pea

soya bean

split pea

lentil

peanut

cashew

brazil

almond

hazelnut

walnut

pistachio

pecan

Nuts
Fruit and nut bars
nut loaf, nut patties –
nut spreads, nutty biscuits [cookies]
peanut butter
peanut cookies
Other uses:
as a garnish or snack *and in*
chop suey
crumble topping
fruit salad, risotto
salads, savouries
stuffings

Potatoes contain valuable protein, as well as starch and fibre. They're extremely adaptable and lend themselves to a wide range of dishes and methods of serving including:
bubble and squeak [fried potato and cabbage]
frikadeller (meat and potato patties)
gnocchi, jacket potatoes
latkes (East European potato pancakes)
potato bread (Irish)
potato salad
Spanish omelette
vichyssoise

Novel protein foods

Some modern foods contain 'texturized vegetable protein' or TVP, which is what vegetable protein is called when it's done up to look like meat. Purists and gourmets tend to look down on it, but it can be virtually undetectable when mixed with normal meat. So long as manufacturers make it clear on their labels that their food contains TVP, it's up to the customer to choose whether or not to buy it.

Texturized vegetable protein is usually based on soya beans, although some other bean, wheat or oats can be used instead. The basis for TVP can be either soya bean meal, or a flour made from oil-free flakes (the flour can be refined so that the product is nearly pure protein). TVP can be processed in two ways. The first, the extrusion process, is similar to that used for spaghetti. The soya bean meal or flour is mixed with water to make a dough, which is then heated and squeezed under pressure through small nozzles. As it comes out of the nozzle, the dough expands and can be cut into chunks or granules. The second process involves spinning vermicelli-like strands of pasta made from the soya bean flour dough into long bundles, which are then baked. The end product looks quite like meat.

Why use TVP? TVP products are cheap, easy to prepare, and involve little wastage, which makes them attractive to catering organizations that serve large numbers. At the moment TVP tends to replace meat, but it's perfectly possible to make synthetic cheese, and maybe other foods, too.

Another plus point with TVP is that the beans on which it's based contain very little fat but quite a lot of fibre. (See pages 100–03 and 109–11 for why low fat, high fibre diets are considered healthy.) Of course, how much fat the end product contains varies. Dry vegetable protein (sold as an extender) is low in fat, but mops up the juices, fats and flavour of whatever it's added to. Reconstituted TVP sold in cans will have had fat (and other ingredients) added to make it seem more like the meat it's replacing. Check where fat comes on the label before buying; ingredients are listed in descending order of weight, so avoid products where fat appears among the first few items.

How safe is TVP? The present ingredients of TVP have been part of the human diet for a long time and therefore should present no special safety problems. The well-known toxins and anti-metabolites present in pulses are destroyed by a combination of processing, cooking and pepsin in the stomach. The standard advice to eat a varied diet should be a safeguard so far as health is concerned.

From the nutritional point of view, TVP is about as different from meat as eggs are from fish. Each is a nutritious food in its own right, although the pattern of amino acids present in one food is not identical with that in any of the others. There is no reason to believe that your health will suffer if you take your protein in the form of TVP (or any other form of vegetable protein) rather than meat and dairy produce. On the contrary, it may benefit from the lower fat and higher fibre intake that comes from eating vegetable protein.

Vegetarianism

Vegetarians are often the butt of jokes, but they may well turn out to have the last laugh. Vegetarians can have several advantages over those who eat meat. Their meals can be cheaper than meat dishes, and their diet is often lower in saturated fats (and so calories) and higher in fibre. Provided the diet is deliberately varied so that it doesn't miss out any essential nutrients or, conversely, overdo any inessential ones, vegetarians who claim that they are eating more healthily may well be right.

The different forms

Most vegetarians avoid only meat and fish, but some of the stricter diets, those followed by vegans, exclude all animal products including milk, butter, cheese and eggs. This can be an even healthier way of eating, as it virtually assures a lower intake of calories and fats. But vegans have to plan meals carefully to be sure of a few nutrients, such as vitamin B_{12}, that are mainly derived from animal foods. A few people choose to be fruitarians, eating fruit and vegetables only, which makes it difficult to eat a balanced diet (if only because you'd have to be eating almost all day long). Macrobiotic diets as originally based on the Japanese style of cooking can be healthy, using brown rice, vegetables (including seaweeds) and fish as staples. They are low fat and low sugar diets. However, nowadays there are many extreme variations, which depart from the original principles of the macrobiotic diet and which, in consequence, can be very dangerous.

Protein

The most important sources of plant protein in vegetarian diets are cereals, nuts, pulses and potatoes. Studies of vegetarian diets in Britain and America have shown they contain adequate amounts of protein, that is, at least 10 per cent of the energy intake comes from these sources. Protein quality in plant foods is not as high as in meat (see page 113), but this does not matter in practice provided meals contain a mixture of protein from different plant sources. Cereals and pulses or nuts complement each other, so a dish like beans on toast, or rice and lentils, or a peanut butter sandwich, is a source of protein of just as high quality as a meat dish. See page 114 for ideas for dishes based on plant proteins.

To use protein properly, the body must have a sufficient intake of energy. This is usually no problem for adults, but it can be for children. There is a risk that a vegetarian diet might be too bulky, and therefore too dilute in nutrients. Certainly, vegetarians tend to have a lower energy intake than people on a mixed diet – largely because plant foods tend to be bulky, low in calories, and more filling than meat.

Fibre

Most vegetarians, especially those who adopt the diet for health reasons, eat unrefined whole foods and get a sizable proportion of their fibre from these. Vegetables are also a good source.

A word of caution: diets that contain a lot of cereal fibre can interfere with the absorption of certain minerals, such as calcium, zinc and iron – but this is likely to be important only in the very young, in vegetarian Asians and in the elderly, who may have little of these minerals in their diet anyway.

Minerals **Calcium:** By far the major part of the calcium in the body is in the bones, but calcium is also important elsewhere – in blood-clotting mechanisms, for example. Although there's quite a bit of calcium in drinking water, especially in hard water areas, most of the calcium in an ordinary diet comes from milk and cheese, so vegans may have a problem getting enough. Nutritionists may recommend supplements of calcium gluconate for vegan mothers during pregnancy and lactation.

Iron: Intakes of iron have generally been found to be good in vegans and vegetarians, although some of the iron in plants is bound up in such a way as to be poorly absorbed compared with iron from animal sources. The body generally adapts to a low iron intake by absorbing more of what's available. Eating foods rich in vitamin C at the same meal also helps the absorption of iron.

Vitamins The vitamin that causes most concern in strict vegetarian diets is vitamin B_{12}, lack of which can lead to anaemia. It is present in practically all foods of animal origin, but cereals, nuts, pulses, fruit and most vegetables don't contain any. The best source for a vegan is kombu or wakame, both types of Japanese seaweed, but yeast extract, TVP and Grapenuts are usually fortified with it, too. Vegetarians who eat cheese and drink milk have nothing to worry about, because these foods are adequate sources of the vitamin, but vegans are advised to take supplements unless they take kombu or wakame regularly. Even vegetarians who boil their milk may be short of vitamin B_{12}, as boiling destroys it.

Plant foods rarely contain vitamin D, lack of which can lead to the development of rickets in children. This is not too serious for those who regularly spend some time out of doors in the sunlight, because the body can make all of the vitamin D it needs as a result of the action of sun on the skin. However, housebound elderly people, who can't get out into the sunshine, and young growing children must have an adequate source of vitamin D in their diet. Fortunately, vegetable margarines fortified with vitamins A and D are acceptable to most vegetarians and, when milk-free, to many vegans.

Are vegetarians healthier? A vegetarian or carefully planned vegan diet can be healthier to follow than one that involves eating a lot of meat. For example, blood cholesterol levels among vegans tend to be lower than those of either vegetarians or meat eaters. (The reason vegetarians don't have a particularly low level is that many rely heavily on dairy produce, which contains large quantities of saturated fats.) Studies have also shown that blood pressure is lower in vegans than in meat eaters. For both these reasons vegans are less prone to heart disease and the other diseases of affluence than people who eat meat.

117

Vitamins and minerals

The natural place to get the vitamins and minerals you need is in food. Provided you eat a varied selection of foods and don't rely on over-processed, over-cooked foods, you'll automatically do so, and there's no need to take vitamin or mineral tablets. There *are*, however, special circumstances where extra vitamins and minerals can usefully supplement what you eat – see Who needs what, when? on page 149. But vitamin and mineral tablets, however impressive the label, are never a substitute for healthy eating, because you also need the right amounts of carbohydrate, protein, fat and fibre. And while a lot is known about some of the nutrients required, there is no perfect diet in a pill.

Despite this, millions of people do take extra vitamins and minerals. Provided these are taken in small amounts, as in a multi-vitamin/mineral tablet, they won't do any harm. But they won't do any good either, if you're getting enough vitamins and minerals from food. These nutrients are essential, but they aren't magic. If your body has enough, it can't use any more. It's just cash down the toilet.

If you're ill, don't try vitamin therapy before getting a proper diagnosis. While extra vitamins and minerals won't hurt you in modest amounts, megavitamin therapy, where you're taking thousands of times the normal amount required by the body, is not necessarily safe: you're using the vitamin like a drug. And you may be completely missing what's wrong with you – allowing illness to develop further because you haven't been properly diagnosed. If, on the other hand, you have a diagnosed chronic problem, such as asthma, eczema, colitis or catarrh, that orthodox medical treatment can't help with except by suppressive drugs, it's worth trying alternative medicine, which may include vitamins and minerals. In any case, try megavitamin therapy only under professional supervision.

Preparing and cooking

To minimize vitamin and mineral loss, follow these guidelines:
- Avoid soaking vegetables before cooking.
- The finer vegetables are chopped, the quicker they deteriorate because more surface area is exposed to oxygen – so chop them up immediately before cooking.
- Saucepans should have close-fitting lids to restrict access of oxygen to vegetables during cooking. Avoid copper pots and pans; these encourage oxidation, and loss of vitamin C.
- Pressure cooking can help by cutting down cooking time. Potatoes cooked this way can keep up to 80 per cent of their vitamin C.
- Keep cooking time as short as possible.
- Use as little water as possible. Bring it to the boil before adding vegetables to drive off dissolved oxygen and cut cooking time.
- Try steaming instead of boiling to avoid vitamin loss into the water.
- Never add bicarbonate of soda to cooking water as it destroys vitamins B and C.
- If you must fry, do it quickly in deep fat, not slowly in shallow fat.
- Eat vegetables as soon as possible after cooking; keeping them warm hastens the vitamin loss.

WHAT YOU NEED AND WHY

The most important column in these tables is the 'source' one. See whether most of the foods are on your shopping list, or recall the last time you ate them. It's easy to fall into monotonous eating habits that exclude main vitamin or mineral sources. You don't need to eat everything on the lists of course — but check that you aren't missing out on too much, especially of the sources of water-soluble vitamins, which the body can't store. Fat-soluble vitamins can be stored for long periods in the body. Research on minerals and vitamins is in full spate — so in a few years, some of our unanswered questions about the optimum amount or how they work will probably be satisfied. (Note: There are 13 known vitamins. Don't be confused by the numbering of the B vitamins — the numbers in between don't exist.)

FAT-SOLUBLE VITAMINS

NAME	SOURCE	FUNCTION	DEFICIENCY/EXCESS	FURTHER COMMENTS
Vitamin A (retinol)	Fish liver oil, liver, dairy produce, eggs. Added by law to margarine in some countries. Carotene, which can be converted to retinol, is in carrots, spinach, and other yellow or dark green vegetables.	Vision in dim light; healthy skin; health of mucous membranes; growth.	**Deficiency:** Causes night blindness and eye lesions in children. Other problems with membranes like those of eyes and lungs may make them more susceptible to infection. **Excess:** Toxic. High dose over a long period can kill. Too much carotene (from which the body can make retinol) can turn skin yellow.	Vitamin A is stored in the liver. A deficiency is likely to occur only after a long period without vitamin A in the diet. Vitamin A may help to protect against many forms of cancer, but it isn't clear whether treatment with vitamin pills (rather than the vitamin as found in food) will do any good.
Vitamin D (cholecalciferol, ergocalciferol)	Fatty fish (herring, salmon, pilchards, sardines) and eggs. Added by law to margarine in some countries. Sunlight on the skin is the most important source.	Absorption of calcium, and used in bone formation and maintenance of blood calcium.	**Deficiency:** Causes rickets in children, bone softening (osteomalacia) in adults. **Excess:** High doses are deposited in kidneys, and can damage them. Calcification of soft tissues in children.	There is a narrow gap between the nutrient requirements and the toxic dose. Can be stored by liver, or in body fat. One good serving a week of foods rich in vitamin D should be ample.
Vitamin E (tocopherols)	Many foods, especially wheat germ, sunflower oil, eggs, wholemeal [wholewheat] cereals, broccoli, breast milk.	Not known what people need it for. Individual animal species have different diseases with a lack of vitamin E: e.g. rats need it for normal fertility; without it cows get muscular dystrophy.	**Deficiency:** Unlikely in adults on a good diet. In premature baby, could lead to anaemia. **Excess:** Harmless — so far as is known.	A vitamin in search of a disease, claimed to help everything from heart disease to sexual performance. No proof what effect it has on humans.
Vitamin K	Leafy vegetables (e.g. broccoli, lettuce, cabbage, spinach), cereals.	Normal blood-clotting.	**Deficiency:** Unlikely to occur.	Can also be made by bacteria inside the intestines. Not sold as a separate vitamin.

119

▷

WATER–SOLUBLE VITAMINS

NAME	SOURCE	FUNCTION	DEFICIENCY/EXCESS	FURTHER COMMENTS
Vitamin B_1 (thiamin)	Many foods, including potatoes and milk, but especially nuts, peas, beans, cereal germ, yeast.	Release of energy from carbohydrates.	**Deficiency**: Beriberi. **Excess**: Excreted in urine.	Cannot be stored in the body. Much of the thiamin in food is lost in cooking. Overcooking or adding bicarbonate of soda to cooking water increases the loss.
Vitamin B_2 (riboflavin)	Liver, milk, eggs, green vegetables, yeast extract.	Utilization of food energy. (This is true of virtually all B vitamins.)	**Deficiency**: In children, may cause poor growth. Rarely, may cause sores around the mouth. Unlikely to occur if dairy produce is eaten. **Excess**: Excreted in urine.	Destroyed by ultra-violet light – so don't leave milk standing out any longer than necessary.
Nicotinic acid (niacin, nicotinamide)	Small amounts in many foods, including meat, fish, wholegrain cereals, pulses, yeast extract, peanuts.	Utilization of food energy.	**Deficiency**: Pellagra (skin becomes dark and scaly, especially where exposed to light). **Excess**: Excreted in urine.	The body can make its own from tryptophan, an amino acid. Up to a quarter present in food is lost in cooking water, and in the juices lost from meat in cooking.
Vitamin B_6 (pyridoxin)	Numerous foods, especially liver, wholegrain cereals, peanuts, bananas.	Metabolism of amino acids; formation of haemoglobin.	**Deficiency**: Rare, but may arise in women taking oral contraceptives containing oestrogen. Depression is a possible symptom.	Has been used successfully in doses of 50 mg a day to relieve pre-menstrual tension.
Vitamin B_{12} (cyanacobalamin)	Animal and dairy produce: meat (especially liver and kidney), eggs, milk, cheese, etc. Not in vegetable produce unless fermented or otherwise contaminated with micro-organisms.	Needed by rapidly dividing cells, such as those in bone marrow and in the gastro-intestinal tract.	**Deficiency**: Causes pernicious and megaloblastic anaemia, and damages nerve cells. **Excess**: Unlike other water-soluble vitamins, excess can be stored in the liver.	Vegans (who eat no meat or dairy produce) should take vitamin B_{12} supplements. Some of this vitamin is lost if an alkali like bicarbonate of soda is added to cooking water. Stores in liver should last a year or two.
Folic (or folate) acid (folacin)	All living matter: liver, leafy vegetables, bread, eggs, rice, pulses, oranges and bananas are all good sources.	As for vitamin B_{12}.	**Deficiency**: Causes megaloblastic anaemia. May arise when body's need for red blood cells rises – as during pregnancy or in diseases that hamper absorption of folic acid in the small intestine. **Excess**: Normally has no adverse effects, but can be toxic if prescribed for epileptics.	Some anti-epileptic drugs and oral contraceptives may hamper the absorption of folic acid. Much folic acid is lost in cooking, and prolonged heating, canning and reheating destroy it too. One helping of fresh fruit or fresh vegetables a day should prevent deficiency.

WATER-SOLUBLE VITAMINS

NAME	SOURCE	FUNCTION	DEFICIENCY/EXCESS	FURTHER COMMENTS
Pantothenic acid	Numerous foods, especially offal [variety meats], yeast, egg yolk, pulses, bees' royal jelly.	Growth; anti-body production; metabolism of fats and carbohydrates.	**Deficiency:** Very unlikely to occur.	Little loss during cooking. In one study, huge doses relieved many symptoms in rheumatoid arthritis.
Biotin	Offal [variety meats], egg yolk, milk and dairy produce, cereals, fish, fruit, vegetables.	Metabolism of fat.	**Deficiency:** Very unlikely to occur.	Raw egg white contains a substance that prevents absorption of biotin – so someone who eats a lot of raw eggs might develop a deficiency. The body can make biotin itself from bacteria in the large intestine, so none is needed in the diet.
Vitamin C (ascorbic acid)	Citrus fruit (oranges, lemons), blackcurrants, green leafy vegetables, green peppers, liver. New potatoes contain more vitamin C than old ones.	Healthy connective tissues like collagen and cartilage in bone; aids the absorption of iron.	**Deficiency:** Causes bleeding, slow healing of wounds, scurvy. May cause death. **Excess:** High doses in pill form over long period may lead to nausea, or to development of kidney stones.	Some lost in cooking, and during storage (so frozen or canned vegetables may have more vitamin C than 'fresh' vegetables picked several days earlier). High doses *may* help protect some people against minor ailments like colds, but this is not really proved.

MINERALS

NAME	SOURCE	FUNCTION	DEFICIENCY/EXCESS	FURTHER COMMENTS
Calcium	Milk, cheese; bread and flour fortified with calcium; green vegetables. Hard water is an important source.	Healthy bones and teeth, muscle contraction, nerve function, activity of some enzymes, normal blood-clotting.	**Deficiency:** In common with vitamin D deficiency, it can cause rickets in children, osteomalacia in adults. **Excess:** Hardening of soft tissues as a result of too much calcium being deposited because of the presence of excess vitamin D.	Absorption of calcium may be hampered by lack of vitamin D, or presence of a lot of fibre in diet.
Iron	Meat, offal [variety meats], oatmeal, wheatmeal, chocolate, treacle [molasses].	Healthy blood: most of the iron you absorb goes to the bone marrow to help the production of red blood cells. Also needed for carrying oxygen round body.	**Deficiency:** Anaemia – women believed to be more at risk than men, because of blood loss during menstruation. **Excess:** A type of anaemia called siderosis. Some alcoholics develop this, and so may people who use iron cooking pots (like the Bantu in West Africa).	Egg yolk and tea hamper absorption of iron; vitamin C helps it. Body stores iron in liver, spleen and bone marrow. Women need slightly more iron than men. Absorption is generally low, except when body stores are depleted. Sometimes prescribed in pregnancy.

▷

MINERALS

NAME	SOURCE	FUNCTION	DEFICIENCY/EXCESS	FURTHER COMMENTS
Sodium	Sodium as salt (sodium chloride) is in most processed foods – e.g. bacon, sausages, smoked fish, canned vegetables, butter, cheese, bread, some breakfast cereals, yeast extract. Added in cooking and at the table.	Sodium is present in all body fluids; needed for maintaining water balance, and for muscle and nerve activity.	**Deficiency:** Muscular cramps – only likely in those losing salt from sweating profusely and drinking large quantities of water. **Excess:** Excreted via the kidneys in adults. Over long period, excess may lead to high blood pressure in susceptible adults (see pages 98–99).	Concentration of sodium in the body must keep within very narrow limits. An adult needs around 4 g of salt a day, which is found naturally in food, but average intake is up to five times higher because of salt added at table and during cooking. Sodium/ potassium balance in body is important.
Potassium	Most foods, especially milk, potatoes, instant coffee, fruit or vegetable juices, yeast extract, milk chocolate, Brussels sprouts, dried prunes.	Health of all cells; complements sodium in body.	**Deficiency:** In extreme case, could cause heart failure. Mild deficiency may arise if purgatives or diuretics are taken frequently. **Excess:** Excreted via kidneys.	Sodium and potassium are very important for maintaining water balance. Potassium may mitigate effects of too much sodium on blood pressure.
Magnesium	Many foods, especially vegetables.	An essential constituent of all cells; present in bones. Needed for functioning of some enzymes.	**Deficiency:** Rare except in case of high losses through diarrhoea.	The body absorbs only around half of the magnesium in the diet.
Zinc	Many foods, especially meat, whole grains, pulses, oysters.	Activity of about 20 enzymes. Also helps wounds to heal.	**Deficiency:** Causes stunted growth.	Phytic acid, present in unleavened bread, hampers absorption of zinc, and some other minerals.
Iodine	Seafood and seaweeds. Amounts in vegetables and meat depend on iodine in soil in area where plants or animals were reared.	Make-up of the thyroid hormones that control level of cell metabolism.	**Deficiency:** Causes slow-down of metabolism and circulation. Thyroid gland in neck enlarges (goitre).	Iodine is stored in the thyroid gland in the neck. In areas where soil is a poor source of iodine, those who eat only locally grown vegetables, and no seafood, may have trouble with goitre.
Fluorine	Drinking water, in many areas; tea and seafood (especially the bones of fish).	Health of bones and teeth; resistance to dental decay.	**Deficiency:** Higher risk of dental decay. **Excess:** Permanent tooth mottling. There are no proven health hazards associated with fluoridation, although the debate is still continuing.	Water in some areas is fluoridated to reduce dental decay in children. Children can be given fluoride tablets, if you live in a low fluoride area.

Salt and your health

Even if you add little or no extra salt to your food at table, your total salt intake will be building up over the day to a surprising extent. Breakfast cereal, toast, butter, biscuits, cheese, bacon – these and many other foods will add little by little to the total quantity of salt in your diet. Most people end up eating between 5 g and 18 g of salt a day; anything over 9 g is probably too much because of the connection between a high salt intake and high blood pressure (see pages 98–99). To stay healthy, try to cut out some of the salt you eat, and to eat rather more of foods that contain potassium, which seems to counter-act the harmful effects of a salty diet. Here are some strategies to try to help you achieve this.

Cutting down on salt

Choosing food:
- Avoid those foods in the top section of the salt league table, particularly if low on potassium too.
- Cut back on processed foods, whose salt content is often unexpectedly high.
- Eat more fresh fruit and vegetables, which are rich in potassium.

Cooking:
- Add less salt, or none, to cooking water and recipes.
- Try adding flavour to home baked bread with grated orange or lemon peel instead of salt.

At table:
- Cut out extra salt by leaving the salt cellar off the table; or if this is too painful, cut back the salt you add at this stage, little by little, so you grow used to the taste of food without it.

SALT LEAGUE TABLE

Foods with a high sodium content

Bacon and other cured meats	Canned meat	Cornflakes	Shellfish
	Canned vegetables	Ham	Smoked fish
Bread	Cheese	Margarine	Tomato juice
Butter	Cheese biscuits	Sausage	Yeast extract

Foods with a moderate sodium content

Beer	Dried fruit	Meat*	Root vegetables*
Biscuits [cookies]	Eggs*	Milk*	Wine
Celery	Fresh fish*	Milk chocolate	
Cream	Instant coffee*	Pulses	

Foods with a low sodium content

Dried prunes*	Fruit juice*	Shredded Wheat
Flour	Green vegetables*	Sugar
Fresh fruit*	Rice (cooked without salt)	Unsalted nuts

Note Foods that contain as much or more potassium than sodium are marked with *

Food processing

The notion of processing food is really nothing new. The simplest methods of preserving food – such as heating, adding salt and drying – have been around for hundreds of years. Modern food processing is an extension of these simple methods. One motive behind it is to keep food palatable for as long as possible. This is especially important nowadays, when so many people live in cities and food has to travel long distances from where it's grown or reared to where it's eaten. Processing also enables the manufacturer to produce and transport food in bulk rather than in smaller, less profitable batches, and extends its shelf-life. It enables the consumer to have a wide range of foods throughout the year, by making available those that are out of season as well as those that can't be grown or obtained locally.

As soon as a plant is harvested or an animal killed, it begins to degenerate. Enzymes naturally present in the food begin to break it down, altering its appearance and flavour. Fats begin to oxidize, and bacteria start feeding off the food and multiply, leading to further degeneration. The bacteria also produce potentially harmful toxins. So to keep the food edible and preserve its appeal, it's processed.

What processing actually involves varies a great deal with different methods. The main ones in commercial use are briefly explained in the chart below, and on the right we show what processing involves for liquid and powdered milk.

THE MAIN METHODS OF PROCESSING

Method	What happens	Nutrient losses	Storage life
Canning/ bottling	The food is quickly heated (or blanched in the case of vegetables) to kill bacteria and enzymes, and sealed in a sterile container.	Vitamin C, thiamin and folic acid are sensitive to heat, and some losses will occur. Slight loss of vitamin C continues during storage.	Very long – one can opened 143 years after sealing was found still to be sterile.
Drying/freeze- drying	Bacteria can't grow in food without moisture. The simplest way to dry is by exposing food to air and sun. Nowadays food is more likely to be dried in ovens or a hot atmosphere. Liquids may be spray-dried. Freeze-dried foods are frozen then placed in a vacuum; the container is then gently heated to make the ice evaporate while the solid stays frozen.	With foods dried in the air, up to half their vitamin C is lost. Thiamin loss occurs during heating and is total if sulphur dioxide is added as preservative. Freeze-drying preserves nutrients well because the food itself isn't heated.	Years rather than months, if properly sealed, with all moisture removed and no fat remaining to go rancid. Opened or permeable packaging may become infested with insects after around six months.
Freezing	The food is stored at or below $-18°C(0°F)$. As bacteria are inactive at $-12°C(10°F)$ this ensures an adequate safety margin. Vegetables and fruit may be blanched initially. Fruit may be frozen in syrup to help preserve its appearance and consistency.	Some thiamin and vitamin C are lost in blanching – but less than if vegetables are picked days before eating. Nutrients are also lost in the juice that drips from thawing meat.	Three months to a year, depending on product. Flavour and appearance may suffer if temperature rises above freezing.

MILK PROCESSING

Untreated cow's milk
Milk contains many essential nutrients, although low in iron, fibre and vitamins C and D. Bacteria present in untreated milk would be a health hazard.

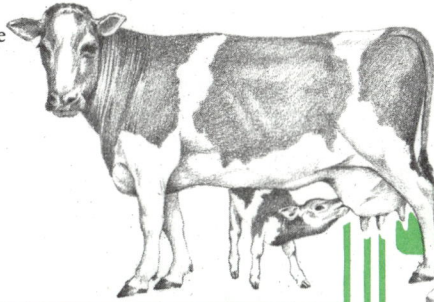

Sterilized
Heated to 120°C [248°F] for 20 to 60 minutes. Thiamin loss 20 per cent, vitamin C loss 60 per cent.

Evaporated
Liquid milk is concentrated at low temperature, then heated to 115°C [239°F] for 15 minutes. Similar nutrient losses to sterilizing.

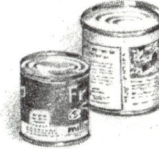

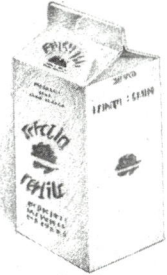

Condensed
Concentrated like evaporated milk, but added sugar means less heat is required to preserve it. Nutrient losses similar to pasteurizing.

Pasteurized
Heated to not less than 72°C [162°F] for 15 seconds. Ten per cent thiamin and 25 per cent vitamin C are lost.

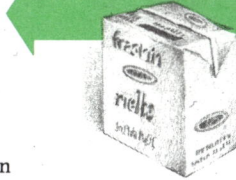

Homogenized
Warm milk is forced through a fine aperture so the fat globules are broken down. Heating and nutrient loss as for pasteurized.

UHT (ultra-high temperature)
Heated to about 130°C [266°F] for one or two seconds. Nutrient loss the same as for pasteurizing.

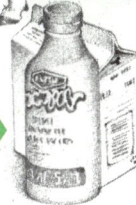

Liquid skimmed milk
Fresh skimmed milk has had most of its fat removed, as well as vitamins A and D. Thiamin and vitamin C losses as for pasteurizing. Some liquid skimmed milks have added vitamins and protein.

Dried skimmed milk
Made from milk from which most of the fat has been removed as well as vitamins A and D. Other losses as for pasteurized.

Milk powder with added vegetable fat
Some dried milks now being marketed are combinations of skimmed milk and vegetable fats. These fats are probably hydrogenated and are therefore saturated.

For and against

In favour of processing:
• It may make food safer to consume, as with pasteurized milk.
• It allows a wider choice of foods.
• Although processing involves some loss of nutrients, this may be no greater than that in 'fresh' food left uneaten for several days. And some processed foods, such as bread, have nutrients added.
• Processed food often needs only short cooking. Apart from being convenient for the cook, this means that the loss of some vitamins during processing may be balanced to some extent by a lower loss during cooking.

Against processing:
• Rapid changes in food technology – such as those behind the chips [fries] on page 126 – mean that even experts find it hard to tell how nutritious some highly-processed modern food is.
• Processed food – particularly snack food like chocolate bars or crisps [potato chips] – tends to be high on fat, salt and sugar.

OVEN-READY FRENCH FRIES

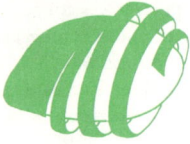

1 Graded potatoes from selected varieties are steam peeled.

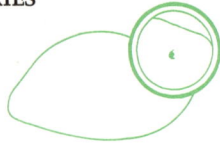

2 Inspected, sorted and trimmed if necessary.

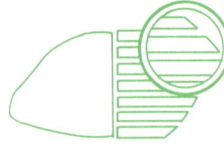

3 Cut into chips [fries] and inspected again.

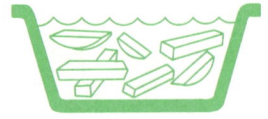

4 Blanched in warm water.

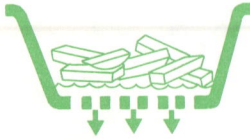

5 Drained and allowed to dry slightly.

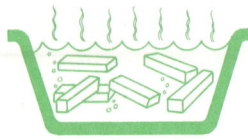

6 Deep fried in oil.

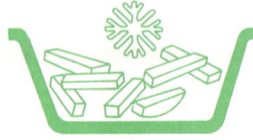

7 Individually fast frozen.

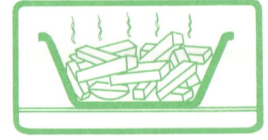

8 Cooked by consumer in oven or under grill.

• When you eat processed foods you give up control over your diet. Unless you read package labels carefully, you won't even realize, let alone decide, what you're buying. The more processed food you eat, the more it makes sense to worry about this.

What to do

• Read the list of ingredients given on food labels. The ingredients are listed in descending order of weight, so the first are the most important. Watch where sugar and fat come on the list.

• Compare different brands for their ingredients and the number of additives (see pages 127–28) they contain. Choose those whose ingredients seem closest to those you would use.

• Buy brands that provide information about the nutritional content of the food – the calories, protein, fat and carbohydrate it contains. Better still, choose those that break down these categories further, and list sugar and starch, or saturated and polyunsaturated fats, separately. Really informative nutritional labelling is lacking in most countries, including Britain, but some manufacturers are making an effort to introduce this type of labelling, which shows that this particular campaign can be won.

• Don't be fooled by products that list 'non-dairy fats' among their ingredients (ice cream, cream substitutes and dried milk are the foods to watch). Even vegetable oils can wind up saturated after processing, and if you want to buy a product that is high in polyunsaturates, look for a label that says exactly that. 'Contains no cholesterol' is misleading, too: foods that contain no cholesterol at all can still raise blood cholesterol by containing saturated fats (see pages 100–03).

• Avoid foods described as consisting of 'meat products' as they usually contain little flesh, but a great deal of fat (together with flour and other ingredients).

Food additives

The vast growth in the use of food additives over the last 150 years is the direct result of larger populations living in cities. Food can't be field-to-mouth – it must travel and be stored before eating.

Food additives have been used for thousands of years in a more limited way: vinegar and salt to preserve, saltpetre to salt meat, herbs and spices to flavour, and more. Now there are about 3,000 additives. Of these more than 2,000 are flavourings, and it's as well to remember that many of these are herbs and spices. However, the new 20th-century flavourings, together with about 30–40 preservatives, 10–20 antioxidants (anti-rancidity agents), 140 or so colourings and over 20 other types, give rise to both anxiety and anger among many people.

The anxiety comes from the feeling that, in spite of Government control, the long-term effects of many additives may be unpredictable or difficult to track back to their cause; the anger from the feeling that food manufacturers may be using their technical expertise to cover up for their products' shortcomings in terms of ingredients and flavour.

Additives can be roughly divided into: the functional – broadly speaking, the preservatives and stabilizers, which reduce the risk of food poisoning and enable food to be stored; and the cosmetic – colourings, flavour enhancers, texture changers and so on. Although functional additives are constantly under scrutiny for safety, ensuring food supply is also an important consideration.

An example is the way sodium nitrates and nitrites have been used for centuries, for both functional and cosmetic reasons, to preserve meats like bacon, ham and tongue. These chemicals prevent the development of potentially dangerous bacteria like *Clostridium botulinum*, and produce the distinctive pink tint and flavour of cured meats. There is considerable debate about the use of nitrates and nitrites because they can be converted by the body into small amounts of nitrosamines, which can cause stomach cancer. Obviously not everyone who eats bacon develops stomach cancer; the degree of risk is unknown, and in fact the incidence of stomach cancer nowadays is declining. And this risk is balanced against the known risk of serious food poisoning if such meat is unprotected. Similar dilemmas result in the continued use of some other additives which, if complete safety alone were considered, might be thought an unjustifiable or unnecessary risk. The antioxidants BHT and BHA, and sulphur dioxide (the most widely used preservative, found in wine, beer, dried and canned fruit, and soft drinks, among other things), come into this category.

Anti-additive campaigners point out that the advent of freezing as a food storage method has reduced the justification for some additives, and that they're often used for the convenience of the manufacturer to give longer shelf-life and safeguard against less-than-perfect hygiene in the factory or shop rather than because of any health hazard. They believe the food industry has too much influence on additive regulation, with consumers running the risk for the sake of manufacturers' profits. When it comes to cosmetic additives, what justification is there for taking any risk at all? The argument against

127

cosmetic additives is strengthened by the fact that several food colours previously considered safe have been taken out of use in different countries because of safety doubts. In the U.K., colours are no longer used in foods designed for infants, for example.

Today, you'll probably eat at least a dozen different additives unless you stick to basic foods. Very little is known about how they interact with foods or with each other. The message: to avoid additives, choose basic, not convenience, foods, and be prepared to pay extra for foods without colours and shelf-life enhancers. Above all, read food labels carefully. Legislation on food labelling varies from country to country, and label reading is a skill that has to be learnt. See the guide below for how to interpret some of the information labels may display.

If you feel strongly about additives, join a consumer lobby for tighter additive control. This is an area where public opinion can be very effective. If people don't buy foods with additives, manufacturers will stop using them.

NUTRITIONAL LABELLING

In the U.S.A. food labels commonly give nutritional information like that on the one below, which makes it easy to see how much fat, for example, a serving contains. But 'carbohydrate' here covers both starch and sugar. And the barrage of technical information this label gives may ultimately confuse rather than help the consumer.

Ingredients: Potatoes, vegetable oil (contains one or more of the following: cottonseed oil, corn oil, peanut oil, partially hydrogenated cottonseed oil, partially hydrogenated soybean oil, partially hydrogenated sunflower oil or palm oil), and salt.

Ingredients must be listed in descending order of weight. Check the position of fat, sugar and salt in the list. For the product above, the mix of oils used will depend on which types of oil happen to be cheapest at the time.

E.E.C. regulations give additives code names (E320 below) which can be identified by checking back to a book. In the U.K. labels need give only the function of an additive (e.g. flavouring, antioxidant) not its name (e.g. oil of lemon, butylated hydroxanisole), and some products, biscuits included, don't yet have to carry ingredients lists at all and do so only for export purposes. In the U.S.A. both the name and the function of additives must appear in the ingredients list.

NUTRITION INFORMATION
(PER SERVING)

Serving Size 1 ounce
Number of Servings 1

Calories.	150
Protein.	2 grams
Carbohydrate.	14 grams
Fat.	10 grams
Cholesterol†. . . . (0 mg/100 g). .	0 milligrams
Sodium. . . . . . (925 mg/100 g). .	260 milligrams
Potassium. . . . (720 mg/100 g). .	205 milligrams

Percentage of U.S. Recommended Daily Allowances (U.S. RDA)

Protein.	2
Vitamin A	*
Vitamin C.	10
Thiamine.	2
Riboflavin.	*
Niacin.	4
Calcium.	*
Iron.	2
Vitamin B₆	10
Phosphorus.	4
Magnesium.	4
Copper.	6

†Information on cholesterol content is provided for individuals who, on the advice of a physician, are modifying their total dietary intake of cholesterol.
*Contains less than 2% U.S. RDA for this nutrient.

Ginger & Fruit Biscuits

INGREDIENTS: WHEATFLOUR, SUGAR, BUTTER, CURRANTS, TREACLE, GOLDEN SYRUP, GINGER POWDER, BAKING POWDER, CARAMEL, SALT, OIL OF LEMON, ANTIOXIDANT E320.

POIDS NET
PESO NETTO   150 g
PESO NETO

BISCUITS AU BEURRE ET AUX RAISINS
INGREDIENTS: FARINE DE FROMENT, SUCRE, BEURRE (17%), RAISINS DE CORINTHE (15%), MÉLASSE, SIROP DE SUCRE, GINGEMBRE (.93%), POUDRE LEVANTE, CARAMEL, SEL, HUILE DE CITRON, AGENT ANTIOXYGÈNE E320. FABRIQUÉ EN ANGLETERRE

BISCOTTI AL BURRO ED UVE DI CORINTO
INGREDIENTI: FARINA DI FRUMENTO (TIPO 00), ZUCCHERO, BURRO (17%), UVE DI CORINTO (15%), MELASSA, MELASSA RAFFINATA, ZENZERO (.93%), CARAMELLA, SALE, OLIO DI LIMONE, CONTENENTE LIEVITO IN POLVERE, BUTILIDROSSIANISOLO. FABBRICATO IN INGHILTERRA.

GALLETAS DE MANTEQUILLA CON UVAS DE CORINTO
INGREDIENTES: HARINA DE TRIGO, AZÚCAR, MANTEQUILLA (17%), UVAS DE CORINTO (15%), MELAZA, ALMÍBAR, JENGIBRE (.93%), LEVADURA EN POLVO, CARAMELO, SAL, ACEITE DE LIMON, AGENTE ANTIOXIDANTE E320. FABRICADO EN INGLATERRA.

A product's name says a lot. Most countries won't let an ingredient feature in the title unless the product contains a significant proportion of the ingredient, as above. The French, Spanish and Italian labels state the exact proportions of the ingredients deemed crucial for their versions of the product title (currants and butter) as well as the proportion of ginger.

Eating naturally

On the time scale of man's existence on earth, patterns of eating in the richer nations have changed radically in a relatively short time. Changes in types and quantities of food have given the body little time to adapt. A dramatic example is the consumption of sugar, which has increased from 7 kg [15 lb] per person per year in the U.K. in 1800 to over 50 kg [110 lb] per year today. Other more subtle changes have taken place over a longer period, for example in the increasing use of dairy products. It's only over the last 10,000 years at the most that people have kept animals in any quantity for milk or meat – a short period in evolutionary terms. Before that, what could be hunted was eaten, but meat was certainly of lower fat content than in modern times, and dairy produce was not a significant part of the diet at all until fairly recent history. Study of fossilized human teeth points to the conclusion that early man's diet was near-vegetarian, consisting largely of seeds, fruits and other plants, mostly eaten raw until the discovery of fire about 300,000 years ago. Man's ability to adapt to eating a wide range of foods has been essential for survival but this doesn't mean that departing from the original near-vegetarian diet has made any positive contributions to health or longevity.

In 1980, the Bateman Catering Organization published a report that highlights the nutritional deficiencies of the majority of British people's diets. Interviews and analysis of meal diaries showed that fewer than 15 per cent of the families surveyed ate a diet providing the minimum nutrient intake, as recommended by the Department of Health and Social Security. Drs. Cheraskin and Ringsdorf, co-authors of *Psychodietetics*, claim that almost 80 per cent of the U.S. population is malnourished, in the sense of being deficient in one or more essential nutrients. Although these figures don't necessarily mean that 80 per cent of the population will show outward signs of deficiency, they do imply that many people may not be getting enough vitamins and minerals to function at their best and to give them the greatest protection against disease. A number of nutritional experts argue that while clinical illness begins to be manifested below a certain intake of essential nutrients, there's an area above that minimum requirement in which there may not be active disease but neither is there optimum health. There's also a great variation between individual requirements of particular nutrients as well as in each person's needs under differing conditions – for example, stress may increase the need for vitamin C. Hence the importance of eating as nutritious a diet as possible.

Unprocessed foods Wholefoods are ones that have undergone a minimum of processing or none at all and therefore, when fresh, still contain all the nutrients (vitamins, minerals, protein and so forth) they possessed in their natural state. For example, wholewheat flour retains the B vitamins and several minerals that are largely refined out of white flour, and although manufacturers of white flour and bread replace some nutrients, they don't replace them all. Similarly, brown rice is a more nutritious food than white rice, which loses some of its B vitamins

129

during milling. Refined sugar of whatever colour is particularly undesirable as not only, in common with other carbohydrates, does its metabolism use up vitamin B_1, but it also provides calories without any nutritional benefits at all.

Organic foods

Another essential part of wholefood thinking is the importance of eating fresh foods and so avoiding additives, such as colouring, flavouring and preservatives (see pages 127–28). Wholefood fruit and vegetables are grown without pesticides, herbicides or inorganic fertilizers. Although many wholefood devotees see vegetarianism as an ideal, not all are vegetarian, perhaps finding it impractical because of their work or social factors; those who aren't seek out meat from animals that haven't been treated with hormones or antibiotics. These specialized foods are supplied by a growing, but still inadequate, number of organic farmers and by meat and poultry producers who avoid using drugs unnecessarily.

Adapting your diet

Below is a guide to wholefood eating, based on the principle of eating natural, unrefined foods and avoiding large quantities of foods that the body finds hard to process.

● At least half the net weight of food consumed should be raw and as fresh as possible.

● Cooking should be conservative – steam or grill rather than boil, fry or roast; undercook rather than overcook fruit and vegetables.

● Protein may come from either animal or vegetable sources – an adequate intake is reckoned to be around 45 g a day. The charts on pages 241–49 will help you to calculate the amount – if your protein comes from vegetable sources (see page 114), which are less concentrated, you'll need to eat more than if it comes from animal sources. If you're not a vegetarian, limit the amount of fish, meat or poultry that you eat to 120 g [4 oz] per day; these animal foods produce toxic acid wastes.

● Chew your food thoroughly. Carbohydrate digestion starts in the mouth when the food is mixed with saliva and unless it's well chewed, only partial digestion is possible.

● Don't eat food that's very cold or very hot, as both extremes interfere with digestion.

● Very fatty food is also difficult to digest.

● Limit foods that have been processed in any way, including items such as bread or cheese, and avoid foods that are salted, smoked, pickled, preserved, artificially coloured or that contain chemical flavour enhancers, such as monosodium glutamate.

● Cut back on sugar and all refined cereals. These are prime examples of foods that have had their nutritive value altered by processing – they're the antithesis of wholefood.

● Replace drinks containing caffeine, such as coffee, tea, cocoa and cola, with herb teas, and don't eat chocolate, as caffeine in any quantity affects nerve function (see page 137).

● Limit alcohol to beer or wine, which are easier to spin out than spirits. Drink real ale rather than normal beer, as it contains fewer additives. Don't drink more than half a bottle of wine or a pint and a half, or 900 ml, of beer [three 12 oz cans U.S.A.] per day (see pages 192–96), and don't drink on more than four days a week.

Eating sensibly and well is one of the easiest ways of improving your health and feeling happier and more energetic. A diet of foods that are as close to their natural state as possible is the first step towards feeling positively well and avoiding the diseases of civilization. Try out the diet below – it's nutritious, contains no undesirable foods and is pleasant to eat and easy to prepare.

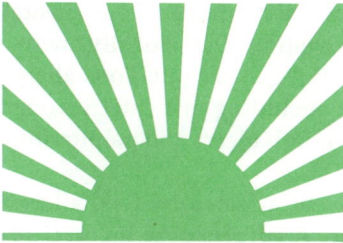

Breakfast
Either cereal, such as oat or millet flakes, soaked overnight in a little water, with dried fruit and seeds (sunflower, linseed or pumpkin), or sugar-free muesli [health cereal]. Add a few nuts, some fresh non-citrus fruit and natural yogurt

Wholemeal [wholewheat] bread and honey; no butter or margarine

Herb tea, dandelion coffee or unsweetened fruit juice

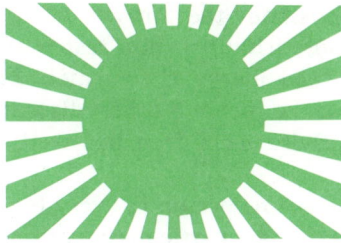

Mid-morning
Herb tea, dandelion coffee or unsweetened fruit juice

Lunch
Mixed raw salad, dressed with vegetable oil, vinegar or lemon juice; add nuts or sprouting seeds for variety

Jacket potato or wholemeal [wholewheat] bread; no butter or margarine

Herb tea, dandelion coffee or unsweetened fruit juice

Mid-afternoon
Herb tea or dandelion coffee

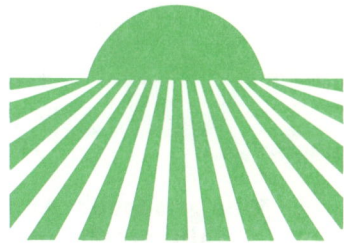

Evening meal
Fish, chicken, meat or a vegetarian cereal and pulse dish

Fresh, lightly cooked vegetables

Fruit

A little wine or beer; herb tea or dandelion coffee

Fasting   Wholefood devotees believe in the importance of fasting, which has long been an essential part of Nature Cure, or curing without drugs. It's seen as a simple and natural way to cleanse and rest the body, allowing the energy normally spent on digestion to be released and used by the body to heal and revitalize itself. If you want to feel spiritually and physically refreshed, try a fast. Take only fruit juice, vegetable juice or spring water; don't spend more than a maximum of three days without food and keep your first meal after the fast small and light. The prospect of fasting may seem very difficult but in fact, after the first 24 hours, you should find that you're no longer hungry. For further reading, see page 250.

131

Problems with food

Food allergy

If the body is invaded by germs, special defence mechanisms are triggered to protect it. The germs act as the antigen, provoking the body to produce antibodies that attack the germs to avert potential danger. With a food allergy, something in the food you eat acts as the antigen (usually some type of protein). A special antibody, immuno-globin, is produced, and attaches itself to sites on cell membranes, sensitizing them to the allergy-causing substance (known as the allergen). This can have various disagreeable results.

What are the symptoms?

There are many possible symptoms. Some are more common immediately after the problem food has been eaten (vomiting, swollen lips, for example); others may take much longer to develop (breathlessness, eczema). Among the common symptoms are migraine (see opposite), runny nose (rhinitis), skin rashes and swelling. Occasionally, with a chronic food allergy, there may be bleeding into the gut. Food allergy may also be behind other disorders, including psychiatric ones, hyperactivity in children, bed-wetting, mouth ulcers and palpitations.

Who gets food allergies?

As many as one person in every ten may be affected by food allergy, and children are particularly susceptible. A surprisingly high 7.5 per cent of young children have been estimated to be allergic to cow's milk. Babies who are breastfed, and aren't given solid food before they're three months old, seem less likely to develop allergies than bottle-fed babies who take solids early. Many children grow out of food allergies by the age of five – but adults may develop them later in life. Susceptibility to allergies, but not necessarily to the same kind, often runs in families.

The common culprits

You can be allergic to almost anything, but some food allergies crop up more often than others. For example, foods containing milk, eggs and wheat come at the top of the list of allergy culprits – possibly because these foods are commonly fed to young infants, at a time when babies are particularly prone to develop allergies. Other common allergy triggers are: bacon, celery, chocolate, coffee, fish, mustard, nuts, oranges, pork, tea and tomatoes. Some food additives are also possible causes of allergy. It's not uncommon to crave a food you're allergic to – so the culprit may be one of your favourite foods.

Tracking down the culprit

Spotting the problem food may be easy, if the symptoms appear very rapidly. The longer the delay between eating the food and the appearance of symptoms, and the more everyday the food, the harder it may be to work out which is to blame.

One way to identify the culprit is to keep a record of what foods you eat, and when any symptoms appear. Over a week or so the foods linked most often with the allergic reaction should emerge. You can then test your theory by eating a little of the suspect foods to see if the allergic response recurs. But *don't* eat a food you suspect of triggering an instant, severe reaction: it could be dangerous (and it's usually unnecessary, too, since the speed and strength of the reaction generally indicate the problem food).

There are other ways of testing for allergies. With a skin test, a small amount of food extract is rubbed into a scratch on the skin, or injected. If an inflamed weal develops at the site of the test, the food may cause an allergy. Unfortunately, this technique doesn't always work. Some foods cause allergies on the skin, but are all right when eaten; others may cause no skin reaction, but still trigger off an allergic reaction in the stomach. An alternative method of testing for allergies is to follow a very bland diet for around a week. This consists of only two foods, such as lamb and pears, that happen to be unlikely to cause an allergy. Other foods are reintroduced into the diet gradually, one by one, until the allergic symptoms reappear. The last food introduced before the allergy appears again is likely to be the cause of it. The trouble with this type of test is that it may have to go on for weeks, and the restricted diet is very dull. It is also possible to test for allergies by recording changes in your pulse rate after you've sampled suspect foods (see page 250 for details of further reading).

If you have an allergy . . . The obvious course is to avoid the food you're allergic to. This is clearly going to be harder if you're allergic to wheat or milk than if you're allergic to oysters, but with care and ingenuity most people manage to cope. And cooking or heating the offending food *may* enable you to cope with it, because this changes the character of the protein. So even if you're allergic to cheese or milk, you may be able to eat them without problems if they have been cooked or heated first, as in a cheese sauce or yogurt.

What about migraine? Migraine is a particular kind of headache that affects around 8 per cent of the (British) population. Although migraine is rarely *caused* by an allergy, certain foods do seem to trigger off headaches. Other common causes of migraine are stress, hormonal changes and low blood sugar. An attack doesn't usually occur unless more than one of these factors is operating, and food is likely to be only *one* of the causes if migraine attacks occur frequently.

The commonest dietary cause of migraine attacks is a substance called tyramine, found particularly in foods that have been allowed to decompose or ferment, such as cheese, game and alcohol. The tyramine content of these foods can vary enormously, so you might eat the same brand of cheese several times before being affected. In one survey of migraine sufferers the foods that most commonly caused attacks were those shown *right*.

Food	Percentage
Chocolate	75%
Cheese and dairy products	48%
Citrus fruits	30%
Alcoholic drinks	25%
Fatty fried foods	18%
Vegetables (especially onions)	18%
Tea and coffee	14%
Meat (especially pork)	14%
Seafood	10%

Food poisoning

Bacteria in food can mar the quality without harming us, but as some moulds may be potential carcinogens, it's best to throw away mouldy food. Don't just cut off the bad bit; the toxins can spread further.

Don't buy

- Swollen chilled food packages (fruit juices, cheese, made-up pastry and yogurt are particularly susceptible).
- Swollen cans or cans that are dented along the seam. Cracks in the seam can cause little openings for invading bacteria.
- Frozen foods containing ice crystals, or packets with chips of ice between them. This usually means they've been refrozen. This isn't necessarily a danger to health but it impairs quality.
- Cheese packed in transparent film with visible mould inside.
- Pulses and dried fruits with visible mould.

How to store food

- Uncooked mince [ground beef], liver, kidneys, poultry and seafood carry many spoilage micro-organisms. Store in the coldest part of the refrigerator (nearest the freezer) for three days maximum.
- Wrapped fresh meat keeps for up to three days in the refrigerator; unwrapped fresh meat for up to five days; whole joints even longer.
- Partly thawed food that still contains ice crystals can safely be refrozen (its quality will suffer, though).
- Cook thawed meat, poultry or fish before refreezing (if desired).
- Cool cooked food as rapidly as possible before putting it in the fridge in a covered container. Some modern fridges can cope with small uncooled items, but check the manufacturers' instructions.
- Keep dried foods cool, in a sealed, dry container.

Preparing food

- Don't let food sit at temperatures that let bacteria grow (see below).
- Never handle cooked and uncooked meat together; the latter may contaminate the former.
- Before cooking, thaw all large cuts of meat and poultry – otherwise after cooking, live food-poisoning bacteria may be left inside.
- If food is to be eaten cold, serve it straight from the refrigerator.
- Wash your hands frequently when preparing food.

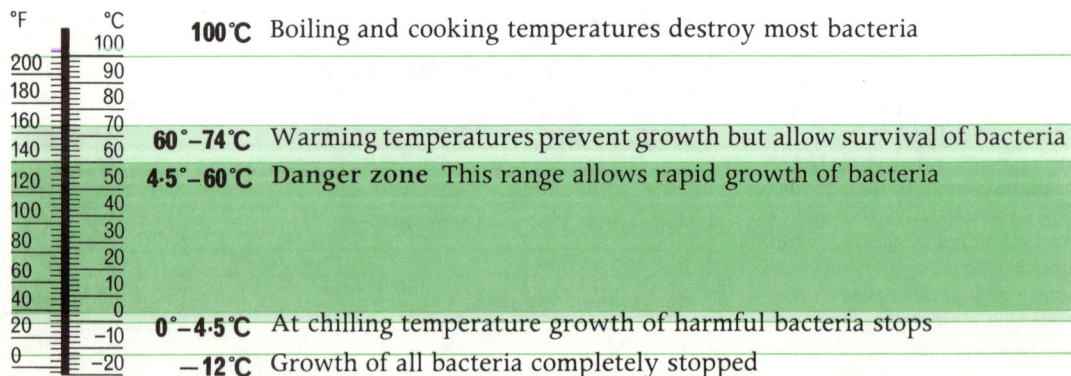

°F	°C		
	100	**100°C**	Boiling and cooking temperatures destroy most bacteria
200	90		
180	80		
160	70		
140	60	**60°–74°C**	Warming temperatures prevent growth but allow survival of bacteria
120	50	**4·5°–60°C**	**Danger zone** This range allows rapid growth of bacteria
100	40		
80	30		
60	20		
40	10		
20	0		
	−10	**0°–4·5°C**	At chilling temperature growth of harmful bacteria stops
0	−20	**−12°C**	Growth of all bacteria completely stopped

Quenching your thirst

Water comprises about two-thirds of the body's weight – the average man, weighing just over 65 kg [143 lb], has about 40 litres [85 pt] in his body. If you lose a lot of water, through sweat, say, the concentration of sodium in the remaining water in your body rises. This triggers the sensation of thirst, which tells you that you need to take in more fluid to restore the concentration of sodium to normal. (Water elimination is regulated in much the same way. When your blood plasma is diluted by the presence of too much water, the kidneys get a signal to work harder to eliminate the excess.)

If you refused to drink, or had no chance to do so, you'd begin to experience quite severe symptoms when your body had lost around 10 per cent of its water; losing 20 per cent of the body's water would mean death. Ten days without water is about the longest you could survive. In normal circumstances, an intake of around 1 litre [2 pt] a day should be enough. If you eat plenty of vegetables and fruit, which are high in water, you'll need less separate fluid. Drink when you're thirsty; don't measure it.

Water   There are no calories at all in water. But what comes out of the tap is not water pure and simple. It may have fluoride added to it to help prevent dental decay (see page 122). It will certainly contain some contaminants from the substances used to disinfect it and from the pipes between the reservoir and the tap, as well as natural trace elements assimilated from rocks and soil.

The most important potential contaminant is lead, which gets into water supplies through the lead pipes often used in houses over 40 years old. In areas where the water is soft, or acidic, the risk of lead contamination increases. Most of the lead accumulates in the water lying overnight in the pipes, and comes out in the first few cups of water drawn in the morning. It's best not to drink this first rush of water: let the tap run for ten seconds or so before filling your glass. Use the tap from the main supply, not from the water tank. Modern plumbing replaces lead with copper.

In areas receiving water from highly-fertilized farm land, the nitrate from fertilizers enters the water supply, too, especially during droughts. Since nitrates are linked with cancer, an unusually high level in water could be a health risk. It's most risky for babies, whose kidneys can't cope with high nitrate levels and who may develop anaemia. There are several devices on sale designed to overcome doubts about the safety of tap water:

● Water filters remove harmful bacteria and chlorine and other disin-fectory traces. Ion exchange filters remove lead and other heavy metals such as cadmium and mercury, too.

● Water softeners remove calcium and magnesium (which are useful minerals) and raise the sodium content of the water – hence it's not a good idea to drink softened water.

● Distillation plants take everything out of water, good and bad, leaving a very flat taste.

135

Soft drinks

Alarming quantities of soft drinks of one sort or another are consumed over the year: for instance over 66 litres [140 pt] of soft drinks were drunk per head of the British population in 1974. In the same year, Americans drank even more: 100 litres [211 pt] per head. Soft drinks have nothing to recommend them nutritionally. They're usually a mixture of sugar, colouring and other additives, sometimes with caffeine-type stimulants, as in cola drinks. As such, they're one of the most obvious products to stop using when you're aiming to improve your diet.

Cola, which is made from extracts of the kola nut, is an active ingredient of one of the most popular soft drinks worldwide. In terms of weight, it's over 10 per cent sugar. Cola drinks also usually contain caffeine – about as much as there would be in a cup of coffee. Since a large amount is drunk by children, who have a lower body weight, the stimulating effect can be high; see also Side effects, opposite.

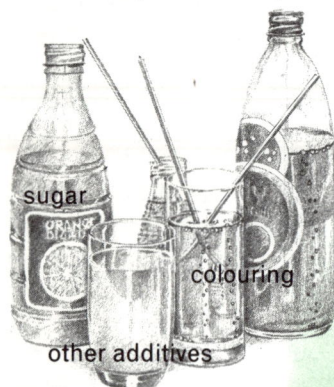

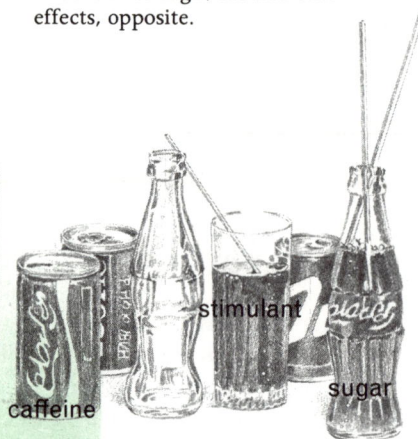

Milk and milk drinks

Whole milk is high in fat, and most milk drinks have sugar added, too. To protect your children's teeth, don't give them sweet milk drinks (e.g. milk shakes, chocolate milk) too often. If you can't sleep after a flavoured milky drink at bedtime, it may be because of the caffeine in the product.

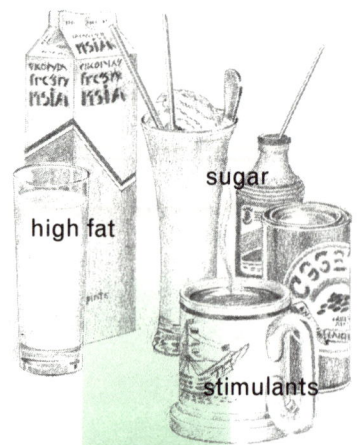

sugar
colouring
other additives
caffeine
stimulant
sugar
high fat
sugar
stimulants

Juice and mineral water

Made by squeezing the whole fruit or vegetable, juice contains roughly the same nutrients as the whole fruit but almost no fibre. Juices contain very little sodium but a lot of potassium (see pages 122–23), so are useful in low sodium diets and for those taking diuretics or recovering from surgery (when potassium tends to be low). Juices are a good source of vitamins, too.

Bottled spring or mineral water is guaranteed free of pollution. Mineral content varies greatly from brand to brand. Low mineral waters have less taste and are suitable for infants. Fizzy mineral water is a good alcohol substitute.

Low fat alternatives

Use fresh skimmed milk (high in protein but low in fat), hot or cold, or skim your own, by pouring the cream off the top of unhomogenized milk. Herb tea, which is drunk without added milk or sugar, is a good substitute for milky drinks at bedtime.

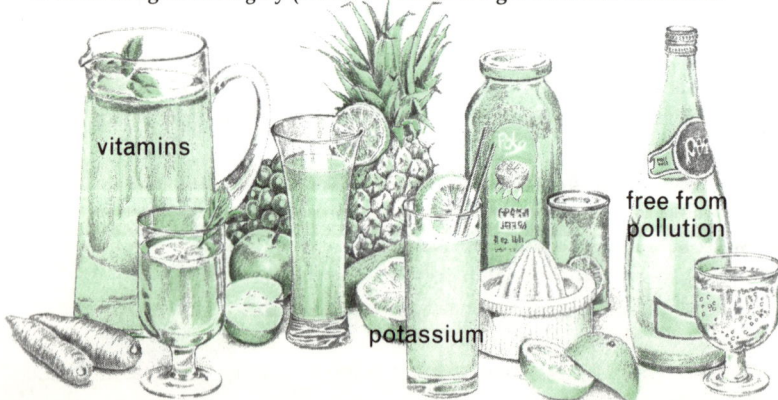

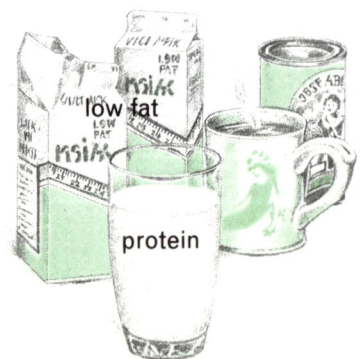

vitamins
potassium
free from pollution
low fat
protein

Coffee

This is made from an infusion of the roasted and ground seeds of the coffee plant. Ordinary coffee contains more caffeine than tea: about 60 to 170 mg per cup. Instant coffee is made from infusions that have been spray- or freeze-dried; the powder contains 20 to 40 mg of caffeine per gram. Both act as a diuretic and a stimulant – and coffee over-stimulates many people.

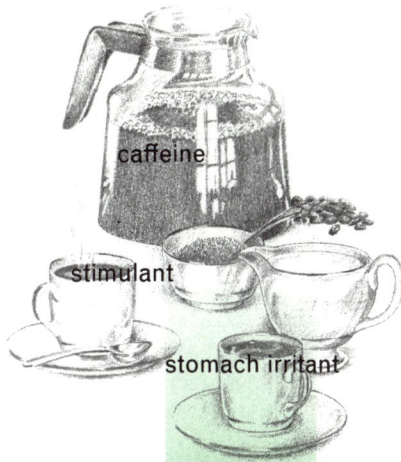

caffeine

stimulant

stomach irritant

Tea

This drink, which probably originated in China more than 2,000 years ago, is now the most popular beverage in the world. In Britain it's particularly popular, accounting for around 65 per cent of total liquid intake (not counting ordinary water); average daily consumption is five to six cups.

Tea contains little in the way of vitamins, although it can contribute some trace elements. But the caffeine tea contains (50 to 80 mg a cup) makes it mildly stimulating and habit-forming. Tea also contains tannin (60 to 280 mg a cup) and some fluoride. It tends to be constipating, and if you drink it with sugar, it's fattening, too.

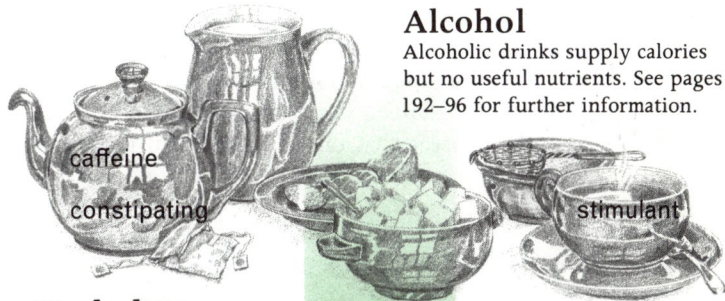

caffeine

constipating

Side effects

Drinking too much tea, cola or coffee can result in side effects such as feelings of anxiety, rapid heartbeat, sleeplessness, changed bowel habits and stomach upsets. If you find you're getting any of these, and there's no apparent medical cause, cut down on the amount of tea, cola or coffee you drink. Sudden withdrawal produces side effects such as lethargy, headaches and sleepiness, but when these wear off, you'll feel and be a lot healthier than you were on a high caffeine intake. In a few cases, people diagnosed as highly neurotic returned to normal after stopping their high consumption of coffee or cola drinks.

Alcohol

Alcoholic drinks supply calories but no useful nutrients. See pages 192–96 for further information.

stimulant

Coffee substitutes

For coffee without the stimulant effect and without the side effects described above, try decaffeinated coffee or coffee substitutes (made from dandelions or grains).

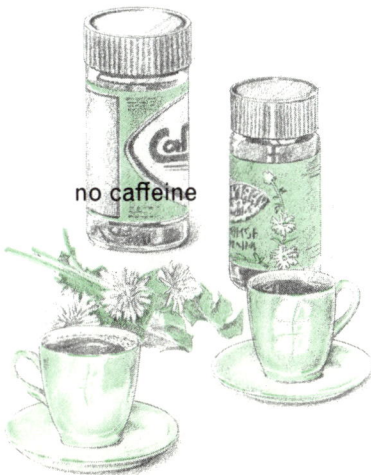

no caffeine

Herbal tea

Several different types of herbal tea are generally available from health food shops, based on fennel, camomile, rosehips and peppermint, for example. Since these are usually free of or low on caffeine, it's worth experimenting with them to find one you like, if you suspect your caffeine intake from ordinary tea and coffee is too high (see above). As a bonus, herb teas need no added milk or sugar.

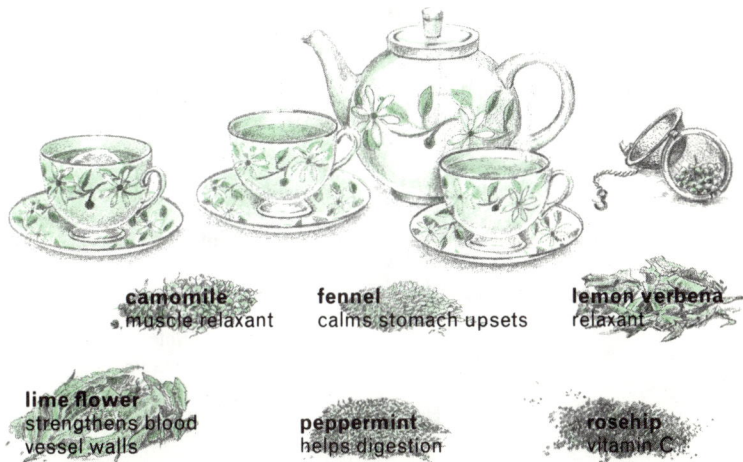

camomile
muscle relaxant

fennel
calms stomach upsets

lemon verbena
relaxant

lime flower
strengthens blood
vessel walls

peppermint
helps digestion

rosehip
vitamin C

BALANCING YOUR DIET : What to aim for

The typical affluent Westerner gets approximately 40 per cent of his calories from fat, 18 per cent from sugar, 12 per cent from protein, 9 per cent from alcohol and 21 per cent from starch. Experts differ on the optimal proportions of these nutrients in the diet, but a number of expert committees have recommended that people should eat no more than 30 per cent of total energy as fat, preferably less; cut sugar consumption by half (or more); and double the amount of starch eaten. So are there any diets in the world that approximate to this?

Good food is good health

In the 1950s Professor Ancel Keys in the U.S.A. set in motion a remarkable number of surveys on seven populations known as 'The Seven Countries Study'. He came to the conclusion that the traditional diets of a number of Mediterranean countries (Italy in particular) came closest to the ideal for good health.

The main difference between Italian and, say, American food is that the focus of the meal is pasta rather than meat. The good thing about this is that eating a plateful of pasta fills you up so that you don't want much meat afterwards. In Professor Keys' opinion, large servings of meat are needed only when a meal is poorly designed and prepared.

The traditional Italian diet is not the only one to provide a healthy balance of nutrients. For example, most Chinese and Indian cuisines are based on rice; Mexican cooking on beans and maize; and traditional Scottish fare includes a lot of soups or broths and oat-based dishes. So the scope for choice of good healthy food is considerable.

Food groups

Most people who learn about nutrition come across the idea of 'food groups', like the meat group, the milk group, the fruit and vegetable group, the cereals group, and the fats and oils group. Foods are classified according to the particular nutrients they contain, and people are told to take so many servings of each group a day. The big drawback of such systems is that because they concentrate on ensuring that people get at least a minimum quantity of nutrients, they fail to prevent *too much* of any one nutrient being consumed. For example, the milk group is often included because it's a good source of calcium. However, many milk products are also rich sources of fat and so anyone who eats something from the meat group, the milk group and the fats and oils group is almost bound to take in too much fat.

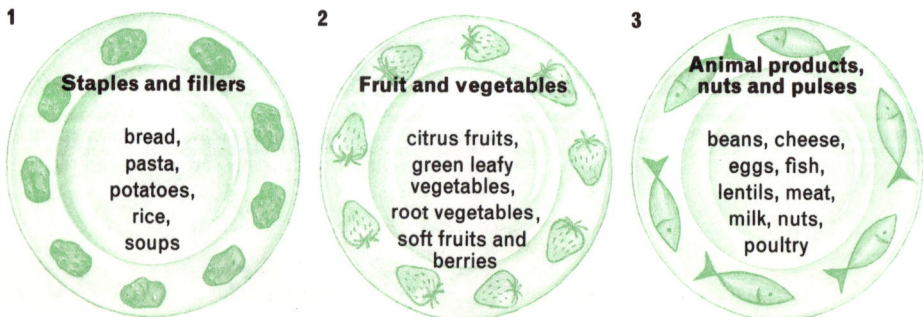

1

Staples and fillers

bread,
pasta,
potatoes,
rice,
soups

2

Fruit and vegetables

citrus fruits,
green leafy
vegetables,
root vegetables,
soft fruits and
berries

3

Animal products, nuts and pulses

beans, cheese,
eggs, fish,
lentils, meat,
milk, nuts,
poultry

A more sensible system is to group foods according to the way they're used to plan meals in 'healthy' cuisines (see opposite). In this system, the fillers come first in planning a meal and the foods in the third group play a minor role, mainly to add piquancy and flavour.

'Healthy' cuisines make a much greater use of pulses – the traditional 'poor man's meat' – seasonings like herbs and spices, and sauces made from fruit and vegetables to moisten and give flavour to the bland filler foods; see also pages 145–48.

Plan meals in this way and you not only meet all the requirements for vitamins and minerals; you also provide more fibre (particularly if wholefoods are included) and, as long as you use oil, cream and butter only sparingly during cooking and preparation, you'll cut down on the amount of fat eaten, too.

The digestive clock

Throughout his evolution, man – a physically weak, small animal – has been a scavenger. He learnt to survive on virtually any foods he could lay his hands on: left-over meat from a predator's quarry, nuts, berries and seeds. So it seems unlikely that in the early days of his evolution he was able to eat regular large meals. With the growth of civilization, however, a system of regular times for eating meals became established, partly because meals are important occasions for people and families to be together and partly because working life has to be regulated with some kind of pattern. Regular meals are important for *social* reasons, but they aren't a biological necessity.

There is no nutritional reason why you shouldn't take all your food each day at one meal, or spread it over several small meals or snacks – provided whatever habit you choose doesn't make you so hungry that you feel lightheaded. What are important are the total quantity and quality of food being eaten over a given period. As far as your digestion is concerned, it doesn't matter whether you eat frequently or infrequently, provided your habits follow some kind of pattern that your body can become accustomed to. Both missing a meal or being forced to eat when you don't want to can make you feel pretty miserable. Possible exceptions are children and people doing heavy, dangerous work. The latter may lose concentration and so cause an accident if they go for too long without food. A child whose last meal comes at six in the evening benefits from taking some food before lunchtime the next day. Hunger may make him feel irritable or lose concentration.

When you eat can make an important difference to *what* you eat. Different kinds of food are thought appropriate for different meals. So eating at one time rather than another can make a subtle and significant difference to your diet. For example, if you prefer a light snack instead of a midday meal, you'll inadvertently be adding to the fat and sugar in your diet if that snack includes a packet of crisps [potato chips] and a jam doughnut. It's important to think about whether you're a snacker or a regular meal-eater, or a combination of the two, and to plan a diet that taken *as a whole* has plenty of starch and fibre but contains much less fat and sugar.

139

Meal planning

A simple rule of thumb when planning meals – or for that matter snacks – is to place greatest emphasis on the staple fillers and fruit and vegetables, to let the more fatty animal and nut products play a minor role, and wherever possible to cut out extras such as salt, fats and sugar.

Breakfast

This is one of the few times in our society when starch-rich foods (such as cereal and toast) are commonly eaten.

Toast Make it from thick slices of wholemeal [wholewheat] bread, with no more than a smear of butter or polyunsaturated margarine. Use sweet spreads only in modest quantities.

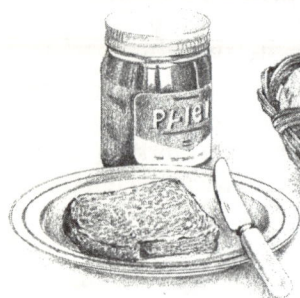

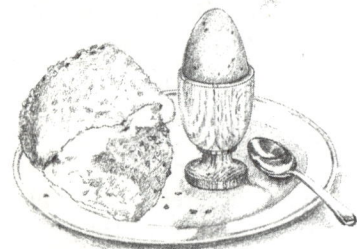

Cereal Eat a wholegrain variety (read the packet to check) or choose a bran-enriched product. Avoiding pre-sweetened breakfast cereals helps you to control the amount of sugar you eat.

Milk Use fresh, skimmed milk, or failing that buy unhomogenized so you can pour the top off (this skims it quite effectively).

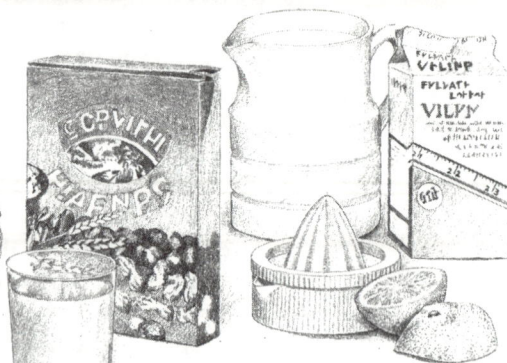

Drink A glass of fruit juice is a healthy way to complete the meal. As a change from the usual tea or coffee, experiment with a herb tea (see page 137).

Cooked breakfast In addition to cereal and toast, try an egg (boiled, poached or scrambled, without salt or butter) or baked beans or grilled mushrooms and tomato. Although grilled bacon is better than fried, it's still high in fat and salt.

If you don't eat breakfast, plan ahead to make up for the starch and fibre you've missed out on. If you get hungry mid-morning, instead of tucking into a chocolate bar, a packet of crisps [potato chips] or biscuit [cookie], have a roll or sandwich (see Packed lunch).

Midday

What you eat at midday very much depends on where you are and what you're doing.

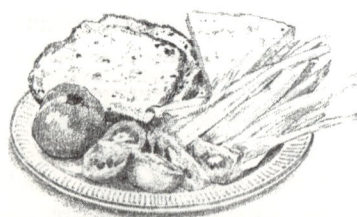

ON YOUR OWN AT HOME
You may not feel like taking the trouble to prepare food. An occasional snack meal doesn't matter, but it's good for morale to plan to eat something you enjoy. Think ahead so you aren't reduced to raiding the fridge or store cupboard when hunger strikes. Planning and eating enjoyable and nourishing meals makes you feel much better about yourself as well as adding variety.

• Cook an extra portion of the previous night's meal so you can reheat it at midday or turn it into something different.
• Keep a supply of home-made soup to eat with good bread.
• Make a quick salad of raw carrots, celery or other vegetable.
• Make a mock pizza: lay tomato slices on bread, top with grated cheese and herbs, and toast under the grill.

EATING OUT

Choose an eating place that offers an imaginative choice of low fat foods (such as fish or chicken dishes or salads). If you like the food, let the management know about it. Let them know if you don't, too. You won't get the sort of food you like served unless there's a demand for it, and eating places won't know there's a demand for it unless their customers express their views.

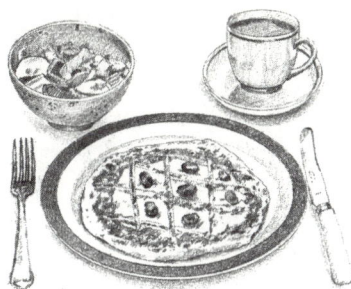

Drink Keep an eye on your alcohol intake: it's hard to say where social drinking, heavy drinking and alcoholism begin and end. Cut out second drinks that you have just to be 'sociable' or out of habit. See pages 192–96 for more on alcohol. If you do round your meal off with coffee, have it decaffeinated and black or with milk, not cream.

PACKED LUNCH

By eating a sandwich or roll you can increase your starch and fibre intake. Sandwiches can be made from different breads (wholemeal [wholewheat] preferably, but brown, wheatgerm, pumpernickel, rye, mixed grain or French, too). Moisten them with cottage cheese, salad or pickle rather than butter or margarine. Salad ingredients also make a good filling with meat, chicken, low fat cheese (see page 104) or a helping of tuna fish. A piece of fruit or salad to go with the sandwich makes up a nutritious, balanced meal (but go easy on oil in salad dressings; instead try a light dressing such as yogurt thinned with milk, vinegar or lemon juice and flavoured with herbs). All this contrasts with bought foods, most of which are very high in fat (especially pies, cake or pastries, and chocolate).

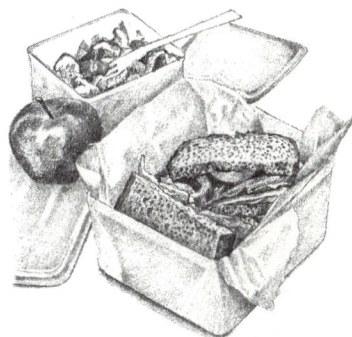

Main course Go for one with the emphasis on the filler, not on meat: shepherd's pie [meat and potato bake], curry, spaghetti or pizza.

Vegetables A low fat salad (not swamped in an oily dressing) is a good choice. If you must have chips [fries], go for thick-cut ones (see page 102), drained of oil.

Puddings/desserts Fat and sugar are the dangers here. See page 143 for some suggestions.

Afternoon/Evening food for children

As a rule, offer sweet foods like cakes and biscuits [cookies] only when the savoury part of the meal has been eaten. With a faddy eater, it sometimes helps to cut out between-meal snacks, if 'proper' food is being rejected. If he's not hungry enough for baked beans on toast or whatever, he's not hungry enough for cakes.

Savoury 'instant' foods for ravenous children are cheese, nuts, or sandwiches made with fish, nut or meat paste, salad, egg, or spreads such as yeast extract. Most children will eat fresh bread on its own – an excellent low fat, unsweetened filler.

Sweet foods As a change from sweet sponge cake, try buns made from yeast dough, plain wholemeal biscuits [wholewheat cookies] or plain fruit cake. Cakes and biscuits are high in sugar but if eaten at, rather than between, meals they do less damage to a child's teeth.

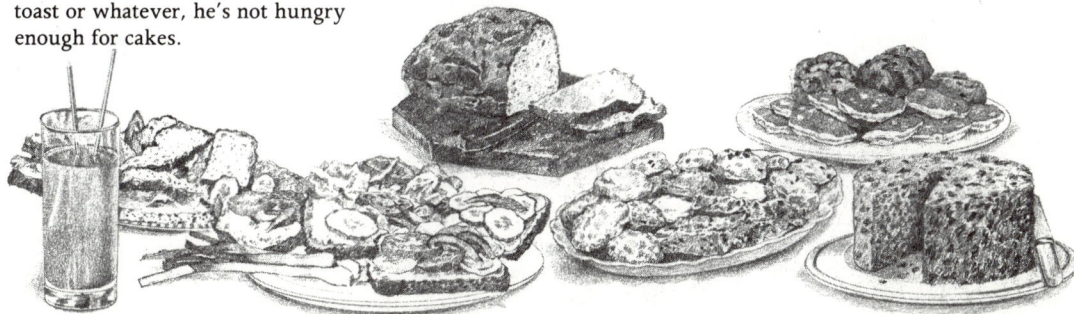

Evening meal

What you eat in the evening often depends on what you and the rest of the family have eaten earlier. But if one of you has had a large business lunch and the other has eaten very little at midday, you'll want different kinds of meals. If you go to the trouble of cooking a meal, you may well feel upset if your partner just picks at it because he or she isn't hungry; but bear in mind that eating a meal simply because it's been cooked is a major cause of overweight and middle-age spread.

STARTERS

Soup A marvellous way of serving vegetables and pulses. The thicker the soup, the more it fills you up. A stockpot can be added to over several days and provided it's adequately reheated, it isn't a health hazard. Compensate for any vitamins lost in reheating by adding new vegetables or eating freshly cooked vegetables or fruit.

Pâté Make your own from lean meats (shop bought ones are often fatty). Natural yogurt, cottage cheese and thick vegetable purées like spinach can be used instead of cream cheese or fat to add moisture and smoothness to a fish or liver mixture.

Salads Vegetables can be served raw or 'à la grecque' (but be sparing with the oily dressing). Poaching vegetables such as mushrooms or onions in a little stock means that you need much less dressing. Try mushrooms and cucumber raw, with yogurt, lemon juice and paprika or fresh mint.

MAIN COURSE

These dishes can be as filling or as light as you want them. Vegetables and fruit are very light because they contain so much water and so can be puréed for soups and sauces or left whole in vegetable stews. Fresh root ginger has a marvellous way of bringing out the flavour of fresh vegetables. Garlic, herbs, spices, wine and good stocks can add an almost never-ending range of tastes and flavours to a dish.

Bread can always accompany a meal. You don't have to eat the same wholemeal [wholewheat] all the time, and it's better to eat bread of any colour than none at all.

Fish Serve grilled or poached, with lemon, wine and herbs. Whitefish provides low fat protein and 'stretches' well (e.g. paella).

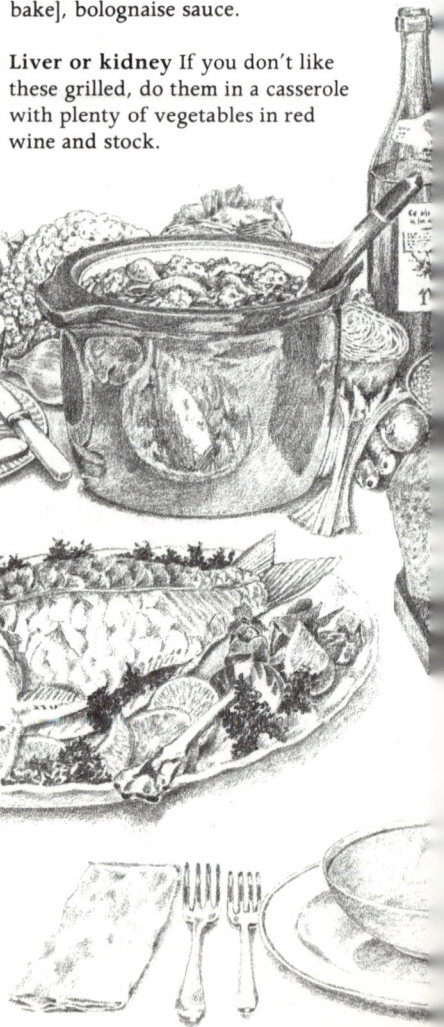

Poultry Remove the fatty skin before casseroling.

Lean mince [ground beef] can go a long way with potatoes, vegetables, herbs and a good stock, as in moussaka, chilli con carne, shepherd's pie [meat and potato bake], bolognaise sauce.

Liver or kidney If you don't like these grilled, do them in a casserole with plenty of vegetables in red wine and stock.

• Cook meals that can be put in the fridge or the deep freeze to be served again another day (which means one less meal to cook later).

• Plan for leftovers. Instead of persuading yourself to finish the last potato or piece of pie use it for the next day's packed lunch or as part of the next meal. Soups, curries, quiches and stews are ideal ways of using up leftovers.

• If you aren't a confident cook, go to classes or try a good simple recipe book. Until you learn to cook you won't have confidence to adapt recipes so that they're lower in fat and sugar and richer in fibre and starch.

Potatoes can be turned into substantial dishes, as in leek and potato pie or potato and bean salad.

Pasta This can be served with a number of sauces, preferably vegetable or a white sauce made with skimmed milk and cornflour. Meat or cheese need be used only in small quantities to add flavour.

Pastry Make it with one part fat to three parts self-raising flour, and use it for tarts like pissaladière (tomato, onion and egg filling); potato, mushroom and tomato quiche; or Cornish pasties [meat and vegetable pies] made from root vegetables, stock, herbs and a little mince [ground beef].

Rice can be used in kedgeree, risotto, paella and curry, with lentils, or for stuffed tomatoes, peppers or aubergines [eggplants].

AFTERS

Fruit, fresh or stewed, or make your own fruit yogurts so you can cut out or reduce the sugar. Yogurt with a little cinnamon or ginger can be an excellent alternative to cream. Egg custard made with skimmed milk is also a low fat alternative.

Fools and mousses can be made using a combination of yogurt and custard, or egg whites.

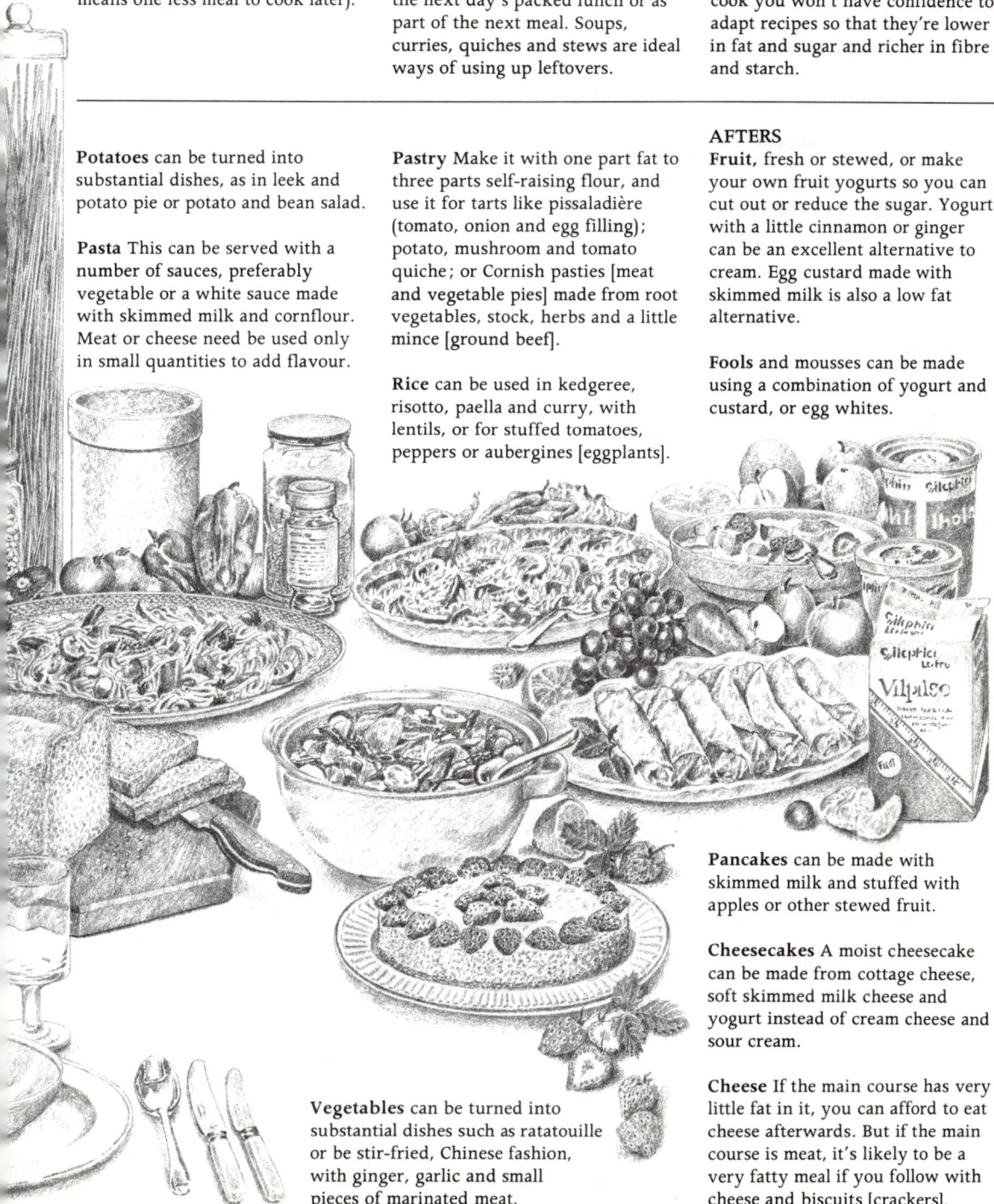

Pancakes can be made with skimmed milk and stuffed with apples or other stewed fruit.

Cheesecakes A moist cheesecake can be made from cottage cheese, soft skimmed milk cheese and yogurt instead of cream cheese and sour cream.

Cheese If the main course has very little fat in it, you can afford to eat cheese afterwards. But if the main course is meat, it's likely to be a very fatty meal if you follow with cheese and biscuits [crackers].

Vegetables can be turned into substantial dishes such as ratatouille or be stir-fried, Chinese fashion, with ginger, garlic and small pieces of marinated meat.

143

Snacks

If you feel hungry or want something to nibble, face the fact that you *are* hungry and try one of the snacks, *right* (or a sandwich).

If your 'hunger' is really a craving for something sweet or salty, the problem has to be handled differently. Rather than try to cut out these foods all at once – and risk giving up and then having a binge – it may be more realistic to set yourself a target limit of one biscuit [cookie], one packet of crisps [potato chips] or whatever. Either nibble at it for as long as you can make it last or save it for a particular time in the day. Knowing you can allow yourself something you yearn for can help control these cravings.

Fresh fruit

Plain low fat yogurt, with chopped fresh fruit if wanted

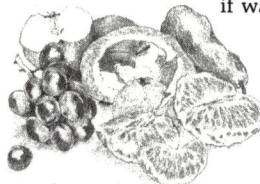

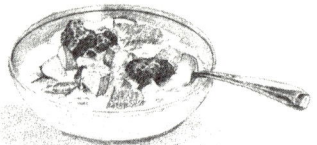

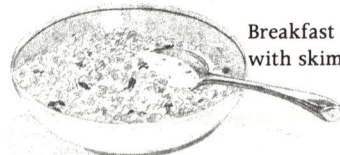

A few dried apricots

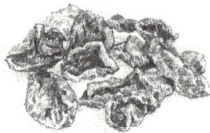

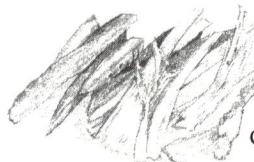

Breakfast cereal with skimmed milk

Toast fingers lightly spread with yeast extract or with cottage cheese

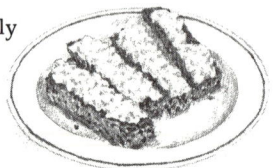

Carrot and celery sticks

Entertaining

There is no reason why any guest should be offended at being served any of the dishes suggested. Instead of spending a lot of money on meat, spend it on fish and good quality vegetables and fruit. If you use traditional recipes from long established cuisines such as Indian, Chinese, Italian or Scottish, nobody will guess you're trying to provide healthy foods. Guests will enjoy it for what it is – good, tasty, attractive food.

If serving up a meal consisting mainly of a large bowl of pasta or rice makes you nervous – because your unenlightened friends will think this is fattening – then instead of serving a three course meal, serve *several* small courses, or have a choice of a number of dishes all at once on the table (Chinese style) so that guests can serve themselves. This way they can sample unfamiliar dishes and come back for more.

Serve a low fat pudding that doesn't need cream added to it, and avoid putting butter or margarine on the table. A good pâté or cheese should never be eaten with butter anyway as the extra fat swamps any subtle or delicate flavour – extra butter in these cases is bad cuisine as well as bad for health. If you feel you *must* put out butter and cream provide very small quantities; this usually inhibits guests from taking large helpings.

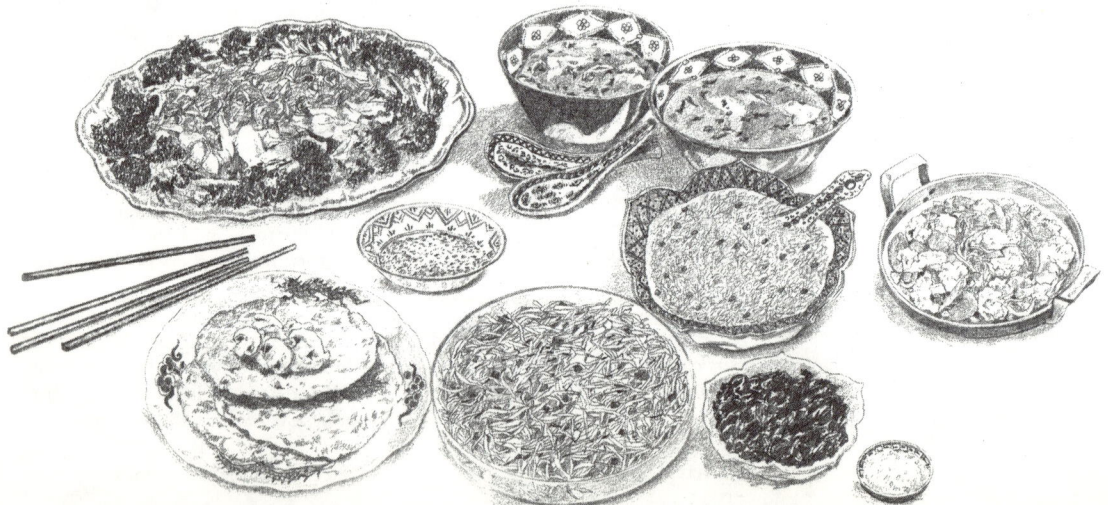

Cooking for health

Traditional healthy cuisines are usually found where people are poor, the earth is fertile, and good food is considered an important pleasure in life. These conditions have taught many people to make the most of the ingredients readily available to them. In the main these are the starchy, staple foods such as wheat, maize, rice and pulses. Locally grown vegetables and fruits may also be in plentiful supply. As meat is expensive to produce, meat and other animal products are used in small quantities for flavouring and garnishing, instead of being the central part of the meal. Chinese and Indian meals, for example, are based on rice and Italian meals on pasta.

Unfortunately, in adaptation a lot of the good of these dishes may be undone, with more emphasis on the highly flavoured side dishes and garnishes than on the staple. Thus a meal that, eaten in the traditional way, would be rich in starch and low in fat becomes the reverse. For example, in the West, Chinese restaurateurs (like all others) aim to give customers what they want. If customers want a greasy Chinese variation of fish and chips, that is what they get. A trip to a Chinese take-away won't produce a healthy, low fat meal if you come away with something like pork in batter and fried rice. Below is a brief guide to some of the cuisines that offer an excellent *choice* of dishes that are healthy and, above all, tasty, even exotic.

Chinese food

The Chinese are reckoned by some connoisseurs to be probably the greatest cooks in the world. Eating is a major Chinese preoccupation and form of entertainment. Despite such well-known dishes as sweet and sour pork there is relatively little sugar in Chinese cooking and rarely any kind of pudding or dessert. Likewise, although stir-fried foods may appear on the menu, Chinese food is generally low in fat, partly because the shape of the cooking vessel – the wok (see page 147) – keeps the amount of cooking fat or oil needed to a minimum, but mostly because the Chinese eat large quantities of rice, which balance the fattier parts of the meal. Chinese meals don't have courses; instead all the dishes – soups, meat, fish, vegetables, eggs, rice and poultry – appear all together in small portions, with each bowl being replenished as and when necessary. The overall result is that the quantity of fat in the diet is small compared with the quantity of rice eaten. (When Westerners complain that Chinese food leaves them feeling 'empty', the reason is usually that they haven't eaten enough rice.)

Liquids, mainly soup and continual fresh cups of tea, play an important role in the traditional Chinese meal, complementing the dryness of the rice and helping to wash it all down. Meat, fish, poultry and vegetables are prepared in a number of different ways so that the meal has a contrasting combination of fried, steamed, dry, smoked and moist foods, which again add interest to an otherwise bland staple.

The Chinese are keen on flavour enhancers like ginger, garlic or onion, soy sauce and monosodium glutamate (MSG), a white crystalline salt. They add these in much the same way as we use salt and pepper. MSG has been used in handfuls for thousands of years in

145

Chinese cooking, as it has an unique way of bringing out all the flavour of anything it's cooked with. (MSG in such large quantities is thought to be the cause of the 'Chinese restaurant syndrome' or 'Kwok's disease' – palpitations, sweating and dizziness brought on in susceptible people; the symptoms do, however, pass, with apparently no long-term effect.) Moreover, one or two naturally salty dishes, such as smoked fish and wind-dried duck, usually feature in a Chinese meal, because such staples of the Chinese diet as rice and vegetables are extremely low in salt. (The Japanese have a similar liking for salty food and their high salt intake is reckoned to make an important contribution to the very high incidence of high blood pressure in Japan today; there is no equivalent information available about the Chinese.)

Indian food

In Indian cuisine all the fat on meat is removed before cooking. Yogurt is much used for absorbing flavours and thickening sauces. Not all Indian foods are low in fat and sugar, however. Cream and rich sweet-meats are popular ingredients – although in the past they probably featured in the diet of wealthy Indians only. In a traditional Indian meal much of the protein is derived from vegetable sources, such as

The two best aids to healthy cooking are a good cookbook and your own ingenuity. But this selection of equipment and gadgets may help you get and stay on the right path.

Fibre in vegetables is highest if you scrub with a **vegetable brush** rather than peel them before cooking. If you do peel root vegetables, use a proper **peeler** so that you take off no more than a thin layer of skin.

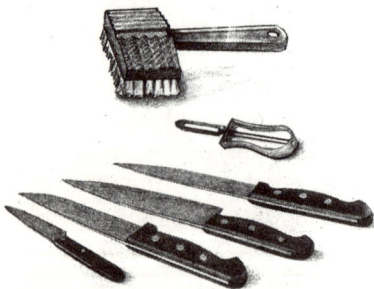

A **mincer [meat grinder]** enables you to mince [grind] your own meat and so cut down on its fat content.

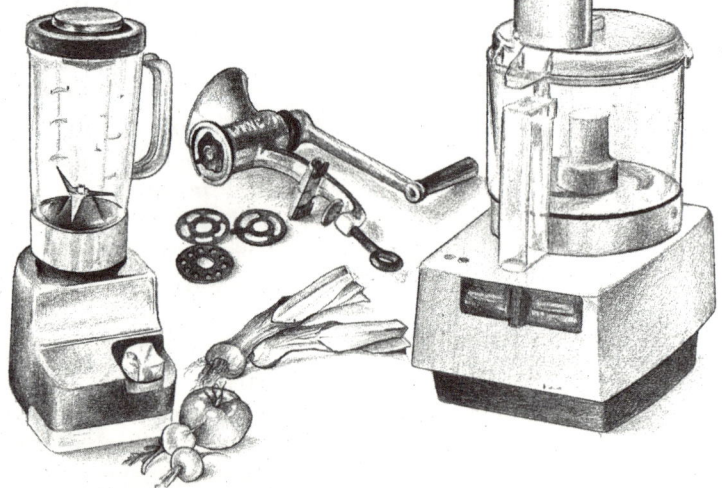

Sharp knives make trimming fat from meat before cooking, or cutting up vegetables, less of a chore.

Use a **blender** to liquidize cooked vegetables for home-made soups and sauces and to make fruit and vegetable juices; it's also good for thickening soups and sauces with vegetable purées rather than with cream or butter.

If you use a blender a great deal or want to make up a lot of salads from raw ingredients, a **food processor** may be invaluable. They're also good for kneading small amounts of bread, and mincing [grinding] meat.

146

rice and lentils, which are also a good source of starch. The dishes are all served at the same time and there might be one of lentils, another of rice, at least three other vegetable dishes, and a choice of pickles, chutney, yogurt, and salad, with meat, fish or poultry playing a relatively minor role. Another nutritional plus is the exclusion of pork, a particularly fatty meat.

Indian food has a similar balance of textures and flavours to Chinese food: dry and moist, bland and spicy, cold and hot, preserved and fresh, light and rich, sharp and sweet. Such contrasts are particularly important in a cuisine that relies heavily on bland, starchy staples.

Italian food

It was the Italians who instructed the French in the art of cookery rather than the other way round – and apparently they weren't impressed by the way their French pupils adapted the original principles!

There is really no such thing as 'Italian' food (or, for that matter, 'Indian' or 'Chinese' food) as their food is highly regional. Florentine cooking is very different from Venetian cooking, and so on. However, one thing that Italians have in common is that meagre resources have taught them to make a little go a long way. Starchy dishes, such as

Steaming vegetables cuts down vitamin loss, and it's easier to do with the proper equipment.

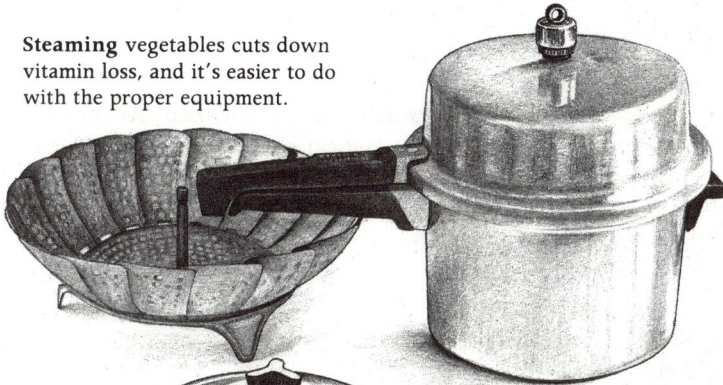

Shorter cooking time with a **pressure cooker** means that there's less temptation to eat a fat- or sugar-laden snack instead of a proper meal. Although some vitamins and minerals are always lost in cooking, the shorter cooking time and steaming baskets or trivets, which prevent vitamins and minerals dissolving in water, make the end result at least as rich in nutrients as other conservative methods of cooking.

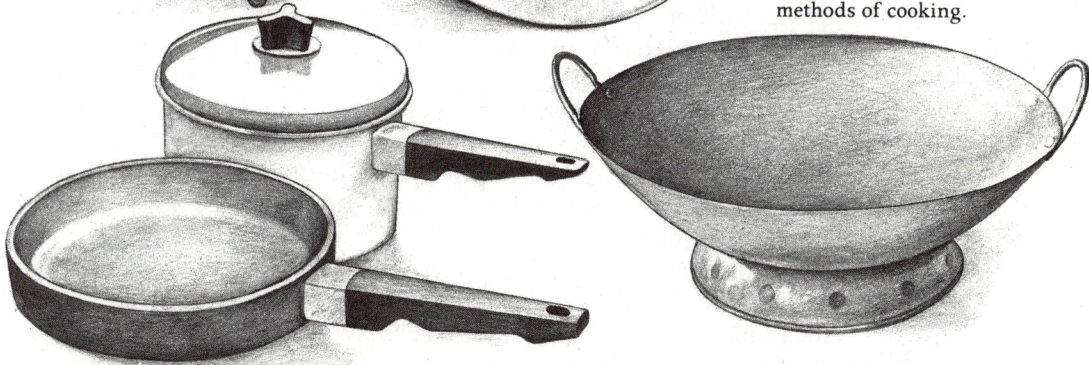

Non-stick pans help cut down on fat used in cooking. They'll last better if you use the proper utensils so as not to scratch the surface.

With its large sloping sides, the **wok** minimizes both the amount of fat needed and, because maximum heat is used, the cooking time. Food cooked in very hot oil

absorbs less fat because the heat seals the surface. Food is usually cut into small pieces and shaken or stir-fried. For the best results, buy a wok with a lid.

147

pasta, pizza and gnocchi (potato dumplings), are an invaluable way of filling hungry stomachs.

The Italians' skill in making a wide variety of meals out of a few basic ingredients is particularly to be admired. It isn't necessarily a complicated cuisine. Pasta may be served on its own with simply a light dressing of olive oil and garlic; a risotto (rice cooked in a good stock) may come dressed with no more than a little Parmesan cheese and butter. Italy has, too, an abundance of good, fresh, flavourful vegetables, which are used in salads, soups and sauces, and excellent local cheeses and salamis, which give flavour to many dishes. The liberal use of garlic may be beneficial to health as the essential oils in garlic have been shown to reduce the 'stickiness' of the blood so that it clots less easily.

Scots cooking

Long neglected by gourmets, Scotland's traditional fare can nevertheless be delicious and nourishing.

One traditional way to cook root vegetables (onion, potato, turnip) would be to simmer them with a little meat to make a broth or soup – a method that has the advantage of reducing nutrient losses, since the cooking liquid is consumed not discarded.

The staple grains for many years were oats and barley, which were used for bread and bannocks (flat cakes). Potatoes were the other mainstay: boiled, cooked in pies or stews, or mashed with flour and cooked to make potato bread on the hot iron plate called the 'girdle'.

The Scots tend to be fish- rather than meat-eaters and many recipes centre on fresh, smoked or pickled cod, salmon, herring and shellfish. The best-known meat dish, the haggis, is really an ingenious sausage, cooked in the stomach bag of a sheep, stuffed with oatmeal, onion, suet, and minced [ground] meat – traditionally the heart, liver and lights of the sheep. This may not sound appealing but according to F. Marian McNeill, author of *The Scots Kitchen*, 'in the haggis we have concocted from humble, even despised ingredients a veritable *plat de gourmet*' – which sums up what good cooking is all about.

Selecting the best

It would be romantic nonsense to make out that cuisines at their most traditional are automatically the most healthy. Italians are frequently overweight; the French complain of their livers (because of too much alcohol); and the Japanese eat too much salt. Anything good, especially food, can be overdone.

It's also important to realize that the meals we so often see abroad or in a restaurant are the *special* meals, not everyday fare. Italians, for example, eating in the traditional way, may eat large platefuls of meat when they go out, but meals at home may be very different.

Look for the best recipe books and scour them for dishes rich in the starchy staples, vegetables and fruit, and that use fats and meat sparingly. If you can't cook, learn. The time you spend learning will pay off in terms of long-term health, since cooking skill allows you to eat what *you* choose, rather than what someone else does.

Who needs what, when?

The body's need for nutrients varies with your stage in life and with special circumstances, such as pregnancy or convalescence. Here is a guide to the main requirements.

Babies

A full-term baby has around a six-month store of some nutrients, such as iron and copper, that aren't in breast milk (a premature baby has less). By the age of six months, the diet has to supply these nutrients, which is partly why mixed foods (cereals, puréed fruit and vegetables, and so on) are introduced around this age. It is not wise to introduce these foods before three months, as the baby may develop a food allergy or become overweight. Drops containing vitamins A, C and D may be recommended from the age of one month. Introducing small amounts of pure orange or tomato juice when the baby is a few months old also ensures a good supply of vitamin C.

Young children

Because of their rapid rate of growth, young children need proportionately more of all nutrients than adults. Food fads are more the parent's problem than the child's: most children thrive even on amazing diets (and grow out of them faster the less fuss is made). Asian children living in northern areas (like Britain) may need to take extra vitamin D, but supplements shouldn't be necessary for other children eating normal food and spending some time outdoors. People living in low fluoride water districts may like to give their children fluoride tablets or drops to fight tooth decay.

Adolescents

The growth spurt during the teens means a greater need for all nutrients; eating a bit more of everything is one solution. The instant snacks many teenagers love tend to be high on salt, sugar or fat, and low on protein, vitamins and minerals.

Adults

People who have to take a lot of meals away from home can go short of the B-vitamins and vitamin C, since food in snackbars, cafés and restaurants may have been cooked some time before it's served. An extra effort to eat nourishing food whenever possible is worth while.

Those who have to take certain kinds of long-term medication may have trouble absorbing particular vitamins and minerals from food, so they should check with their doctor whether a vitamin or mineral supplement is advisable. During convalescence the need for all nutrients is higher than it is in normal health.

Women need more of all nutrients during pregnancy and while breast-feeding. Really bad vomiting in early pregnancy may make vitamin and mineral supplements advisable. A good intake of fibre is particularly important through pregnancy, because all the body's muscles are slacker then, and constipation is often a problem. Iron and folic acid supplements are prescribed for women who are anaemic and are sometimes given routinely as a preventive measure. Women with particularly heavy periods may benefit from iron supplements. After the menopause women may benefit from supplements of vitamin D. Bone fractures, so common after the menopause, are partly due to the change in hormone balance. Women taking some contraceptive pills may become low on vitamin B_6, folic acid and zinc, vitamin C and vitamin B_2, and may feel fitter if they take a multi-vitamin preparation.

The elderly

Many elderly people (especially those living alone) find it too much bother to buy, cook and eat nourishing food – but the elderly need vitamins and nutrients as much as younger people. In fact they need *more* not less nourishing food because in old age the body begins to work less efficiently and absorbs nutrients less well. If they eat a lot of fibre, the elderly may have difficulty in absorbing calcium, and should drink an extra 300 ml [$\frac{1}{2}$ pt] of milk (or yogurt) a day to compensate. Vitamin D is the most likely deficiency and it's advisable to take vitamin D tablets or cod liver oil, or eat more oily fish such as sardines. Cod liver oil tastes awful, but it's easier for the body to absorb than a vitamin D tablet. Sitting in the sun – even by an open window – helps build up vitamin D stores too.

See also vitamins and minerals chart on pages 119–22.

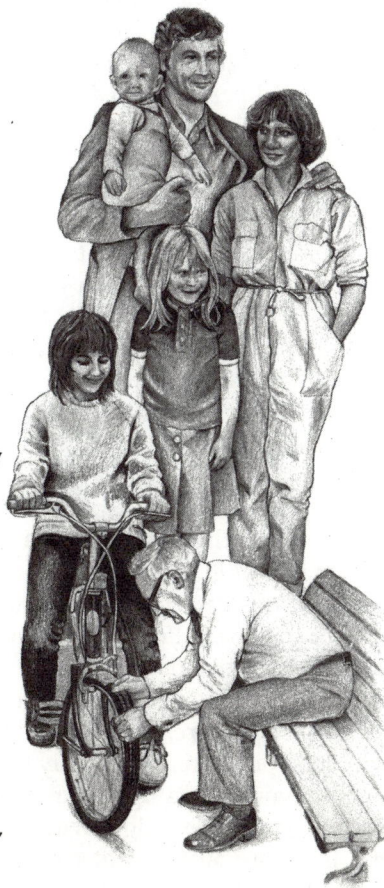

149

BALANCING THE SCALES: Overweight...?

Everyone has some fat – it's needed as an energy reserve – but obese people have an excess of it. Although this may seem obvious enough and most people will reckon they can easily recognize that someone is overweight, there is no simple way of measuring body fat, nor even a generally accepted definition of overweight or the point at which it becomes obesity.

Women have more body fat than men: it makes up about 25 per cent of a woman's weight, and only 15 per cent of a man's. Two-thirds of the fat lies just under the skin – the rest is distributed internally. One way in which a doctor assesses whether a patient is overweight is by measuring the thickness of his or her folds of skin with a pair of calipers. The theory is that the depth of the fat lying just under the skin is a predictable guide to body fat. However, fat is not distributed evenly and different people put on extra fat in different places. Moreover, you can't use this method to measure your own excess fat, since the skinfold that gives the most reliable measures lies just below the shoulder blade and is virtually impossible to get at yourself.

The simplest method is to measure the body weight in relation to height, sex and frame size, although even this may not be an absolutely reliable guide. The extra weight of an athlete or boxer could well be owing to bigger, heavier muscles. Frame size, too, can be difficult to assess: someone with a small frame who is overweight may look like a moderately sized person with a medium frame.

Weight charts The most widely used method of assessing overweight and obesity is derived from data collected by the Metropolitan Life Insurance Company of New York. Obese people die younger, which means that their life insurance benefits have to be paid out sooner, so the M.L.I.C. found it useful to work out which weight ranges are associated with a higher death rate, and, conversely, those that go with longevity.

The drawback to these charts is that they relate weight to death only, not to ill-health in general. Overweight people are prone to a number of discomforts and illnesses that, although not fatal, can make life pretty miserable. Nor are insurance company figures necessarily representative of the population as a whole: life insurance may be taken out by people who suspect that they are at particular risk. However, these are the only figures available and they have proved useful, if not infallible, in practice.

A review of the data from life insurance companies in both the United States and Great Britain has come to the following broad conclusions. The risk of death is increased at all ages by significant overweight, although young people who are obese seem to run a particular risk. The heavier you are, the greater the risk. If you have hypertension (high blood pressure), or a family history of heart disease, and you are also obese, you have a significantly higher chance of earlier death than someone of average weight with similar health problems. Among the obese, there are 50 per cent more deaths from heart and kidney disease, and death due to diabetes is four times more common.

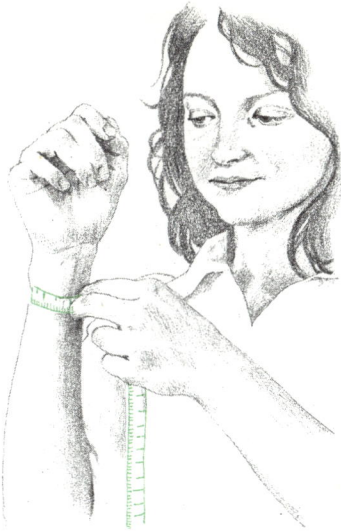

Working out your frame size
A suggested guide to frame size is your wrist-width. On the hand you use most, measure the wrist at its slimmest point – just below the knob of bone. For women, 13.9 cm [5½ in] or less indicates a small frame; 16.5 cm [6½ in] or more, a large one. Anything between gives a medium frame. For men, 16.5 cm [6½ in] or less gives a small frame; 17.8 cm [7 in] or more a large one.

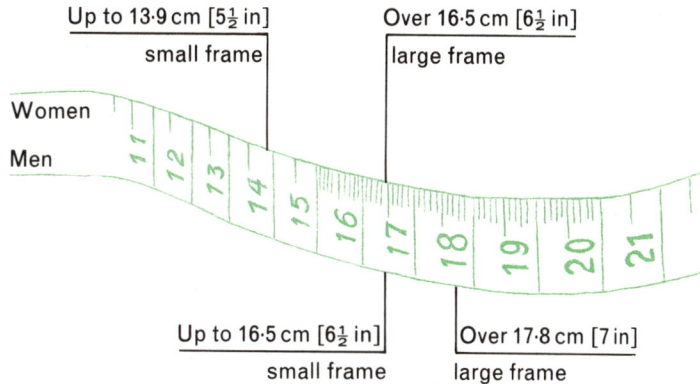

Up to 13·9 cm [5½ in]
small frame

Over 16·5 cm [6½ in]
large frame

Women

Men

Up to 16·5 cm [6½ in]
small frame

Over 17·8 cm [7 in]
large frame

How much should you weigh?

The chart overleaf will help you to work out your 'ideal' weight range. Overweight has been described as being 10 per cent above your ideal weight; you're obese if you're 20 per cent or more above the ideal.

Ask someone else to estimate your type of frame. If you think you really do have 'big bones', get your partner to feel whether your bones are near the surface of your skin. If they're not, you're deluding yourself about your frame size – you're overweight. Your hands and feet are a good guide to your frame: if they are small and neat, you're probably small-framed. Measuring the width of your wrist provides a similar guide. Or look at a picture of yourself when you were at your slimmest and compare your shape with that of other people in the picture – an old school or college photograph can be useful for this.

Are you fat?

If you were slim at 25 and are now middle-aged, do you still take the same clothes size? Middle-age spread may be an accepted norm, but it isn't a healthy trend and is usual only in affluent societies. Since the metabolic rate does gradually slow down with age, it's important to reduce your intake of energy to accommodate this, and to exercise regularly.

Your doctor will probably be the most objective source of advice as to whether you're overweight. Family and friends can be as subjective as you are, especially since they may actually prefer you to be fat.

The most unsparing way to assess overweight is to stand naked before the mirror and to look at your figure as impartially as you can. Jump up and down and see whether the fleshy parts of your body – such as stomach, hips, thighs and upper arms – quiver. If they do, they're probably fat.

A child between age two and puberty is overweight if you can't see the outline of the ribs when he or she is naked.

WEIGHT CHARTS	height without shoes cm	small frame kg	medium frame kg	large frame kg	height without shoes ft in	small frame lb	medium frame lb	large frame lb
Men	155	48	53	58	5 1	105	117	128
	157	49	54	60	5 2	108	120	132
	160	50	56	62	5 3	111	123	135
	162	51	57	63	5 4	113	126	139
	165	53	59	65	5 5	117	130	142
	167	54	61	67	5 6	120	134	147
	170	56	63	69	5 7	124	138	152
	172	58	64	71	5 8	128	142	156
	175	59	66	73	5 9	131	146	161
	177	62	68	75	5 10	135	151	166
	180	63	70	78	5 11	140	155	171
	183	65	73	79	6 0	144	160	175
	186	67	74	82	6 1	148	164	180
	188	69	77	84	6 2	152	169	186
	191	71	79	87	6 3	157	174	191

	height without shoes cm	small frame kg	medium frame kg	large frame kg	height without shoes ft in	small frame lb	medium frame lb	large frame lb
Women	142	39	44	48	4 8	87	97	106
	145	40	45	50	4 9	89	99	109
	147	42	46	51	4 10	92	102	112
	150	43	48	53	4 11	95	105	116
	152	44	49	54	5 0	97	108	119
	155	45	50	55	5 1	100	111	122
	157	47	52	57	5 2	103	115	126
	160	48	54	59	5 3	106	118	130
	162	50	56	62	5 4	110	123	135
	165	51	58	63	5 5	114	127	139
	167	53	60	65	5 6	117	131	144
	170	56	62	67	5 7	121	135	148
	172	57	63	69	5 8	125	139	152
	175	58	65	71	5 9	128	143	157
	177	60	67	73	5 10	132	147	161

How dangerous is obesity?

It has become an accepted creed that obesity predisposes to coronary heart disease, but this is now being questioned more closely and the truth is by no means so clear cut. It seems that the effects of obesity are very much related to those of such other risk factors as aging, raised blood pressure and cholesterol levels, and smoking. The contribution that obesity makes on its own is hard to assess. It may be that the diet's content, and in particular its saturated fatty acid content, is more important than obesity alone. It has certainly been shown that in the younger age group – people around the age of 30 – overweight is significantly related to a much higher rate of heart disease, particularly that resulting in death.

The available information suggests that an excessive intake of energy may be more dangerous than obesity itself. For example, a consistently thin man may keep his weight down by burning up more energy in the form of heat, while still having increased levels of, probably harmful, fats in his blood. On the other hand, when an overweight man reduces his energy intake in order to slim he may also reduce his blood fats, and thus run a lower risk of heart disease than the thin man.

There is still much to be understood about the relationship between obesity and heart disease, but it's always a good idea to slim, if you're overweight, as this reduces the other problems associated with heart disease, such as the tendency to diabetes and hypertension.

Although experts differ as to the relationship between obesity and the development of hypertension, studies have shown that a combination treatment of dieting and salt restriction can control moderately high blood pressure. It was noted that food restriction during the Second World War substantially reduced blood pressure. Fat young people are more likely than thin ones to suffer from hypertension as they get older. Men who are 14 kg [30 lb] or more overweight at 20 are three times more likely to have a stroke. In fact, quite a small gain in weight, together with modestly raised blood pressure, will increase your chances of suffering a fatal stroke. However, since blood pressure is also influenced by heredity, weight gain may affect it only in certain individuals.

Exercise causes blood pressure to rise higher in an obese person than it does in someone of average weight, so measuring blood pressure at rest only may give quite a false indication.

Further hazards of obesity

As weight increases, the body makes more cholesterol, which is excreted into the bile. The bile can't deal with this excess and becomes supersaturated with it. Eventually, the cholesterol, together with mineral salts, is converted into gallstones.

Obesity can cause diabetes (see pages 96–97). If your veins have weak valves, excess weight exerts pressure to weaken them further, which will result in varicose veins. Carrying extra weight can strain the weight-bearing joints, such as the knees and hips, and lead to osteoarthritis. Obesity increases the hazard of medical operations, since a greater amount of anaesthetic will be required. It also interferes with thorough medical examination since it's extremely hard for a doctor to check what's going on under a thick barrier of fat. Obesity can also make you avoid the physical activity that is so vital for good health. Statistics show that overweight people seem to have more accidents. An obese woman may be infertile, and even if she does conceive, she'll be more likely to have a difficult pregnancy and to have a stillborn baby.

However, the cheering thing to note is that if, from being fat, you succeed in reducing, and keeping down, your weight, your health risks immediately decrease, too, and your life expectancy rises.

153

What causes overweight?

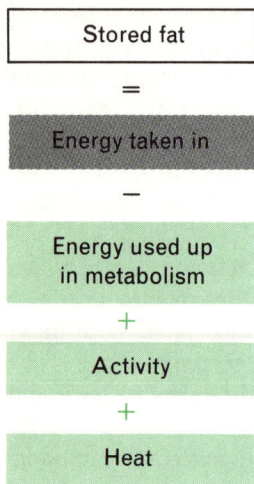

Stored fat

=

Energy taken in

−

Energy used up
in metabolism

+

Activity

+

Heat

Although the short answer is that overweight is caused by eating too much, it's not quite as simple as that. It is common knowledge that two people can eat an identical diet, yet one will put on weight while the other will stay slim. There *are* cases in which obesity is caused by sheer gluttony, but it more often occurs in those whose food intake does not seem particularly excessive. Such people do eat more than they need, but they need less than everyone else. Since any energy taken in but not used is laid down as fat, they become overweight.

The energy that you eat is used in three ways. It may be used to fuel the chemical reactions that keep you alive – the metabolic processes; or to give you the energy to move and work; or to provide the fuel to keep you warm – in other words, heat.

Until recently most weight-losing regimes have concentrated on reducing the amount eaten. Some have also encouraged more exercise, although not all experts agreed on the value of this. The other two elements of the equation – metabolism and heat – have had relatively little attention, but recent research suggests that people differ in their ability to produce heat, and that this may affect whether or not they become obese.

Appetite and energy balance

It is largely appetite that regulates the amount you eat. Some obese adults eat fewer meals a day than others, but they eat more at each meal and they eat it more quickly. In one trial obese people were found to eat more food than those of average weight when it was readily available, but less than average when they had to overcome barriers to get at the food. It has been noted that heavy newborn babies respond to the availability of food rather than to their own feelings of hunger. It's beginning to seem likely that these babies, and obese adults, have some appetite defect.

Exercise has not always been advised by dieting experts, since the number of calories used up during activity is comparatively small. A brisk 30-minute walk, for instance, burns off only about 150 calories – equivalent to those provided by a piece of buttered toast. It was also feared that exercise would stimulate the appetite. Evidence now, however, suggests that a little exercise can actually suppress the appetite, and certainly helps to regulate it. Moreover, it offers a further benefit in that being fit makes you feel happier and more resolute in sticking to a sensible diet. Eating less, combined with exercising more, is the most efficient way to lose weight, and the exercise should tone up your muscles and improve your shape.

Brown fat

Perhaps the most exciting discovery in obesity research has been that a particular type of tissue, brown fat, seems to be implicated in the way that the body burns off surplus energy.

In a series of experiments, a group of rats were offered a free choice from a range of processed foods that included cakes, biscuits [cookies] and pâté. On this diet, they ate as much as 80 per cent more than their usual intake, and although some became obese, others, remarkably,

ENERGY USED UP IN 30 MINUTES' ACTIVITY

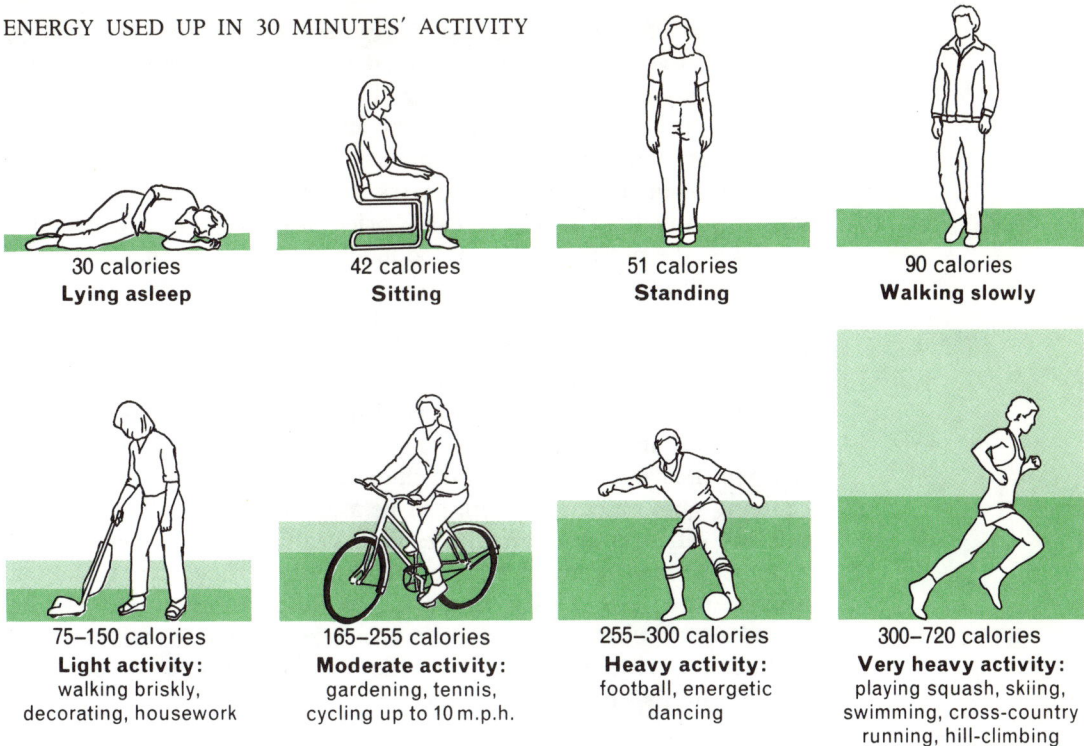

30 calories
Lying asleep

42 calories
Sitting

51 calories
Standing

90 calories
Walking slowly

75–150 calories
Light activity:
walking briskly,
decorating, housework

165–255 calories
Moderate activity:
gardening, tennis,
cycling up to 10 m.p.h.

255–300 calories
Heavy activity:
football, energetic
dancing

300–720 calories
Very heavy activity:
playing squash, skiing,
swimming, cross-country
running, hill-climbing

stayed the same weight. Measurements showed that these rats were burning off their excess energy. It was two Canadian researchers who realized that this burn-off was occurring in deposits of brown fat – which, in fact, was already known to be the tissue responsible for rewarming hibernating animals.

Brown fat is found in several places, particularly between the shoulder blades and around the kidneys; altogether it usually makes up only 2 per cent of the weight of the body. It can produce heat rapidly after being stimulated with noradrenalin. The rats that stayed slim while eating the sweet, fatty foods developed three times as much brown fat between their shoulder blades during overfeeding as a control group on a normal, less appetizing diet. Obese rats were found to have defective brown fat that didn't work as well as that in lean rats.

It seems that man has a very similar mechanism to control his weight. This opens up fascinating possibilities for treatment: new drugs, for example, could be developed to speed up the working of 'lazy' brown fat tissue in obese people.

Eating patterns today

Obesity is more common nowadays, despite the fact that people actually eat less, on average, than a generation ago. This apparent paradox is probably the result of the advent of television and labour-saving technology, particularly the family car; taking less exercise means that people burn up less energy, and so appetites are smaller. Although the overall amount of food eaten has dropped, there has been no cut back on the high energy foods.

The body is good at regulating the amount of energy laid down as fat, but even the best mechanisms can become strained when challenged too much or too often. Today's efficient food industry provides virtually any food at a reasonable price. As this food is constantly available, the problem is one of too much choice rather than too little. You don't have to overeat vastly in order to tax the regulatory mechanism. One more slice of toast than the body needs or can cope with each day can, over the years, lead to obesity.

People often eat more – and therefore put on weight – when they give up smoking. This is partly because nicotine acts as an appetite suppressant and partly because they still feel the need to have something in their mouths. Sugar-free chewing gum, or nicotine-flavoured chewing gum on prescription, can be a great help. Don't go back to smoking – it's far more harmful to your health than overweight.

Some women seem to put on weight when they start to take a contraceptive pill. This is often due to fluid retention and can be remedied by changing to a different form of pill. It may also be because, in preventing ovulation, the pill also prevents the surge of metabolism that normally follows it.

Eating and stress

People often find that they overeat when they're under stress or feel anxious or insecure. They may eat too much when facing a difficult decision, going through a personal crisis, or when changing job or moving house. Usually when the crisis has resolved itself, craving for extra food goes – although there's a danger that the habit of overeating may be difficult to shed. Some people react to overwork and mental exhaustion by losing their appetite; others, in the same situation, may overeat, making up for a drained mind with a filled stomach. People also tend to eat more when they're bored. In a survey by Britain's Consumers' Association, more than half the dieters questioned said that they ate more when they were depressed or worried, and 37 per cent said that they ate more when lonely. It seems that many people eat as a way of comforting themselves. The situation can become further confused when overweight itself causes anxiety, especially in fat children, who may feel they are social outcasts.

Weight gain after pregnancy

Some women find that their weight problems start during pregnancy. The normal average weight gain at this time is 13 kg [28 lb], although it can vary a great deal. A healthy woman who was previously slim should have no difficulty in losing this without dieting, particularly if she breastfeeds her baby. But although some of the extra fat gained in pregnancy is used up in breastfeeding, part of it may be kept as a reserve and this may not finally disappear until lactation has stopped. Moreover, a woman who is breastfeeding still has in her blood some of the pregnancy hormone that relaxes the muscles and ligaments, so

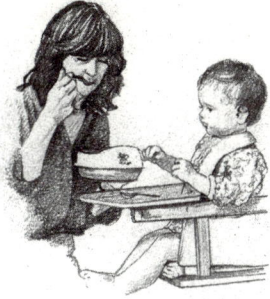

It's only too easy to gain weight by eating up the baby's leftovers.

that her hips are actually wider. This will make it very hard for her to get back into her old clothes, until she resumes her normal shape.

It's not clear why some women should have difficulty in losing weight after they've had a baby, since there doesn't seem to be any permanent change in the hormone balance (although women who've had miscarriages can find it especially hard to lose the extra weight they've put on). But having a baby does change your life enormously. If you're at home, instead of at work, you'll have permanent access to the food cupboard. Even though previously little-used muscles may be aching from lifting babies and carry-cots, you may still not be taking as much exercise as you used to. And some women, while they complain about being fat, may subconsciously prefer a 'mother-earth' figure, feeling that it's more appropriate to their new role.

Do fat babies make fat adults?

Obesity runs in families, possibly because overeating may be a habit ingrained from childhood rather than a result of some specifically inherited factor, although it may be a combination of the two.

About one in four babies under the age of one gains weight at an excessive rate. Among the suggested causes are the decline in breast-feeding, the availability of artificial infant food and the early intro-duction of non-milk solids (usually unnecessary below three months). In breastfeeding the baby takes only as much milk as he or she needs, while a baby given artificial food may eat too much if encouraged to drink everything in the bottle. If a formula feed is too concentrated, it can make a baby thirsty; he or she will therefore demand more milk and a vicious circle will be set up. The highly undesirable practice of adding cereals to feeds may also make a baby put on extra weight.

It is a received truth that fat babies grow into fat children who grow into fat adults. The suggestion is that you have a fixed number of fat cells laid down in babyhood; if you are overfed as a baby, more fat cells are laid down and will remain into adult life. Although this theory is often quoted, the evidence for it is not very conclusive. There are quite a number of fat babies, but far fewer fat adults — indeed, only one in five fat babies is still fat by the time he or she starts school. However, most fat adults were also fat babies. The theory may still turn out to be correct, but since it's difficult to count fat cells, it's at present not possible to prove or disprove it. So don't underfeed a baby with the idea of preventing it from becoming an overweight child; but don't fall into the trap, either, of overfeeding children as a way of showing your love. If children become used to eating when they're not hungry, the normal development of feelings of hunger and satiety may become confused until eventually they may not recognize when they need to eat and when they should stop.

Is it your glands?

Although 'glandular' or endocrine disorders are sometimes blamed for causing overweight, genuine instances of this are rare. In the over-whelming majority of obese people, routine tests show that their glands are functioning normally.

157

How to lose weight

No one knows precisely how many people are trying to lose weight at any time, but it may be as many as one in ten. For many people it's a constant problem since, if they're prone to overweight, reducing their weight to even an acceptable level is only one part of the challenge. Keeping it at a suitable level thereafter is equally hard, because it's so easy to slip back into old eating habits without realizing it and to put weight on again.

There is no magic formula that will guarantee weight loss. The only answer is to take in less energy and to use up more: if you take in fewer calories than your body burns up, you'll lose weight. If you want to maintain that lower weight you'll have to alter your eating habits permanently.

● Don't be over-ambitious. Unless you're grossly obese, it's better for your health if you aim at a small but steady weight loss of, say, 1–1.5 kg [2–3 lb] a week, rather than trying to lose all your excess weight in a week or two. The weight loss in the first two weeks will be greater anyway, so don't get disillusioned when this slows down in succeeding weeks. In fact, some of the initial weight loss is caused by loss of water rather than of fat tissue, which makes it very easy to regain. Fat is unlikely to come off evenly – it often comes off first from those areas that weren't especially fat in the first place. However, as you maintain your diet, the balance between your proportions will return to normal. You can't rely on losing weight from a particular spot, although well-chosen exercises will help to firm the area up. Don't forget that good posture (see pages 12–15) can improve the appearance of your figure.

● Motivation is all-important. Although many people recognize that they're overweight, and want to slim, the success rate isn't very high. American surveys have shown that while about 25 per cent of men and nearly 50 per cent of women realize that they're too fat, only about 10 per cent are actively trying to reduce their weight. The rest clearly haven't been motivated sufficiently to make them *want* to lose weight. It's a good idea to familiarize yourself with the health risks attached to being overweight (see pages 152–53). Some people, particularly those in the younger age group, are motivated by a desire to improve their appearance; others by the realization that their clothes no longer fit them properly.

● Start by taking a long hard look at your present eating habits. Make a list or keep a chart of what you eat during a normal day, when you eat it, and why. Remember to include any snacks between meals and the occasional drink before dinner. This will give you a clearer idea of your eating patterns, and by studying it you may well spot areas in which you could cut down without much effort.

● If you're only a little overweight, it may be sufficient to do without sugar in your coffee or to stop eating that mid-morning chocolate bar. If you regularly eat just 300 calories more than your body needs each day – equivalent to a 60 g [2 oz] bar of plain chocolate, or two slices of bread and butter – you'll put on about 30 g [1 oz] a day, which can soon

Writing down everything that you consume, as precisely as you can, is the best way to keep track of your eating habits.

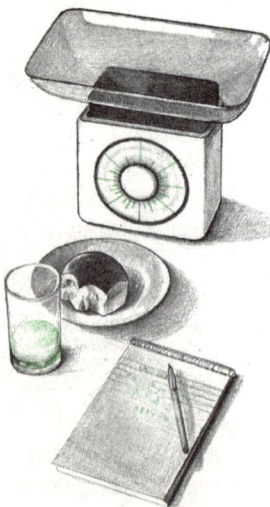

lead to noticeable overweight. If you're 3kg [7 lb] or more over-weight, you'll probably need to make a rather more systematic attempt to lose weight.

• Some people overeat because they are overpowered by the sight and smell of food, and eat even when they know that they aren't hungry. If you're one of these people, it's important to recognize it and consciously avoid coming into contact with food too often. Take a detour so that you don't pass the pâtisserie window, with its mouth-watering chocolate cakes. If you simply must have a treat, make it an infrequent one, and ensure that it fits in with the rest of your diet by making a sensible allowance for it.

• Some people may become overweight through sticking to three regular meals a day. When they see that the clock indicates a meal time, they automatically get hungry and expect to eat. If you're such a person, you need to train yourself to look out for your body's signals of hunger rather than to watch the time. Some people are better off on only two meals, or even one meal, a day, while others do well on several small ones or snacks. Either way the total food intake shouldn't exceed your set target. Eating early in the day rather than later allows you to burn up more of the energy in activity; if you go to bed soon after a meal, you'll use up fewer of the calories you've just taken in, leaving some to go towards your store of body fat.

• Recognize that your desire to get slim is battling with your desire to eat, and that it will require strong control every moment of the day if you're to succeed fully. It's all too easy to have that firm resolve for most of the time and then to let your guard slip for a few moments. If you allow yourself to gorge during those moments, you'll undo much of the success you've achieved.

• Occasionally your sensible, controlled diet may well go out of the window and you'll find yourself on a binge. This isn't unusual and although it may set back your progress, don't be too depressed by it – and don't let it make you lose heart and, to find comfort, continue to eat more than you should. Come to terms with the guilt feelings after a binge, and learn from your experience, by writing down what you ate and the circumstances that led up to the binge. You'll then know what to avoid next time. Physical exercise is an excellent antidote to guilt, and will go a little way to burning up the extra food you've eaten. It's a good idea to develop an absorbing hobby that will fill your leisure hours and your mind, and stop you thinking about food.

• Don't weigh yourself more than once a week. Weight can fluctuate considerably day by day, and you could get depressed if it seems to have gone up instead of down. Always weigh yourself on the same scales at the same time of day and in the same weight of clothing.

• A woman shouldn't diet while she's pregnant, and, after the birth, not until she's finished breastfeeding (which in itself uses up several hundred calories a day). The only exception would be a woman who was very fat at the time she conceived, in which case her doctor might put her on a special diet during pregnancy.

159

Which diet?

Of the several different diets you can follow, all are basically aimed at reducing the number of calories you eat without leading to an unbalanced diet. A good diet should be founded on sound principles so that once the weight has been lost, you can adapt the diet to become the basis of your permanent eating habits. It should be flexible enough to allow for the demands of your social life – dinner parties or meals out; otherwise you'll only be tempted to break it.

If you have much weight to lose, you may prefer to shed it in stages. Aim to lose 6.5 kg [14 lb] in a couple of months, then give yourself a rest. Eat to maintain your weight at this new lower level for a month or two before starting on the next bout of dieting and then aim to lose another 6.5 kg [14 lb].

Calorie-counting

The method that most regular weight-losers choose is the calorie-counting diet. It can take some getting used to since it involves estimating and then restricting the number of calories in everything you eat. To start with you'll need to weigh and measure all your food and drink and refer to calorie charts (see pages 241–49), but once you've learnt the calorific values it takes far less time. Always write down all the calories you eat, so that you can't cheat.

On a calorie-counting diet you aim to take in fewer calories than you're using up. By referring to the chart opposite, you can estimate roughly how many calories you use up during the day. Your energy requirement depends on a number of factors – men use up more energy than women, young people use more than the middle-aged and elderly, and, of course, if you have a sedentary job you'll use up less than if you're constantly on the go. Once you know roughly how many calories you're burning up, you can calculate your diet to leave an energy gap of, say, 500 or 1,000 calories a day, which your body will make up for by using its store of energy in the body fat. Thus, you should get slimmer. For example, a moderately active middle-aged man may use up, on average, 2,750 calories a day. To cut his intake by 1,000 calories he should devise a diet that gives him 1,750 calories a day. If you find that, having set yourself a calorie allowance, you're eating *more* on this diet than you usually do, you probably have a slow metabolic rate. Cut your calorie allowance further, but don't go below 800 calories per day, since it's dangerous to go below this level for extended periods except under medical supervision.

Every 3,500 calories saved by dieting represents about 450 g [1 lb] of fat, so a diet that saves 500 calories a day will result in a weight loss of 450 g [1 lb] of fat in a week. This may not sound much, but over weeks and months it amounts to a reasonable weight loss. A diet that saves 1,000 calories a day, giving a weekly weight loss of 1 kg [2 lb] of fat, is what the average dieter should aim at – anything more will make the diet too restrictive to be easily followed. A strict diet would mean a reduction to an intake of about 1,000 calories a day.

Adapt your diet to your lifestyle. Planning your calorie intake on a weekly, rather than a daily, allowance can be a help. If you're very

APPROXIMATE ENERGY REQUIREMENTS

Age	Men	Calories	Age	Women	Calories
18–34	Sedentary	2510	18–54	Sedentary	2000
	Moderately active	2900		Moderately active	2200
	Very active*	3350		Very active*	2500
35–64	Sedentary	2400		Pregnant	2400
	Moderately active	2750		Breastfeeding	2750
	Very active*	3350			
65–74	Sedentary	2400	55–74	Sedentary	1900
	Moderately active	2750		Moderately active	2150
75+	Sedentary	2150	75+	Sedentary	1680

*Professional athletes may require even more energy

Energy needs depend on sex, age and lifestyle. 'Moderately active' means exercising daily or having a physically active job, such as gardening. 'Very active' is to have a physically demanding job, e.g. mining, or play frequent strenuous sport. Even spending 24 hours in bed uses up 1,200–1,500 calories.

active at weekends, you may be tempted to eat more then, so if you've set yourself a 1,500-calories-a-day diet and find that you eat 2,500 on both Saturday and Sunday, be stricter with yourself during the week to make up for those extra 2,000 calories.

Aim to get most of your calories from valuable foods like bread, cereals, lean meat, pulses, fruit and vegetables, but, within your allowance, set aside, say, 150 calories a day to be taken in the form of your favourite food treat – preferably one like cheesecake (see page 143) that isn't just fat and sugar.

Low carbohydrate diet

Another well-known, but less desirable, method of losing weight is the low carbohydrate diet. Instead of counting calories you limit your carbohydrate intake. The attractions of this type of diet are that you spend less time with your pocket calculator adding up calorie values, and that in cutting down carbohydrates you also cut down on other foods – for example, cutting down your bread intake means you reduce your butter intake, too.

Essentially you cut down on or avoid altogether foods that contain sugar and starch: including jam, honey, potatoes, cereals, bread, biscuits, pasta and alcohol. You can either eat less of everything, or you can avoid certain foods as far as possible. The first method requires much will power and careful judgement. The advantage of the second method is that you always know when you're cheating, and if you've made public your decision – to cut out potatoes, for example – your friends and family know you are, too.

A low carbohydrate diet has two main disadvantages. First, you may find yourself eating more of everything else and thus end up losing no weight at all. This has happened to people who've followed this diet

161

over a period of years. Second, cutting out bread, potatoes and other starchy carbohydrate foods makes an unbalanced diet, low in fibre and with a high proportion of fat. If you're losing weight for health reasons, there seems little point in taking up unhealthy eating habits.

Low fat diet

A recently developed diet, which many nutritionists believe is healthier than the low carbohydrate one, and more effective than an unstructured resolve to eat less, is the low fat diet. As easy to follow as the low carbohydrate, it's better balanced since it encourages you to eat plenty of roughage – bulk and fibre – and restricts fats and sugars. Since fats provide at least twice as many calories as carbohydrate, this makes a lot of dieting sense. Reducing fat intake has the added benefit of cutting cholesterol levels in the blood and thus the risk of heart disease, see pages 98–103.

For this diet, foods are graded according to a fat rating, so that only a limited amount of fat is consumed each day. In general the foods that contain a lot of fat are also those that contain the highest number of calories: foods such as cheese, cream, nuts and fatty meats. There are a couple of additions to the low fat rule. Sugar also must be limited because it contains a lot of calories while having no other nutritional value. Alcohol, too, (as on a low calorie diet) is restricted. You can eat as much as you like of the foods that contain no fat: bread, fresh fruit (except avocadoes), most vegetables, pasta, rice, and most breakfast cereals.

Following these rules it's not difficult to stick to a diet containing only 1,000 calories a day. Trials have shown that this diet is effective and easy to keep to: dieters have lost as much as 13 kg [28 lb] in a couple of months. It also has a psychological advantage since you know that if you're hungry you can always fill up with foods that contain little or no fat – tomato or cucumber sandwiches (made without butter or margarine, of course), or a plateful of potatoes. Dieters often complain of feeling empty and missing those satisfying fillers – the low fat diet actually encourages you to eat them.

It's possible to slip up on this diet if you're not aware of the amount of fat that may have been added to the food in the cooking process so see pages 103–04 for tips on cutting down on fats.

On a low fat diet, avoid the foods with high or moderate fat content. See pages 241–49 for a more precise breakdown of the fat content of individual foods.

High fat	Moderate fat	Low fat
Avocado pear; most nuts; fried foods, chips [fries]; sausages, bacon, ham, pork, beef, tongue, lamb, goose; mackerel, herring, canned tuna, kippers, sardines; whole milk, cream, cream cheese, processed cheese, hard cheese, Camembert, butter, margarine, lard, oils; biscuits [cookies], cakes, pastries; pâté, French dressing, mayonnaise, ice cream.	Chick peas [garbanzos], soya beans, olives; chicken, duck, turkey, veal, rabbit, kidney, liver, sweetbread; pilchards, salmon, trout; eggs; soya flour (full fat); fish paste, meat paste, peanut butter, creamy soups.	Fruits (except avocado), most vegetables (except chick peas [garbanzos], soya beans); tripe, venison, snails; whitefish, shellfish; buttermilk, skimmed milk, cottage cheese, yogurt; wheat- and cornflour, bread, breakfast cereals, spaghetti, rice, oatmeal; tomato ketchup, clear soups, herbs and spices, low calorie soft drinks.

Behavioural therapy

This is an alternative method of encouraging weight control, widely used in the United States. Treatment takes place over three to four months and much time is spent counselling the overweight patient. Of the various approaches tried, there isn't enough data so far to show which has the most long-term effect. All encourage the patient to get to know himself and his own body's signals.

It has been suggested that the amount of trouble you take over what you eat may be related to the extent of your self-esteem; the greater the care, the happier you feel about yourself. So the therapies encourage the individual to eat more slowly and ceremoniously. Surveys have shown that many fat people eat their food very fast, often while they're doing something else – talking, watching television or working. By the time they begin to be aware of and to enjoy the flavour of the food, they've finished it, so they reach out for more to satisfy the taste buds. Patients who usually do this are told to put any food they're going to eat on a plate, to sit down, look at the food and savour it, and then to chew it slowly, so that they get the maximum conscious enjoyment out of it. This should lessen the desire to go on to a second helping, and is a helpful idea for every dieter.

A typical therapeutical approach starts with self-monitoring. Patients write down everything that they've eaten and drunk, when and where they consumed it, what they were doing, how they felt, how hungry they were, and so on. By discovering the conditions that encouraged them to eat they can learn to break the associations between the environmental stimulus and eating – some people resort to a packet of biscuits [cookies] to work out their feelings of frustration every time they feel that they've been imposed upon, for example. Once people are aware of this type of habit, they usually eat less food, although it may take several months to lose the automatic response of feeling hungry.

Patients are also encouraged to find something else to do whenever they feel the urge to eat. Hunger pangs can be forgotten if there's a sufficiently distracting alternative activity available – reading a good book or knitting a complicated pattern. They're also taught relaxation techniques and how to cope with others who press them to eat. It's common for friends and family (consciously or not) to encourage a patient to stay fat. Losing weight often changes relationships and fat people and/or their families can't always cope with this and with the new stresses imposed upon them. Fatness may then be preferred as the familiar devil as opposed to the unknown one.

Weight-reducing drugs

Drugs that suppress appetite are available only on prescription. They aren't a substitute for a diet but are designed to help you to keep to a regime. Although fairly effective, they have many drawbacks – the main one being that once you stop taking them you'll put back on all the weight you've lost, unless you've also altered your eating habits. Since these drugs are mostly related to the amphetamines, they have all the side effects of that group. You may suffer sleep disturbance and faulty concentration, or be overstimulated, and you can get addicted.

Tests show that amphetamine-related drugs, especially diethyl-propion, fenfluramine and phentermine, do reduce food intake, at least to begin with. In a lengthy trial, in which people took a particular drug for 36 weeks, the average weight loss was about 12 kg [26 lb]. But by the end of the trial period the dieters' weights had stabilized; it seemed that even if they'd continued to take the drug their weight wouldn't have been further reduced. The drug treatment was combined with a food intake of only 1,000 calories a day. The drug, by cutting the appetite, helped the reducers to keep to their diet.

In studies on dieters who used behavioural therapy and/or drugs, although those using drugs lost more weight in the early weeks, after a year those who had used behaviour modification alone were slimmer.

So don't rely on drugs to help you diet. You must realize that your weight will come down if you eat less – and will increase again if you eat more – than your body needs. Using drugs won't help you to find out *why* you have a weight problem, although it can be a help to get you started if you're grossly obese.

Dietary aids

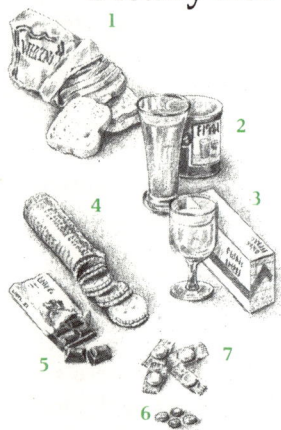

1 Dietary bread. 2 Meal in a glass of milk and 3 in water. 4 Meal replacement biscuits [cookies] and 5 chocolate bar. 6 Bran and 7 other bulking agent tablets.

Some dietary foods can be helpful – particularly the low calorie ones – but it's important not to be misled by advertising claims.

Of the foods that are claimed to curb the appetite, some take the form of tablets available from the chemist [druggist], over the counter. Most of them contain cellulose, which is supposed to expand when it's in the stomach and to make you feel full. Besides containing only small amounts of cellulose, they also provide a lot of calories. Moreover, tests have shown that the bulking effect can be achieved only if large amounts of bulking agent are used – this would also mean taking in large numbers of calories.

Some dieters find the substitute meals – the meal-in-a-drink, for example – useful. However, once again, these won't help you to improve your eating pattern, they're low in fibre, and are not a balanced diet. Indeed the meal-in-a-biscuit [cookie] type tend to be sweet, which only perpetuates poor eating habits.

The various brands of special dietary bread should be treated with scepticism. Weight for weight it contains about the same number of calories as ordinary bread, although because it's generally smaller and lighter in texture, one slice doesn't weigh as much as a slice of ordinary bread. Some dieters find dietary bread helpful, but, of course, the whole benefit will be lost if you proceed to pile it with butter and jam.

Crash diets

The various crash diets that come in and out of fashion are unhealthy and have only a short-term effect. Most of the weight loss is water, which easily goes back on again. They are, in any case, hard to keep to, since they tend to allow only a tiny range of foods.

Avoid any diet that limits fluids – too little liquid is bad for you. Water, on its own or with a meal, has no calories and isn't fattening. Indeed, by helping to fill you up it can reduce your appetite.

Brief fasts

Some people prefer to eat what they like for six days, then fast for one day, on which they take in only calorie-free or low calorie fluids. This doesn't do the body any harm, although you should take care not to fast on a day on which you need to do a lot of important things, since it can make you quite lightheaded. However, it's not a certain method of weight control, since there's a temptation simply to eat extra on the day after the fast, to make up for it.

Starvation

Starving to lose weight is used only in severe cases of obesity as part of hospital treatment. Weight losses have sometimes been impressive, but are seldom long-term. Although effective, it is dangerous, since when the body loses weight at a faster average rate than 1 kg [2 lb] a week, as well as losing fat, it loses lean muscle tissue, which is used to provide glucose from the breakdown of proteins. This tissue can be lost from any part of the body – if it happens to come from the heart muscle, the result can be fatal. Therefore a small quantity of glucose is always given as part of the treatment, in order to prevent this loss. Clearly, starvation should never be undertaken without close medical supervision.

Dieting groups

Groups and clubs can be beneficial to those who can't lose weight on their own. Most offer useful information, guidance and moral support, and many people find both the discussion of shared problems and the element of competition a great help. There is, however, some evidence that when the dieter leaves the group, the weight loss is not maintained. In other words, if a group is what you need, you may have to keep going to it for life, to keep your weight down permanently.

Localized weight-reducing aids

The only way to lose weight is to use up fewer calories than you consume. Passive machines (see page 56) and creams that are claimed to reduce weight just do not work. Nor do any of the supposed remedies for that controversial substance, cellulite.

Dental splinting

For those with a very serious weight problem, and who haven't been helped by dieting, it's possible to wire up the jaws. This prevents you from eating anything, although you can drink liquids and liquidized food. It's sometimes successful, but once again when the weight has been lost – and the jaws are unwired – the patient tends to start eating as before and to put all the extra weight back on.

Surgery

When obesity threatens a patient's life, doctors may advise surgery, during which part of the intestines, from which much of the food is absorbed, is removed. While this does produce weight loss, complications are common and can be extremely serious.

In a form of cosmetic surgery – an apronectomy – extra fat is cut away from the abdomen. This operation is both costly and ineffective, since if fat is put back on again afterwards (as is usually the case), it doesn't go on smoothly, but in unsightly lumps and bumps.

165

Helping overweight children

Always try to serve a nutritionally balanced diet, so that children learn sound eating habits.

If your children show a tendency to tubbiness, avoid giving them sweet, fatty foods like cakes and biscuits [cookies]. Don't give them sweets [candies]; if they develop a liking for them anyway, make sure that they have a strictly limited number, say once a week, and preferably eaten after a meal. Try substituting sugar-free chewing gum or fruit. If the children insist on drinking sweet fizzy drinks, these should be of the fruit juice and soda water variety. Never use food as a reward – a hug and a word of praise are a much better way of showing affection and thanks. Although *you* may not give sweets as presents, many elderly people do. It can be very hurtful to reject their kindness, so instead, where possible, explain the situation to them and suggest an alternative gift. For example, a child might be encouraged to start a scrapbook or a collection of postcards; grandparents could give interesting items to add to it – cheaper and more lasting presents than bags of sweets [candies].

Don't give your children large amounts of food. Wait until they ask for more before giving a second helping. Don't make them eat food just because there's only a little left and you want it finished. Throwing it away will be better for your children's health and happiness.

Encourage children to take up extra physical activity. This may need tact since many fat children are acutely embarrassed that they can't run as fast as their peers. They can feel sadly conspicuous in shorts and vest, so loose, comfortable tracksuits are a better idea.

If a child is fat, one (or both) of the parents is likely to be fat, too. It's a good idea for parent and child to diet together, each giving the other moral support, and facilitating the family catering.

If you're worried that your child is seriously overweight, seek medical advice. A child is still growing and should never be put on a strict diet without medical supervision. Most dieticians and doctors aim to keep weight constant, or to reduce the rate at which weight is gained so that as the child grows taller, he or she gets slimmer.

Puppy fat
Overweight children are often described as having 'puppy fat'. Some children do become plump just before puberty and the subsequent growth spurt. However, they don't 'grow out' of this stage automatically. They'll either burn up more energy for some reason – going on to a secondary school where more sport is played – or eat less, and so lose weight. Unfortunately ice-cream vans and take-away food shops on or near school premises can make losing weight hard for children.

Adolescent eating patterns
Parents have to be careful about reacting to adolescent eating habits. While these sometimes seem bizarre, the few studies done on them show that they can be surprisingly balanced. So if your teenagers live on hamburgers and baked beans for a while, it's not necessarily bad for them. Adolescents are trying to stand on their own feet and guidance on such matters as food is often seen as interference.

Underweight

While the majority of weight problems are connected with overweight, there are some people who would actually like to weigh more. These people are naturally slightly built, and find that, however much they eat, their weight hardly fluctuates. They seem to have a super-efficient weight-controlling mechanism that automatically burns off whatever extra calories they eat, with the result that they remain thin. Nutritionists generally agree that there is nothing that a person who is naturally thin can do to put on weight.

It should be noted that a large, unexplained weight loss must always be investigated by a doctor.

Food and the mind

Psychologists have recently become aware of a range of problems, found almost exclusively among girls and women – generally those in the middle classes – which have been grouped under the name of 'diet manipulation'. These problems tend to begin during or just after adolescence. One such problem is the cycle of dieting and bingeing, in which the sufferer alternates between trying to stick to an unrealistically restricted diet and gorging enormous amounts of food. These binges may or may not be followed by vomiting and/or the use of laxatives to counter the effects of the overeating. The sufferer becomes obsessed with food. There are various theories about the causes of this behaviour but it does seem to be found in those who have difficulty in forming close relationships and have doubts about their ability to control their own lives. Extreme and continuous dieting becomes a way of demonstrating some kind of control; when the sufferer then goes on a binge, what she sees as her lack of self-discipline causes her agonies of self-disgust.

To break this cycle, sufferers are encouraged to relearn how to recognize and respond to the signals of their own bodies – to eat only when they're hungry. Many people get over these problems on their own – for those who feel that they can't, counselling and self-help groups can be greatly beneficial.

Anorexia nervosa

This is an extremely serious, and nowadays fairly well-known, form of diet manipulation. About 90 per cent of sufferers are girls and young women – while it does occur in young men, this is relatively rare. Anorexia is characterized by a terror of weight gain and as a result, a sufferer will go to extraordinary lengths to reduce her weight and to keep it well below what it should be. The anorectic person, apart from being extremely thin, will probably show other signs and symptoms. Once she goes below a certain weight, about 41 kg [91 lb], menstruation, ovulation and thus fertility cease; indeed, it's suggested that an anorectic may be attempting to return to the pre-pubescent state. Her breath may smell of vomit, or of acetone from fasting, her body may become covered in downy hair, and she may also go through phases of bingeing. Vomiting can cause her tooth enamel to be eroded by stomach acid. Above all, she becomes determined to avoid eating any food, and especially carbohydrate.

167

Girls from middle-class homes are particularly vulnerable to anorexia; it is rarer in girls from less wealthy backgrounds. A British study of schoolgirls over the age of 16 from affluent homes showed that one in 100 had the disease badly. It also noted that many of the other girls showed some form of diet manipulation behaviour at some stage in their adolescence. The disease is probably equally as common in young women who have left school.

The anorectic may begin by believing that she is overweight, and starting to diet. Refusing food, even though she's hungry, turns out to be easier than she'd expected. She may take pride in being able to control her food intake so well. After a period of severe starvation she may find that she becomes a little 'high' – which she may like. She will continue to lose weight, even though her weight may now be well below what is considered normal. Sometimes when she does eat what she thinks is a great deal she'll make herself sick afterwards in private: or she may use laxatives in large amounts, in order to avoid absorbing the food that she's just eaten. Most anorectics can think of nothing but food, which causes them much anguish.

Anorectic girls sometimes say that they were influenced to start dieting by a parent's, or a friend's, comments that they were too fat. It does seem that, in some cases, this sort of chiding or teasing can trigger off a predisposition to excessive dieting. Studies show that many adolescent anorectics fear, or are conscious of, being a disappointment to their parents.

The fact that a girl has become anorectic is often concealed from family and friends very successfully. She may become extremely secretive about food, doing her best to avoid eating with other people. She may go to great lengths to hide her thinness by wearing loose, baggy clothes. She may give the appearance of eating a good deal – pushing her food around on the plate, saying that she's already eaten a huge meal, spending hours preparing elaborate meals for others while eating nothing herself.

Anorectics often can't see that they're unduly thin, because they have distorted images of their own body shapes. They'll look at their emaciated bodies in the mirror and complain about how fat they are.

The condition can last for months or even years, and in some cases can lead to suicide or to metabolic disorders with fatal results. The patient may literally starve herself to death. Repeated vomiting can result in potassium loss, which can cause heart failure. Anorexia must be classed as a serious disease, and treated seriously by all those involved. There are those – perhaps 10 per cent of sufferers – who recover well, after a few months of treatment. For the rest anorexia can be a lifelong problem, with periods of illness and remission. Treatment is difficult and involves not only feeding the patient up, but attempting to uncover and alleviate the psychological problems that have led to her weight phobia. Even after she has left hospital a patient must be given proper outpatient support while she re-establishes a normal eating pattern.

MIND
AND
BODY

STRESS IN YOUR LIFE: The choice is yours

Stress is both externally and internally generated: in the former case usually by change, in the latter by conflict between our real and fantasy worlds. Throughout this chapter the word 'stress' is used to mean any stimulus that harms the body but it must be emphasized at the outset that stress isn't always harmful. Indeed, a *degree* of stress is necessary to rouse and maintain enthusiasm for activity; too little stimulus results in a sense of flatness, which can lead to inertia or apathy. Not only can the right amount of stress help to raise performance level, but it can be both enjoyable and exhilarating. A challenging job, for example, is a stimulus in itself and its successful completion resolves the stress factor. It's only if the pressure goes beyond a healthy stimulus that problems arise.

While it's impossible to determine the optimum amount of stress people in general can take – even the death of a loved one will produce very different degrees of response from different people – it's important to get to know your own tolerance level. That may sound easy but in practice it can be difficult because the relationship between any stress factor and you is a highly complex one, governed by all kinds of variables, including individual attitudes and beliefs. It is of course difficult to evaluate your own attitudes and beliefs honestly and objectively. But the way you cope with stress depends on them to a great extent and you may well need to re-examine and change them if you are to avoid serious harm to your health.

Fantasy versus reality

If there's a close degree of harmony between the world as it is and the world as you feel it ought to be, stress is absent. If reality and your fantasy differ widely and wildly, then stress is present and a number of reactions are possible. There may be mild irritation. To take an example: you're waiting for a train and the train's late; your reaction is that it shouldn't be. Reality as it's perceived is that the train is late; reality as fantasized is that trains should always be on time: your irritation results from the failure of reality to match your fantasy. The greater your degree of helplessness, the stronger your reaction. If nothing can be done and the delay means you will miss an important appointment, then the amount of stress created may be extremely high. Lack of opportunity for releasing these pent-up emotions produces harmful consequences. If, however, you can telephone and explain why you will be late, you will reduce the stress. If you can – and do – take another form of transport, and thus avoid being late altogether, although you may remain annoyed, the stress will have disappeared.

The key to avoiding the harmful effect lies in recognizing whether or not you can do anything to resolve the situation and if so, doing it, and if not, accepting reality.

Living in the present

Uncertainty about the future is a common source of stress. The future is unknown; therefore whatever you fantasize becomes, in your own mind, reality, and you can generate enormous degrees of stress worrying about events that, in fact, may never happen. Part of the solution to this lies in learning to live in the present and, while paying due regard to practical preparation for future events, not allowing your imagination to start drifting towards 'what if such and such happens...'. Concentrate your attention on present activities; meditation can help with this (see pages 238–39).

A matter of choice

Everyone has the ability to react to external stresses in a variety of ways. The response is always a matter of personal choice, even though it might appear to be otherwise. You can choose to feel angry, jealous, guilty, bitter, hating and so on, and you can choose to be happy, giving, forgiving and loving, whatever the external stimulus may be. At the very worst you can learn to accept what can't be altered and to tackle constructively what can be changed. Suggestions for ways of learning how to alter responses are given on pages 197–202.

Relationships

Personal relationships are fraught with stress pitfalls. Misunderstandings, unconscious expectations, feelings of inadequacy or of being taken for granted all generate emotional tension. It's never possible to solve all interpersonal problems since the other person may not be open to reasonable overtures. However, the important thing is to deal with others as you would want to be dealt with; again turn to pages 197–202 for ways of preventing or dissipating emotional tension.

External sources of stress

Apart from the list of factors in the table overleaf compiled by Drs. Holmes and Rahe of Washington Medical School, other external stress factors exist which, while not difficult to identify, are less easy to put on a scale. These include excessive noise; excessive heat or cold; repetitive occupations; and such experiences as commuting on an unreliable transport system or having to drive in heavy traffic for hours every day. Extreme external stress factors are often endured by people in potentially dangerous jobs.

Environmental stress

Research is currently being done into two aspects of what might be called environmental stress. These are the effects of positive ions in the atmosphere and lack of full spectrum light.

Ions

The air contains electrically charged molecules, known as ions. Some are negatively charged, others positively. In the main these ions are inhaled but some are absorbed through the skin. In fresh country air there are usually between 1000 and 2000 ions per cubic cm with a ratio of positive to negative of about 5 to 4, the normal balance between positive and negative ions. In cities, however, there are often fewer than 100 ions per cubic cm and the ratio of positive to negative ions increases to about 2 to 1.

Ions are destroyed by smoke, atmospheric pollution, dust and breathing, and can be trapped by synthetic carpets, television screens, man-made fibres, and air-conditioning and heating units; negative ions are particularly susceptible.

171

Generally speaking, people feel better in areas of high negative ion concentration, for instance at the seaside or in the mountains, and rather worse – heavy, lethargic and depressed – when there's a high concentration of positive ions, as in a smoky, centrally-heated room, before a thunderstorm or during seasonal wind periods such as the mistral of southern France.

It seems that although most people cope with ion imbalance, for some, excessive positive ions can bring about hormonal changes in the body. For instance, they may stimulate the over-production of

STRESS OF ADJUSTING TO CHANGE OVER PREVIOUS SIX MONTHS

Events that bring change are the source of most external stress factors. In the U.S.A. a sample list has been compiled by Drs. Thomas Holmes and Richard Rahe of Washington Medical School.

Scores are added up to give a 'stress level'. Differences in individual personalities and behaviour must be borne in mind when assessing scores. A score of 160 or more on this list indicates a high probability of health being affected. The key word here is 'probability'. It cannot be over-emphasized how very differently people react to stress. In some cases scores of 400 plus have been shown to have no apparent effect on health.

Remember it's not just one situation but continual stress that leads to problems, so if it's feasible, space your changes as much as you can. Often, however, you won't have control over events, so the objective is to adapt your response to them. This section of the book is designed to help you learn how to go about doing that so that you can minimize the effects of stress and so avoid stress-induced ill health.

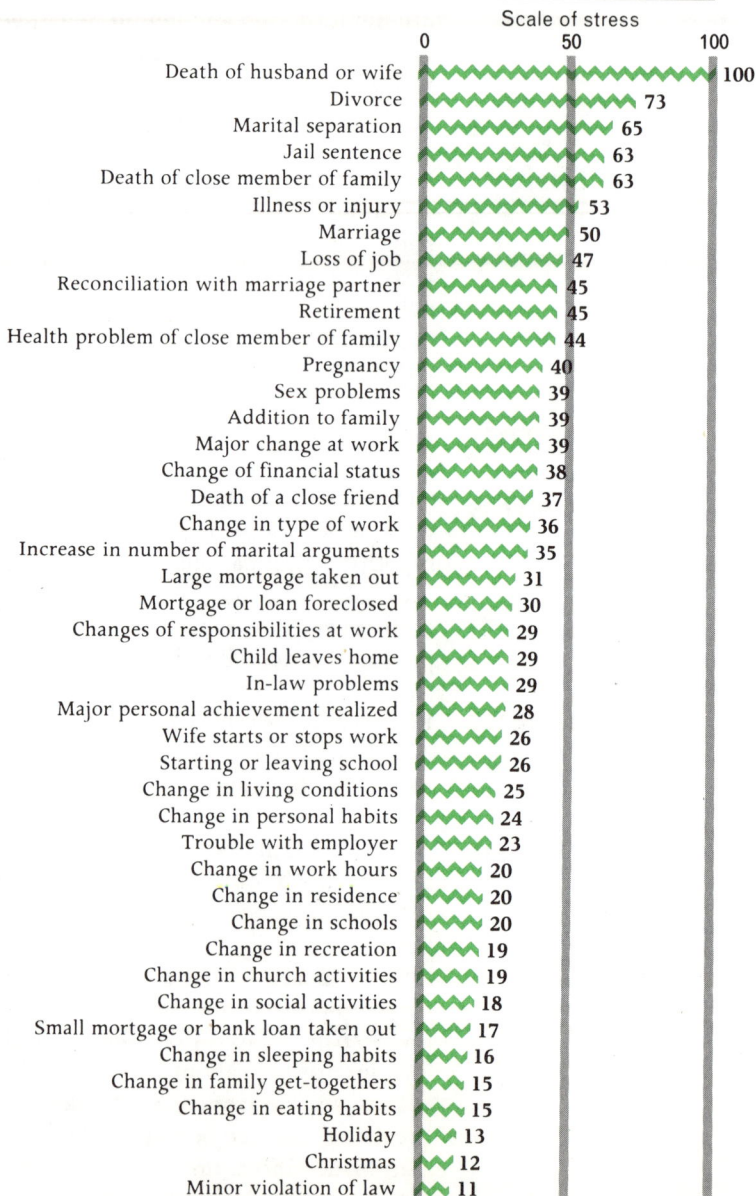

Scale of stress

Event	Score
Death of husband or wife	100
Divorce	73
Marital separation	65
Jail sentence	63
Death of close member of family	63
Illness or injury	53
Marriage	50
Loss of job	47
Reconciliation with marriage partner	45
Retirement	45
Health problem of close member of family	44
Pregnancy	40
Sex problems	39
Addition to family	39
Major change at work	39
Change of financial status	38
Death of a close friend	37
Change in type of work	36
Increase in number of marital arguments	35
Large mortgage taken out	31
Mortgage or loan foreclosed	30
Changes of responsibilities at work	29
Child leaves home	29
In-law problems	29
Major personal achievement realized	28
Wife starts or stops work	26
Starting or leaving school	26
Change in living conditions	25
Change in personal habits	24
Trouble with employer	23
Change in work hours	20
Change in residence	20
Change in schools	20
Change in recreation	19
Change in church activities	19
Change in social activities	18
Small mortgage or bank loan taken out	17
Change in sleeping habits	16
Change in family get-togethers	15
Change in eating habits	15
Holiday	13
Christmas	12
Minor violation of law	11

Two types of ionizer for home or work (1) and (2) and a smaller model for the car (3).

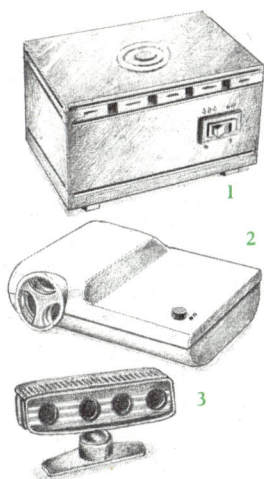

histamine, the hormone that increases liability to allergies. They may also increase the production of serotonin, a hormone that creates mood changes and affects sleep and nerve function; an excess results in insomnia, breathlessness and headaches. Although most people are capable of neutralizing this excess, in some the effects are very upsetting. (It should also be pointed out that too little serotonin, as well as too much, can produce insomnia; see page 206.) Another change that can take place, if exposure to the ion imbalance in the atmosphere is prolonged, is the gradual build-up of adrenalin. Although a little adrenalin is beneficial and promotes a sense of well-being and alertness, a build-up over a period of time can produce all the classic stress symptoms (see pages 175–79).

For people who are affected by a lack of negative ions, replacing them by means of a machine called an ionizer can be the answer. These machines are relatively cheap, small and can be carried around and plugged into any room. Anyone who has a generally low level of health that fails to respond to improved nutrition, exercise and relaxation, as outlined in this book, would do well to investigate this simple answer to a complex problem.

Full spectrum light

Like any other nutrient, light can be refined and the result will be, for some, ill health and a greater susceptibility to stress. Light consists of waves of radiant energy that is measured in wavelengths. Sunlight contains all the wavelengths, including those of all the visible colours plus infra-red (heat) and ultra-violet. These provide the total electromagnetic spectrum but with the development of artificial light and the tendency to spend a great deal of time in an environment where only parts of this spectrum are available, access to full spectrum light has diminished. Windshields, spectacles and glass in windows all block part of the spectrum, and further distortion is caused by tinted glasses and contact lenses as well as a polluted atmosphere.

At the University of Michigan, Dr. Joseph Meites has found that the retina contains photoreceptor cells that convert light into chemical energy, which is transmitted, via neurochemical pathways, to the pineal and pituitary glands. These control the entire hormone-producing system of the body.

Dramatic behavioural improvement was noted among hyperactive children when full-spectrum fluorescent lighting was installed in place of standard lighting. General health improvements were also noted. Full spectrum light does appear to be a vital need of the body and it's advisable to spend at least half an hour outdoors each day without glasses. If this isn't possible, being by an open window during daylight is the next best thing.

Minimizing the load

Because stress is cumulative, a relatively minor event, when added to a large existing stress load, will often prove to be more than the body's adaptation processes (see pages 175–77) can cope with. The smooth functioning of these processes can all too easily be undermined by

173

abuse of aspects of daily life that everyone can in fact control: personal habits and lifestyle, the amount, or quality, of exercise, nutrition, rest, relaxation and sleep.

Sleep The value of rest and sleep cannot be overestimated. Their importance is explained on pages 204–06 but it's worth emphasizing here that while stress can result in disturbance of the regular sleep pattern and lead to insomnia, the converse is also true – sleep disturbance creates stress and promotes depression.

Muscle tension This may result from emotional stress but it may also be caused by lack of exercise, poor posture or habitual working positions such as hunching over a desk all day. Such muscular tension feeds back impulses via the nervous system and activates the central nervous system so that mental relaxation is prevented. In other words, just as mental states can create physical tension, so a prolonged degree of muscular tension can influence the emotional or mental state. Physical exercise, as well as relaxation techniques and deep massage or manipulation of the soft tissues, can reduce such tension (turn to pages 208–10 for methods of muscle relaxation and to pages 221–35 for massage techniques).

Diet Imbalanced nutrition is all too often a root cause of a general feeling of being below par and can lower the body's resistance to stress. Despite this, in the developed world the principles of a balanced diet are often ignored. For example, sugar consumption has shot up over the past 100 years or so; not only does sugar provide a lot of calories without any nutrients, but the over-consumption of foods containing highly refined sugar can lead to the condition known as hypoglycaemia (low blood sugar), which produces wild swings in mood and behaviour. Characteristic symptoms include: hypersensitivity, irritability, argumentativeness, dizziness and fatigue. If your blood sugar count is low, you will react unpredictably to external stress factors.

Too low an intake of fresh, unprocessed foods especially vegetables, fruit, pulses, whole grains and nuts (the diet may be the same as that leading to hypoglycaemia) can result in a vitamin deficiency, in which a string of interrelated vitamins, minerals and enzymes is lacking. This creates an internal environment that prevents the body from countering stress adequately and also lowers general levels of bodily function to such an extent that a whole range of apparently unrelated minor symptoms coincide to produce a general feeling of unwellness, which is in itself a stress factor. Such a feeling is often accompanied by insomnia, poor appetite, depression, nervousness and oversensitivity (see pages 178–79). Turn to pages 129–31 and 138–49 for guidelines on how to balance your diet and so counter or prevent such symptoms.

By taking care of these aspects of your daily life, which are the easiest to alter, you'll be going a long way towards equipping yourself to counter stress.

How the body reacts to stress

The body strives constantly to be efficient and to attain an equilibrium, known as homeostasis, in which the various body systems work harmoniously in response to the demands made on them, whether the demands are generated internally or externally. Should such demands be noxious or potentially harmful to the body, they're generally called stress factors. These range from such obvious stimuli as excessive noise, heat or cold to more subtle, internal worries such as imagined threats, or fears that result from prolonged anxiety.

Fight or flight reaction

Whatever the stress factor, the body's response follows a predictable pattern. This response has been called the 'fight or flight' reaction because what the body is doing is preparing either to fight or to run away. Along with a rapid increase in metabolism, hormonal, physiological and biochemical changes take place, almost instantaneously.

During the 'fight or flight' reaction, the muscles of the body tense, as if preparing for activity. The part of the brain known as the hypothalamus, which is a coordinating centre for the multitude of body functions not normally under voluntary control, receives the alarm message and calls into play the hormonal function of the master gland, the pituitary (also in the brain). The hormones produced by the pituitary gland mobilize other hormone-producing areas, notably the adrenal glands, which release adrenalin and noradrenalin to keep the 'fight or flight' reaction going. These, in turn, bring about a series of physiological changes that are necessary for activity to take place in response to the stress stimulus.

So that the muscles can work properly they need glucose, and the liver responds to this by releasing some of its store into the bloodstream, which carries it to the muscles. The glucose has to be transformed into energy, so the blood also carries the necessary oxygen. The heart, of course, has to pump harder for the blood to reach the parts where it's most needed, which leads to a rise in blood pressure. Breathing becomes faster so the lungs can take in extra oxygen.

As the amount of blood in the body is limited, it has to be diverted to the priority areas – muscles, heart, lungs and brain. Consequently, there's a temporary 'shutdown' in other areas: for example, the digestive system slows up or stops altogether; the salivary glands dry up; the blood vessels in the kidneys and abdomen constrict; the immune system, which deals with infection, becomes less active.

Changes take place in the skin, too; see page 176 for details of this and further changes.

All this is appropriate if the stress factor is best dealt with by physical action. For instance, if the source of stress is a hostile dog running towards you, you'll need all the help your body can give, and fast, as you dash for safety. Once you're safe, the body swiftly reverses the process and no harm is done. But today physical responses such as running away may not be appropriate and when the whole complex mechanism is brought into play repeatedly by a form of stress incapable of being physically – or even psychologically – resolved, then

175

The fight or flight reaction

This is the body's initial reaction to stress. If the problem is solved and the tension released, all is well. But if stress occurs repeatedly without resolution the result can be great damage to health.

1 Muscles tense – as a reflex action.

2 The hypothalamus, a complex of nerve cells in the brain, receives the message of danger and acts to coordinate body functions. It stimulates the pituitary gland, which activates other glands, notably the adrenals, to produce hormones.

3 The hormones produce the bodily changes shown below.

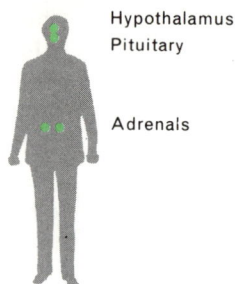

Hypothalamus
Pituitary

Adrenals

INCREASED ACTIVITY

Eyes
The pupils dilate.

Lungs
The lungs need to take in more air, to provide extra oxygen for the tense muscles, and to get rid of more carbon dioxide, so breathing speeds up.

Heart
The heart pumps more vigorously to get blood round the body to the tense muscles. Because the heart is working harder and pumping faster, blood pressure rises.

Liver
The liver releases some of its store of glucose to provide the necessary fuel for the muscles; this reaches them through the bloodstream and is transformed into energy by oxygen.
It may also overproduce cholesterol, discharging this excess into the bloodstream.

Skin
The skin gets ready to cool down; in anticipation of overheating, which will result from conflict, the skin sweats. There's also a tendency to turn pale as a result of blood being diverted to muscles and of the capillary blood vessels, near the skin's surface, constricting.

Muscles
The tense muscles give off lactic acid, so increasing the amount in the blood and heightening anxiety.

DECREASED ACTIVITY

Saliva
The salivary glands stop producing saliva, so the mouth dries up.

Kidneys
The blood vessels in the kidneys constrict.

Digestive system
Digestion slow down or stops altogether. The stomach and intestines stop working.

Rectum
The sphincter muscles at the end of the rectum close, to prevent urination or defaecation. Sometimes, however, the reverse happens, and there's involuntary urination or even diarrhoea. This results from an overreaction by the parasympathetic nerves, the part of the nervous system responsible for restoring the body to normality after the emergency.

Immune system
The immune system is subdued – in its normal active state, it would be a hindrance rather than a help in a situation calling for fighting or fleeing.

the 'fight or flight' mechanism can become the cause of great damage to the body. Build-up without resolution means there's nothing to trigger off the wind-down to normality and you stay wound up. Although the 'fight or flight' reaction has been part of man's survival kit throughout history and has enabled those equipped with the best response to survive, it hasn't itself adapted to the more subtle form of stress reaction required in a modern competitive society.

Adaptation stage

The stress spiral
The slide down the spiral begins when acute reactions start to be chronic. The exhaustion stage at the bottom of the spiral is reached when the body's adaptive powers can keep going no longer. However, the downwards slide need not be inexorable: there's a lot you can do to get back to the top. The nearer the top you start, the easier it is.

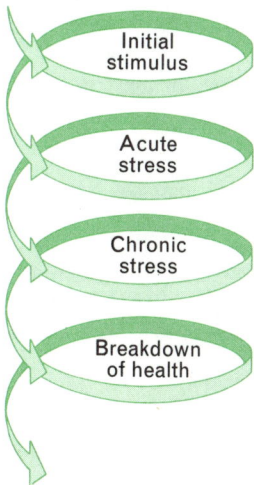

Initial
stimulus

Acute
stress

Chronic
stress

Breakdown
of health

When stress occurs repeatedly over a long period without resolution, a second stage of stress – the adaptation stage – is reached. Many of the changes that took place in the acute 'fight or flight' phase become chronic – they take place all the time – so that they're working against, rather than for, you.

The maintenance of constricted blood vessels and high blood pressure can lead to the high blood pressure (hypertension) becoming permanent; circulatory problems involving the heart may start to appear. Since your digestive system functions more slowly or stops altogether when stress arousal occurs, there is a tendency in the adaptation, or chronic, phase for such conditions as stomach or duodenal ulceration, colitis, diarrhoea or constipation to develop. Chronic muscular tensions can produce a multitude of musculoskeletal aches and pains as well as severe headaches. The sustained or repetitive stress stimulus impairs the working of the body's defence mechanisms, which makes infection and allergic symptoms more likely. The likelihood of nervous symptoms such as phobias also becomes greater. For a fuller discussion of stress-related conditions, see pages 180–83.

During the adaptation phase there is a dramatic contrast between what the individual intends to achieve and what the now malfunctioning system is capable of achieving. There is a general level of 'underperformance', which can, of course, lead to feelings of guilt, self-doubt and insecurity. Job performance declines, libido will often disappear and personal relationships are strained. All of this creates further stress at a time when the person is least able to cope with it.

Just how long this phase can go on without a major mental or physical breakdown depends upon inherited constitutional factors; basic health habits such as diet and exercise; and the degree of emotional support provided by family and friends. The adaptation phase can last 10, 15 or 20 years, or it may be brief, depending on many different factors, such as the ones mentioned above.

Exhaustion stage

If action can be taken at the adaptation stage to alter either the stress factors or the reactions to them, then the final exhaustion phase can still be avoided. However, if action isn't taken before the adaptation phase ends, exhaustion follows; the body, no longer able to cope, collapses into disease of one form or another. Being able to recognize the signs of stress and knowing how to escape from the vicious acute-adaptation-exhaustion spiral is therefore of the utmost importance.

177

Signs of stress

Some of the symptoms below may derive from causes other than stress, but if several are present concurrently, stress is probably a major factor in their origin. Remember that the mind and body are inter-related to such an extent that mental symptoms are unlikely to be present without physical ones too. Before looking at these early physical and mental signs of stress, note the commonest signs of dietary deficiency; if there is such a deficiency, the likelihood of stress damaging the system is greater.

If you're in any doubt about the significance of any of the symptoms – dietary, physical or mental – consult a suitable practitioner. If that practitioner advises tranquillizers or other medication aimed at masking the symptoms, insist on seeing a health professional who will attempt to unravel the causes.

Symptoms of dietary deficiency
1 Changes in skin texture such as dryness and tendency to crack and flake, especially on thighs and lower abdomen
2 Tongue and inner lips bright red instead of a softer pink colour
3 Cracks at corner of mouth
4 Scaling of skin at wings of nose
5 Ridged nails that become brittle or soft
6 Receding gums that bleed easily after brushing
7 Thin and lifeless hair with scurfy scalp
8 Tendency to swelling of lower legs, especially on inner surface
9 Increased tendency to bruise
10 Diminished vitality as evidenced by apathy and listlessness
11 Cuts and grazes that are slow to heal

Physical symptoms of stress
1 Lack of appetite
2 Craving for food when under pressure
3 Frequent indigestion, such as heartburn
4 Constipation or diarrhoea
5 Insomnia
6 Constant tiredness
7 Tendency to sweat for no good reason
8 Nervous 'tics' and tendency to touch face, hair, moustache repeatedly
9 Nail-biting
10 Headaches
11 Cramps and muscle spasms
12 Nausea
13 Feelings of breathlessness without exertion
14 Fainting spells
15 Frequent crying or desire to cry
16 Impotence or frigidity
17 Inability to sit still without fidgeting
18 High blood pressure

3+

2+ Warning
If more than three of the dietary deficiency symptoms are present plus two or more of the physical symptoms, the adaptation stage is operating (see page 177) and it's time to take appropriate action.

5

3+ Warning
If more than three of these symptoms are present at the same time, you could well have a deficiency problem.

Action 2
First analyse the causes of the symptoms (see pages 170–74). Then turn to pages 197–202 for advice on how to adjust your lifestyle in order to minimize and counteract stress. This advice, combined with a sound and balanced diet, adequate exercise, and regular practice of relaxation techniques, provides a starting point for tackling most stress conditions successfully.

Action 1
All these can be remedied by balancing the diet as suggested in Eating naturally, pages 129–31, or as outlined on pages 138–49.

Do you see anything familiar about these? If any of them remind you of yourself, you could be in trouble. The time to tackle symptoms of stress is as soon as you're aware of them – the longer you ignore them, the harder it will be to restore yourself to a state of relaxed well-being. The checklists on this and the previous page will help you spot such symptoms.

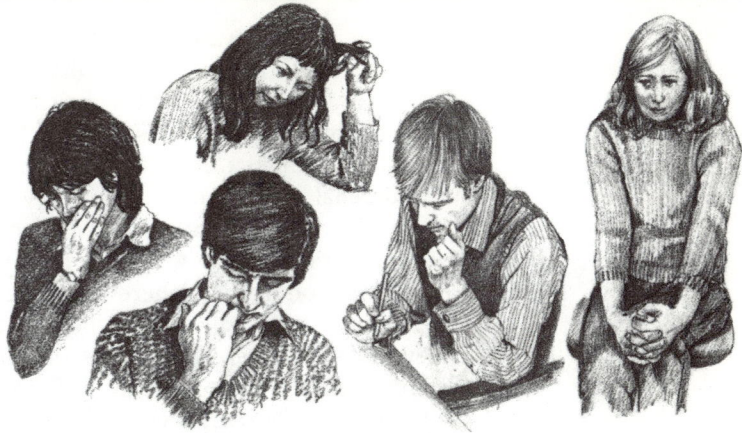

Mental symptoms of stress

1 Constant feelings of irritability with people
2 Frequent feelings of helplessness and being unable to cope
3 Lack of interest in life
4 Constant or recurrent fear of disease
5 A feeling of being a failure
6 A feeling of being bad, including self-hatred
7 Difficulty in making decisions
8 A feeling that your appearance has altered and that you are ugly
9 Loss of interest in other people
10 Awareness of suppressed rage or anger because of inability, for whatever reason, to show your true feelings
11 Difficulty in letting go and laughing
12 A feeling of being the target of other people's animosity
13 A feeling of having been neglected or let down by people you rely on
14 Dread of the future
15 A feeling of having failed as a partner or parent
16 A feeling of having no one whom you can really confide in
17 Difficulty in concentrating
18 The inability to finish one task properly before having to rush on to the next
19 An intense fear of open or enclosed space or of being alone

5 **5**

Warning
If five symptoms from either the mental or physical category are present, or if there is a combined total of five symptoms, remedial action is essential.

Action 3
There's still a great deal that you yourself can do to restore your mental and physical state to normal, because in all probability no irreversible changes will yet have occurred. So, follow the action plan outlined in Action 2, all of which is intended to be complementary to psychotherapy, whether on an individual or a group basis, should this be necessary.

Above all, if you can regard the symptoms in a positive light, as a warning, a challenge to be met, you'll gain real benefits from tackling the causes of stress.

When illness signals red

Long-term stress results in ill-health which can take the form of physical or mental disease, or both. Stress, and the way the body adapts to it, is one of the major causes of such chronic illnesses as heart and circulatory disease; hypertension (high blood pressure); asthma; rheumatoid arthritis; eczema; migraine; depression; colitis; gastric and duodenal ulcers, and digestive dysfunction in general. A link is also suspected between mental attitudes related to stress and the development of cancer. Although it's by no means the only cause of any of these conditions – there's often an inherited tendency towards a particular problem, and other factors, including imbalanced nutrition, lack of exercise and infection are involved in the production of chronic disease – stress is an ill-defined common factor.

The degree of stress to which the body is exposed and the way it reacts often depend upon personality traits. There is mounting evidence of the role of personality and character in the development of serious ill-health.

Cancer Dr. W. Herberger, the German cancer specialist, has noted that chronic anger, disappointment, fear and the inability to cope with misfortune all play a role in the development of cancer. Further research into the attitudes of cancer patients has shown that a disproportionate number display a tendency to dwell on past bereavements and real, or imagined, misfortunes. They also seem to have little sense of the future when compared with other patients who are seriously ill but not suffering from cancer.

Dr. Hans Moolenburg, a Dutch physician who has done a great deal of work with cancer patients, found that such people had often been buffeted by fate, having endured a series of personal shocks and emotional disasters. Indeed, some psychologists have gone so far as to describe cancer as 'a socially acceptable way of committing suicide': a way of escaping from the stresses of life without actively destroying oneself. However, while this may be true of some cancer patients, it's certainly not true of all. Dr. Hans Nieper, head physician at Silbersee Hospital, Hanover, and an international expert on cancer, speaks of the need for cancer patients to display intelligent and positive co-operation in their treatment. In his experience, this marks out the patients who recover from cancer, or in whom the disease is controlled, from those who simply fade away. Similarly, when the radiologist Dr. Carl Simonton was chief of radiation therapy at Travis Air Force Base in the U.S.A., he observed that some patients, for no obvious clinical reason, made better recoveries than others; after analysis he found that the patients who recovered were those who possessed a stronger will to live and a more hopeful attitude towards both the disease and life itself.

In general, four main types of attitude have been defined among cancer patients: aggressive motivation towards cure; bland denial of the disease; stoic acceptance; hopelessness and helplessness. Good recovery is significantly more common among patients who have responded in either of the first two ways; and research is currently trying to discover what it is that promotes or prevents these responses, with the aim of helping patients to develop them.

Whether or not there is a 'cancer type', the evidence points to stress and, more importantly, the way stress is reacted to, as being instrumental in predisposing a person towards serious illness, be it cancer or anything else.

Hypertension

Stress plays a more obvious role in some conditions than others – in high blood pressure, for instance. As has been discussed in the section How the body reacts, long-term stress results in the quite normal raising of blood pressure, in response to a stimulus, becoming chronic, simply by virtue of constant repetition. However, more than 40 per cent of those affected can control their condition – once the causes have been understood – by changing their lifestyle and embarking on a regime that includes adequate rest and sleep.

According to Dr. Peter Nixon, senior consultant cardiologist at Charing Cross Hospital, London, pharmaceutical drugs are unsatisfactory in the treatment of hypertension because, while they may reduce blood pressure, they don't deal with the underlying causes of exhaustion and over-arousal. If the causes aren't tackled, the patient faces the prospect of taking, for the rest of his life, drugs with considerable side effects.

Digestive disorders

Most people have experienced minor digestive upsets or diarrhoea as a result of an upset or anxiety – the connection between emotions and the digestive system is clearly recognized. A variety of symptoms may be the result of long-term stress and anxiety. These include derangements of bowel function such as constipation or diarrhoea, or more often an alternation between these two extremes. There is often spasmodic, colicky pain anywhere in the abdomen but more frequently low in the bowel. Many people experience a feeling of abdominal fullness and nausea. Another common symptom is difficulty in swallowing and a feeling of a 'lump in the throat'. All these symptoms of digestive disorders are often accompanied by other evidence of stress.

Once organic disease has been ruled out and obvious dietary factors have been eliminated as a cause, the most successful treatment of these conditions begins with a discussion of the lifestyle of the person and any stressful relationships. This can be done with a sympathetic friend or doctor. The next step is to bring about an improvement in lifestyle and normalize any relationships that are causing stress. According to Dr. John Fielding, a consultant physician at Jervis Street Hospital, Dublin, drug therapy in such cases is on the whole disappointing. He does, however, emphasize that it's important for the patient to realize his condition is not 'all in the mind' simply because there's no evidence of actual organic disease. Indeed Dr. Fielding urges that the distinction made by many doctors between organic and

181

functional (psychosomatic) disorders be re-examined, because many problems that begin as functional end up as organic. Gastric and duodenal ulcers are the most obvious examples of early functional problems becoming organic lesions.

Multiple sclerosis

This disease, together with clinical depression (see below), serves to illustrate the effects of stress on the central nervous system. In multiple sclerosis, which runs a variable course, there's often a connection between relapses and stress caused by over-exertion, infection or emotional upsets. Strange as it may seem, even going on holiday can produce sufficient added stress to provoke a relapse. It should be recalled that all change presents a degree of challenge to the body's adaptive mechanisms and this is stressful. Adequate sleep and rest periods during the day will, however, minimize such risks in multiple sclerosis patients.

Clinical depression

Reactions to stress are frequently the underlying cause of clinical depression. In this withdrawn state of mind any effort on the part of the patient to regain normal health becomes impossible and professional help is necessary. A battery of symptoms may be present, ranging from palpitations, tingling legs and arms, hot flushes, headaches, digestive disturbance and lack of appetite to uncontrollable weeping and a tendency towards intense self-pity or self-blame.

The depression may result from an inability to cope with life's demands: it will almost certainly reduce the ability to cope with life. People can become depressed when they distort events, infer self-blame from them and draw illogical and unfavourable conclusions about themselves. As discussed on pages 170–71, much stress is the result of a mis-match between the physical and psychological demands of life and the individual's ability to deal with them, a mis-match that in turn often stems from a discrepancy between the world as it is and the world as the individual thinks it ought to be.

Some cases of depression can be thought of as a way of opting out of what is seen as an intolerable situation. Collapsing into a depression appears to be one way of avoiding the problem: the act of suicide is an even greater act of avoidance.

Depression causes changes in behaviour as the person attempts to cope. The new behaviour replaces the normal pattern of behaviour and may be accepted by those near to the individual. It may attract sympathy and in consequence be more difficult to change. Phobias and neuroses can grow out of such a situation. If, because of anxiety, a particular situation is avoided, then a phobia might well develop by repetition of this action. 'I might faint, therefore I won't go out where people might see me' results in avoidance of going out. The same (unconscious) thought, repeated each time the possibility of going out of the house is mentioned, results in an intense fear of going out, a phobia. The true fear is perhaps of fainting and making a spectacle of yourself, but the fear becomes transferred to going out.

Understanding the cause of this type of irrational fear is part of the cure. The actual cure comes when the individual learns to modify behaviour, to do gradually what is feared and, finding that no harm results, abandons the fear. This takes time, patience and the use of relaxation and other 'mind' exercises.

Drug therapy can control clinical depression (for another form of depression known as endogenous depression, caused by a chemical imbalance in the body, drugs are the only effective means of control – even then there's a likelihood that the illness will recur). In the long run, in cases of clinical depression, only a coming to terms with reality will bring about a cure. Counselling or psychotherapy may be required to effect self-understanding and a recognition of the relationships between behaviour, attitudes and stress.

To sum up, although stress can't be pinpointed as the sole contributory factor in the chronic illnesses and disorders discussed above, it does play a major role, in some cases influencing the duration and direction of the illnesses. It makes sense therefore to recognize this potential for harm and to take steps to counter stress and tackle it positively. When the early stress signs appear, the chance for successful remedial action is at its best. When a breakdown, either physical or mental, has occurred, the task is harder and expert professional advice is essential. Even then, however, there's still an enormous amount you can do. Indeed, there's always something you yourself can do if you're prepared to make the effort – after all, it's your life.

Various systems have been developed linking certain personality traits with tendencies towards particular diseases and ailments. One such system is that evolved by Dr. Ray H. Rosenman and Dr. Meyer Friedman of California, who have linked certain behaviour patterns with proneness to coronary heart disease. They divide people into two categories, Type A and Type B, on the basis of their behaviour, Type A people being three times more prone to heart attacks than Type B. However, Type A people can lessen the risk of heart attacks dramatically by changing their behaviour so that it more closely resembles that of Type B. Below is a selection of the main characteristics of the two types. If half or more of the type A ones fit your personality you're a Type A.

Type A	Type B
1 Eager to compete	1 Not competitive (in sport or business)
2 Forceful personality	2 Retiring and easygoing personality
3 Gets things done quickly	3 Does things methodically and slowly
4 Constantly striving for promotion in business or advancement in society	4 Content with present position in business and social life
5 Eager for public recognition	5 No desire for fame or public recognition
6 Easily angered by people and events	6 Slow to anger
7 Gets reckless when idle	7 Enjoys periods of doing nothing
8 Speaks quickly and explosively	8 Speaks slowly
9 Thrives when thinking and being involved in more than one thing at a time	9 Copes well with only one thought or activity at a time
10 Moves, walks and eats quickly	10 Moves, walks and eats without rush
11 Impatient and angered when delayed	11 Not upset by delay
12 Very time-conscious, likes to have deadlines and to beat them	12 Not time-conscious, ignores deadlines

THE COMMON PROPS : Smoking

Why, despite the mounting evidence that smoking is a health hazard, do people continue to smoke? Although very little is known, still, about the underlying causes, there are a few clues worth noting.

The most frequent reasons given by young people for starting to smoke are: they wanted to satisfy their curiosity; they wanted to be like their friends; and they were 'offered a cigarette'. A connection has been established between children beginning to smoke and the smoking habits of the immediate family: children of parents who are smokers are twice as likely to smoke as children of non-smokers, or ex-smokers.

Social and cultural factors are a major influence in smoking, as they are in other habits such as drinking tea, coffee and alcohol. Smoking is a social lubricant, among other smokers.

Smokers claim that smoking produces a sense of relaxation and that it aids concentration. Whereas the latter claim has been almost impossible to test experimentally, it's been shown, as stated in the British Royal College of Physicians report (1977), that inhaling tobacco smoke 'reduces tension in voluntary muscles, making them less responsive to reflex stimulation'. Feelings of fatigue are certainly reduced, but only very slightly, as a result of the release of catecholamines, neurotransmitters, which are hormone-like substances, produced in the nerve endings and the adrenal medulla. This apparent benefit is, however, short-lived. Tests to determine differences in speed of intellectual reaction between smokers and non-smokers seem to show that the subjective attitudes and personality of the smoker are of more significance than any direct pharmacological response. Moreover, if the smoker believes the cigarette will make him more alert, or relaxed, then it will, briefly. The belief is reinforced by continuing the habit.

Psychiatrists have suggested various unconscious forces that may cause smoking. These include: oral gratification; for men, the impression that it's macho to smoke, an impression heavily reinforced by advertising, the cinema, and TV; and feelings of deprivation after breastfeeding ceased. It's also been suggested that some people have a behavioural compulsion to set fire to things, which may have something to do with the attraction of smoking. It's thought, too, that starting to smoke when young may be a rebellious act of defiance.

Personality types

Heavy smokers (those who smoke more than 20 cigarettes a day) tend to be restless, intense and energetic as compared with the more dependable, steadier and quieter non-smokers. This correlates with Type A and Type B personalities (see page 183). American surveys have shown that smokers change jobs, enter hospital and take part in sport more often than non-smokers. This increased likelihood of participation in sport also correlates with Type A competitiveness. A U.K. survey has shown that, among smokers, cigarette smokers tend to be more extroverted and pipe smokers more introverted. It has also been suggested that both smoking habits and liability to lung cancer might result from hereditary predisposition.

WHY DO YOU SMOKE?

The reasons smokers give for smoking can be divided into six basic categories, given in bold type. (Note: Most smokers are cigarette smokers, but throughout the smoking section the general references to cigarettes apply to pipes and tobacco, too.)

To find out your main reasons for smoking, grade each statement accordingly:
5 always true
4 frequently true
3 occasionally true
2 almost never true
1 never true

Eleven or more in any one category is high; seven or below, low; in between, average. If your score is high in several categories, your motivation for smoking is complex, and stopping will be harder. If none of your scores is high, giving up should be relatively easy.

Stimulation
To stop myself slowing down.
To stimulate myself.
To give myself a lift.

If your score is high, a substitute activity such as vigorous physical exercise will help to break the smoking habit. By working even a short period of exercise into your daily routine, you'll feel more refreshed and alert mentally and physically.

Handling
I enjoy handling the cigarette.
I enjoy the various steps leading to lighting up.
I enjoy watching the smoke.

If this is your major reason for smoking, try other ways of keeping your hands busy – doodle or play with a pencil, key ring or worry beads.

Relaxation
Smoking is relaxing.
Smoking gives me pleasure.
I want a cigarette most when I'm relaxed and comfortable.

Smoking for relaxation or as a source of pleasure can be nullified by an honest consideration of the harmful and dangerous effects of the habit. An even more concrete way to stop is to practise one of the relaxation techniques on pages 208–40.

Tension
I smoke when I'm angry.
I smoke when I'm upset or uncomfortable.
I smoke if I'm feeling down or want to forget my worries.

If relieving tension is the motivating force, physical activity, together with a relaxation technique that you can draw upon in any periods of tension, will help.

Habit
I smoke automatically, and am not even aware of it.
At times I light up when I have a cigarette going.
I've smoked without remembering I've lit up.

If smoking is merely a habit, with little or no other motivation, awareness of what you're doing to yourself each time you light a cigarette will help you to become conscious of the futility of the habit and to break it.

Addiction
If I run out of cigarettes, I find it unbearable.
I'm conscious of the fact when I'm not smoking.
I yearn for a cigarette when I haven't smoked for a while.

If this is what keeps you smoking, you'll need to be strongly motivated to give up. You can reinforce your motivation by smoking double or even treble the quantity you normally smoke for several days beforehand to nauseate yourself with the poisons involved and then actually sweat out the withdrawal symptoms until the craving has gone. Severe withdrawal symptoms don't generally last longer than six weeks: most people are fine after three or four weeks. Remember, the symptoms *do* pass, the craving *does* go.

185

Hazards of smoking

Whether you opt for a pipe, cigar, filter-tip or non-filter cigarette, all forms of smoking have some things in common:
● There is always tobacco smoke. This is a complex mixture of gases and droplets containing nearly 1,000 identified chemical compounds.
● *Some* smoke, albeit very little in the case of pipe smokers, is always inhaled, even though the smoker might insist that he or she doesn't inhale.
● About half the inhaled smoke is retained in the lungs; some minute droplets are deposited directly on the walls of the bronchial tubes.
● While the constitution of tobacco smoke varies according to the type of tobacco and how it's processed, it always contains carbon monoxide, which, inhaled, displaces oxygen in the blood; tar, which in turn contains nicotine; and hundreds of other toxic chemical compounds. The lower the tar, the less of all these compounds – and nicotine – you take in. According to the British Government definition, a low-tar cigarette is one containing less than 10 mg of tar.

One cigarette produces between 1 and 3 mg of nicotine, depending on its composition and size, and on the variety of tobacco. The smoker who inhales absorbs as much as 95 per cent of this, whereas the would-be-non-inhaler may absorb as little as 10 per cent.

Effects of nicotine

Nicotine causes the surface blood vessels of the limbs to constrict and raises the blood pressure while speeding up the heart rate so that more blood leaves the heart faster. The digestive system and the muscular movement of the bowel at first speed up then slow down.

Nicotine impairs the absorption of vitamin C and, according to the Canadian scientist Dr. Omer Pelletier, destroys vitamin C already present in the blood; Dr. Pelletier suggests that 25 mg of vitamin C are needed to replace that lost by smoking one cigarette. Nicotine constricts the blood vessels of the mouth and prevents the phagocytes in them from working, thus increasing the chance of infection. (Phagocytes are the body's first line of defence against bacterial invasion.) It has been estimated that one cigarette puts this part of the defence mechanism out of action for 15 minutes.

Nicotine intake causes the pituitary gland to produce an anti-diuretic hormone, which reduces the quantity of urine passed. Adrenalin is also produced. (The temporary rise in the level of adrenalin produced by heavy smoking is between 27 and 77 per cent; individual reactions depend on a variety of factors, not least general state of health and regularity of smoking.)

Links with other common 'props'

Research evidence links smoking with an increased desire for caffeine and sugar. Smoking has also been linked with alcohol consumption: there are twice as many smokers among regular drinkers as among non-drinkers.

The combination of coffee, tea (and other caffeine-containing substances) or alcohol with a nicotine intake of 20 or more cigarettes a day places a marked strain on the body's ability to control and balance the blood sugar level. If the level is too high, the result is diabetes. For the effects of low blood sugar, see page 174.

Long-term dangers

Clearly, even moderate smoking impairs health. But the deleterious effects described above pale into insignificance beside the long-term dangers, probably the best known of which is lung cancer. The risks of suffering from this and from the other serious conditions listed below and overleaf are greatest for cigarette smokers, with the exception of cancers of the lips, mouth and tongue, where the risk is greater for pipe and cigar smokers.

Even though there's some argument that the link between smoking and heart disease may be coincidental, the diminishing risk (see table page 190) for those who give up cigarettes points particularly strongly to the direct effect of smoking on the health of the heart and arteries. In the U.S.A. the decrease in the number of deaths from heart disease since the mid-1960s is almost certainly due in part to a 25 per cent fall in the numbers of male smokers.

Despite research findings (see below), there are arguments against the link between lung cancer and tobacco, the principal one of which maintains that since only one in eight heavy smokers develops lung cancer, the case is weak. This argument supposes that cigarette smoking is the only contributory factor and this is obviously not so. Diet is thought to play a role in predisposing towards certain forms of cancer; there's a strong suspicion of a link between personality and outlook and the development of the disease; there may be an inherited tendency towards cancer, including that of the lungs, in certain people; and environmental factors, such as asbestos, may be implicated in some cases. However, although other factors may also play a part, this does not minimize the dangers of smoking.

Lung cancer
Research in numerous hospitals and clinics throughout the world has revealed that: the increase of lung cancer parallels the use of tobacco; inhaling tobacco smoke is associated with cancer of the trachea and lungs; the quicker a cigarette is smoked the more benzpyrene is produced. Benzpyrene is present in all tobacco smoke. It's contained in tar and is toxic. It covers the mucous surface of the breathing apparatus from the nose to the lungs and paralyses the cough reflex, which would normally cause an immediate cough in response to hot smoke being breathed in. In the morning, before the first cigarette is smoked, this reflex is functioning again, and the hacking and spitting characteristic of the 'smoker's cough' go on until the first cigarette suppresses the cough reflex. Ninety-five per cent of lung cancer patients are smokers and 70 per cent smoke more than 20 cigarettes a day. The chance of getting lung cancer increases dramatically as the rate of smoking goes up. Among non-smokers there is an incidence of about one in 220. In smokers the rate goes up to one in eight. The duration of smoking, that is, the age at which you start and how long you continue to smoke, also greatly affects the risk.

Chronic bronchitis
Heavy smokers are five times more likely to be admitted to hospital with chronic bronchitis than non-smokers. Although more men are afflicted than women, among men and women with similar smoking habits, the pattern of bronchial infection is much the same. There are other contributory factors, but cigarette smoking is a major one.

Emphysema
The cigarette smoker also takes in cadmium, a toxic metal, which can produce this chronic respiratory disease. Lung tissue loses its elasticity, and breathing becomes difficult.

Coronary heart disease
People who smoke a pack of cigarettes a day are twice as likely to die from coronary heart disease as non-smokers, and the greater the number of cigarettes smoked, the higher the risk. The greatest danger is for middle-aged men, but studies in the U.K., Ireland and Sweden have also shown a much higher proportion of smokers among middle-aged women who have had heart attacks.

The three leading causes of heart disease are high blood pressure, high levels of cholesterol in the blood and cigarette smoking, and a combination of these factors multiplies the separate risks. So it's especially important for smokers with high blood pressure or cholesterol to stop. However, if other risk factors are low, for example in physically active smokers with low blood cholesterol, the danger of a heart attack is slighter. It's also much lower in cigar and pipe smokers who inhale very little.

Thromboangiitis obliterans
Smoking is a major contributory factor. The blood flow, especially to the legs, is impaired; it often leads to gangrene, necessitating amputation. King George VI, a heavy smoker, suffered this fate.

Gastro-intestinal diseases
Smoking is seen as a perpetuating and irritating factor rather than the cause. One of the most obvious effects of smoking is the damping down of hunger pangs: it tends to reduce the secretion of gastric juices, the churning of the food in the stomach and the movement, by peristalsis, of material through the bowel. A study of patients suffering from such conditions as heartburn, nausea, flatulence and abdominal discomfort has shown that symptoms were greatly alleviated by stopping smoking. Extensive hospital studies have concluded that smoking interferes with the treatment and healing of gastric ulcers, thus making them more chronic and potentially more dangerous. Smokers who have ulcers are three times more likely to die as a direct result than non-smokers.

Cancer of the bladder
A definite link has been found – in men – between smoking and cancer of the bladder. Cigarette smokers who inhale deeply are most at risk. There's also evidence linking cigarette smoking with cancer of the prostate gland.

Stillbirth/low birth weight
Expectant mothers who smoke tend to produce children of lower birth weight than their non-smoking counterparts, with a higher incidence of neonatal deaths. There's also strong evidence that smoking mothers have a significantly greater number of pregnancies resulting in stillbirth. According to one research project quoted by the U.S. Department of Health, Education and Welfare, one out of every five unsuccessful pregnancies would have been successful if the prospective mother hadn't been a regular smoker.

Other conditions ranging from cirrhosis of the liver to a rare form of blindness (tobacco amblyopia), as well as cancer of the lips, tongue, palate, tonsils, pharynx and larynx, have also been associated with smoking.

Safety measures   It's more hazardous to smoke a high-tar brand of cigarettes than a low-tar one. Whatever the form of smoking, it's safer if there's no deep inhalation. Quite logically, the fewer cigarettes smoked the less risk. Certainly from the viewpoint of lung cancer and heart disease, it's safer to smoke cigars or a pipe. However, while pipes and cigars are not as harmful in this respect, they do carry risks, notably cancer of the lips, mouth and tongue. The relative reduction in overall risk for pipe and cigar smokers seems to stem from less deep inhalation.

Dangers for non-smokers   Even granting that there are ways of making smoking slightly less dangerous, evidence of the link between lung cancer and other serious illnesses and smoking is overwhelming. Moreover, recent reports indicate that there are dangers to the health of non-smokers in inhaling smoke 'secondhand'; living or working in an environment where others smoke is potentially hazardous. Lung cancer among non-smokers who live with a heavy smoker (and therefore breathe in a certain amount of tobacco smoke) is, according to some studies, twice as high as among people who live in homes where no one smokes. Close exposure to other peoples' cigarette smoke involves between a third and a half of the risk factor attached to smoking the cigarette yourself. The effects are even worse with pipe smoke, which releases a great deal of benzpyrene. For a non-smoker, an hour in a room with a heavy pipe smoker is equivalent to smoking four cigarettes. Non-smoking spouses of heavy cigarette smokers are shown to die on average four years younger than non-smoking spouses of non-smokers – although they don't necessarily die of lung cancer.

To sum up, the benefits of smoking are illusory. The smoker puts at risk not only himself but those around him at home or at work. Breaking the habit isn't easy, but it's far from impossible.

How to stop smoking

The real key to finding the desire and the will to stop smoking lies in understanding why you smoke, combined with a really strong dislike of the habit itself. Admittedly, as discussed earlier, there's no simple answer to the reasons why people in general, or you in particular, smoke but the previous section should give you some clues and help you work out your own reasons for doing so.

Because, in general, the reasons are so diverse and complex, there's no one straightforward formula for giving up or cutting down. Many people find a quick decisive rejection of the habit the best way to stop. Some, however, find a gradual reduction the best route towards giving up completely. Yet others give up smoking often, boasting that they can break the habit early, but in fact they start again. It would appear that it's not giving up that they find the problem but maintaining the abstinence.

Getting to dislike the habit

Once you've worked out your reason, or reasons, for smoking, you need to work up a – literally – healthy dislike of smoking. Here are some of the reasons that can reinforce the aversion: the habit itself; its expense; the exploitation of human weakness by cigarette manufacturers; the fundamental uselessness of smoking as a source of pleasure, relaxation or extra energy; the 'dirtiness' of the habit – the stain of nicotine on your fingers and teeth, the smell that lingers on your hands and clothes and in your hair, and the bad taste it leaves in your mouth; the silliness of putting a lighted weed into your mouth and breathing in the smoke; and, most important of all, the physical harm you're doing to yourself and to those around you. Bolster your determination to stop by thinking positively about the many benefits that giving up smoking brings (turn to the table overleaf).

189

THE BENEFITS OF GIVING UP SMOKING

- Increased life expectancy.
- Reduced risk of contracting smoking-related illnesses, or suffering from conditions such as the following. The time it takes for the risk to decrease to approximately that of the lifelong non-smoker and/or other benefits are:
cancer of bladder: seven years.

cancer of mouth and larynx: 10–15 years.
chronic bronchitis and *emphysema:* lung function may improve and rate of deterioration slow down.
coronary heart disease: ten years, with sharp decrease after one year; relapse less likely after a coronary in those who stop.
lung cancer: ten years.

stillbirth or *low birth weight:* risk eliminated if a pregnant woman stops smoking before the fourth month of pregnancy.
- Greater resistance to many other illnesses, including coughs and colds.
- More efficient heart and lungs.
- You'll look, and smell, better and have more money to spend.

Anti-smoking aids

There are various aids to stopping smoking, including tablets that make cigarettes taste foul, ordinary chewing gum (preferably non-sugar) and gum containing nicotine, available on prescription only. Recent research has shown the nicotine gum to be very successful. Progressively more effective filters help to reduce the quantity of smoke, and nicotine, that gets through to you, which is useful as long as you don't start smoking more cigarettes to compensate. Acupuncture has also been found helpful; it's thought to work by stimulating the release into the brain of endorphins (the body's own painkillers), which reduce the withdrawal symptoms.

There are, too, a lot of people and organizations around to help you attain your goal. Tell your friends and colleagues that you're giving up smoking, so that fear of losing face if you fail bolsters your will power. Health education departments or organizations can provide advice on how to give up; and you can also turn to your medical adviser, anti-smoking clinics or groups, or go to a hypnotist. Talk to successful ex-smokers, too. In the end, though, no one else can give up for you; stopping smoking is a personal decision, which requires determination and intelligent action. If you can't make a quick, clean break, turn to the table opposite for suggestions on how to cut down.

Picking your time

Before you give up, make a note of the occasions when you smoke, of the situations that trigger off a desire for a cigarette, whether it's driving to work, socializing, or before a difficult phone call. When you start to give up smoking, use this information to avoid the danger times and situations. Adjust your routine if necessary; even if you can't, being aware of the trigger will help you to fight the cigarette urge. Keep away from smokers as much as you can.

Some people find holidays a good opportunity to give up. The pattern of the normal day, which may well be linked with your smoking pattern, doesn't apply and you should be under less strain than at work. Pick your best time, without procrastinating unnecessarily.

Withdrawal symptoms

However you make the initial break, you're bound to experience some withdrawal symptoms, and you won't be able to rule out the possibility of a relapse for some months. Trembling, sweating, irritability, anxiety and insomnia are all usual to a greater or lesser degree; in general, the symptoms may be more severe and prolonged the greater your addiction, but severe symptoms are unlikely to last more than a month to six weeks and may be gone sooner. If your dependence on smoking is purely psychological – you're convinced you need to smoke but you're not physically addicted – the symptoms, while unpleasant, will wear off, say, in three or four weeks. However, psychological dependence can be as strong a factor as physical addiction. This usually relates to the ritual and habit of smoking and may be tied to the belief that smoking produces relaxation.

You might also find that you want to eat more, which may, in part, be a physiological response to the previously depressed appetite, and in part a replacement activity. Sometimes this passes fairly quickly but some people find a craving for food lasts months. In general, if your diet is balanced and you eat nothing between meals, you should find that your appetite becomes healthier and that your digestion functions more efficiently. Any initial marginal increase in weight should gradually disappear. Chewing a non-sugar gum is a help if you're craving for food. During the withdrawal phase many smokers find it helpful to take large supplemental doses of vitamin B complex, which has a calming effect, and of vitamin C, which helps to compensate for that lost in smoking.

HOW TO CUT DOWN

If you can't stop smoking cigarettes – at the moment – try to cut down in the following ways:
• Remember that the unburned part of the cigarette acts as a filter. If you can put the cigarette out before it's half smoked, you'll avoid taking in a significant amount of toxic material.
• Don't inhale. If you do, don't inhale deeply.
• Ration yourself and stick to the ration. Make sure you smoke fewer than 15 a day – any more and it's soon a pack a day.

• Try a pipe or cigars instead of cigarettes, and don't inhale.
• Smoke the lowest tar cigarette available.
• If you smoke a pipe or cigar, ration yourself. Use filters; if you're a pipe smoker, use less tobacco, if a cigar smoker, buy smaller cigars.
• Concentrate on one of the trigger situations at a time. For instance, give up smoking after meals to start with. Once you've managed this, go on to the next trigger. Treat yourself to some-

thing as a reward for progress. Have a definite timespan in mind for stopping completely – don't make it too protracted or your enthusiasm and will power may wane.
• If even this proves hard, work out the times of day or situations when you most need to smoke and allow yourself to do so then, but only then.
• Above all, don't be disheartened if you don't manage to give up the first time. It may take several attempts.

In people who stop smoking (whether pipe, cigars or cigarettes) rather than cut down, there's usually a marked reduction in craving after a week or so whereas, unfortunately, for those who cut down, even by up to 60 per cent, the craving remains unchanged. If, however, over a period, the body can get used to a lower intake of nicotine – if you smoke fewer cigarettes and switch to a lower tar brand, say – it becomes progressively easier to break the habit.

Whatever method you use, it takes determination to see it through. But the sense of achievement and overwhelming improvement in your health that giving up smoking brings are more than ample reward.

THE COMMON PROPS: Alcohol

ONE DRINK =

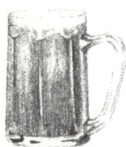

½ pt or 300 ml [or 12 fl oz can (U.S.A.)] beer or lager

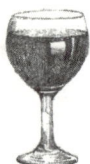

1 glass of table wine

1 small glass of fortified wine

1 measure/30 ml [1 fl oz] spirits

Alcoholic drinks have been made throughout recorded history. They've never been treated lightly – while specific drinking practices vary, there have always been conventions regarding alcohol's consumption.

In those countries where alcohol is permitted, not everyone, of course, drinks it. In the United Kingdom about 20 per cent of adults won't have had a drink during the past month; in the United States the figure will be nearer 40 per cent. Nevertheless, many people do drink alcohol, because throughout the ages it has given pleasure and satisfaction. Taken in moderate amounts, it stimulates the digestive juices, loosens the tongue a little and encourages a sense of well-being.

Manufactured alcoholic drinks are based on ethyl alcohol, a compound of carbon, oxygen and hydrogen. It is a clear, colourless liquid with a burning taste and very little odour – the distinctive smell on a drinker's breath is due to congeners, the by-products and additives in the drink. The precise amount of ethyl alcohol in a drink varies from country to country, but is about 3–6 per cent in beers and lagers; 8–14 per cent in table wines; 15–20 per cent in sherry and other fortified wines; and 30–40 per cent in most distilled spirits.

Alcohol is absorbed into the blood via the stomach and intestines and quickly and uniformly distributed throughout the body water. If a pregnant woman drinks it, it crosses the placenta into the foetus's bloodstream; it will pass into breast milk. One drink a day is probably the most a pregnant or lactating woman should take.

Most of the alcohol is eliminated from the body by metabolism in the liver, where enzymes break it down ultimately to carbon dioxide and water. A little, perhaps 3–5 per cent, is excreted unaltered via the kidneys, skin and lungs. Although the amount excreted on the breath is so tiny, it indicates the total concentration in the body, which is why some countries use breath-testing equipment to check drivers' blood alcohol levels.

Blood alcohol concentration

The level of alcohol in your blood – the blood alcohol concentration (B.A.C.) – determines your immediate physical state and, on occasions, your legal status, too. B.A.C. is usually expressed as milligrams of alcohol per hundred millilitres of blood, or mg%. It is mostly determined by three things: the amount of alcohol consumed, the speed of drinking and your body weight. To make a realistic assessment of your own B.A.C. level you must take all three into account. The longer the period over which the alcohol is drunk, the lower your B.A.C. The precise rate of absorption is influenced by various factors. If the concentration of alcohol in a drink is high, it's more rapidly absorbed; so alcohol is absorbed more quickly from spirits than from beer. The sugar in sweet drinks retards absorption, while the carbon dioxide and bicarbonate of sparkling wines and mixers accelerate it. If you eat a meal before you drink, it can delay absorption. Women, because of their lower level of body water, absorb alcohol slightly more quickly than men of the same weight. Since their body weight is generally lighter, women will have higher B.A.C. levels if they drink

Moderate drinking level
=
No more than 24 drinks in one week, with a maximum of 6 drinks in one day. Spread the drinks over the course of the day. Don't drink on more than four days in a week.

as much as men. But whatever its rate of absorption, the alcohol still has to be metabolized. This takes place at a fairly uniform rate, equivalent to breaking down the alcohol in 600 ml [1 pt] of beer every hour and a half. There's no way of speeding up metabolism and no cure for a hangover. The 'hair of the dog' remedy – taking more alcohol – merely extends the period of the hangover. Nor will drinking coffee help, since recent studies have shown that caffeine interacts with alcohol to prolong the disruptive effects of alcohol on perception and reaction times – with obvious implications for drinking drivers.

The only way to avoid a high B.A.C. level with all its adverse consequences is to drink moderately, although you must remember that any drinking that raises B.A.C. level above 20 mg% increases the risk of accidents and misjudgements. The fact that you don't *feel* drunk – you may even pride yourself on your 'hard head' – is no guide to your actual B.A.C. level, which could well be high. The maximum amount you can drink without suffering alcohol's serious penalties is no more than six drinks on any day, distributed throughout the day – not in one sitting and certainly not in one hour. You could consume this, at most, on four days in one week.

B.A.C. LEVELS
The figures in bold, *right*, are approximate B.A.C. levels. Your B.A.C. level will vary according to your body weight, the amount of alcohol you've consumed, and the speed at which you've drunk it.

As your B.A.C. level rises, you'll suffer its effects, *below*.

Number of drinks	55 kg [120 lb]			70 kg [155 lb]		
	Hours taken to consume drinks			Hours taken to consume drinks		
	1	2	3	1	2	3
1	30	10	0	20	0	0
3	80	60	40	60	30	20
5	130	120	100	100	80	60
7	190	180	160	140	120	110
9	250	230	220	180	170	150
11	310	290	280	230	210	200

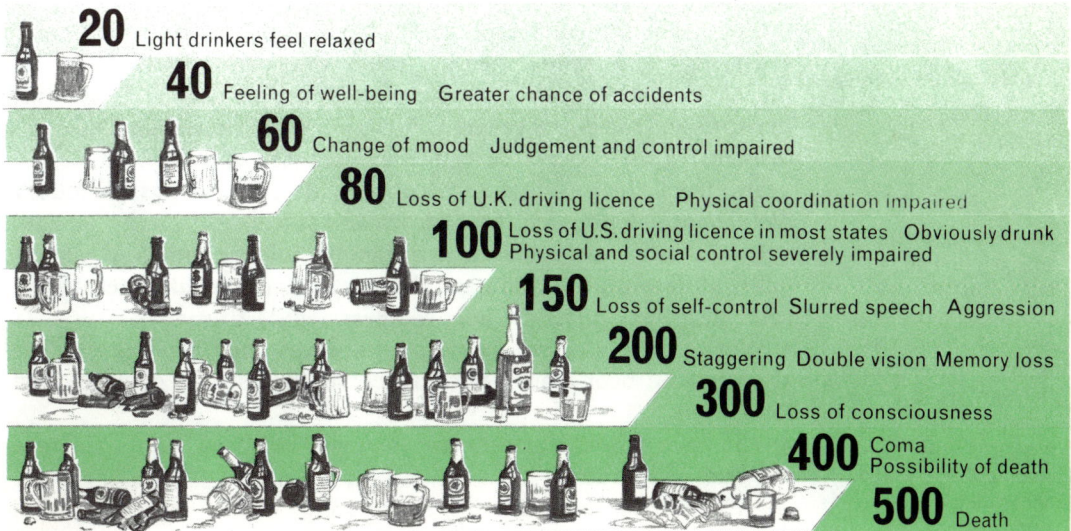

20 Light drinkers feel relaxed

40 Feeling of well-being   Greater chance of accidents

60 Change of mood   Judgement and control impaired

80 Loss of U.K. driving licence   Physical coordination impaired

100 Loss of U.S. driving licence in most states   Obviously drunk   Physical and social control severely impaired

150 Loss of self-control   Slurred speech   Aggression

200 Staggering   Double vision   Memory loss

300 Loss of consciousness

400 Coma   Possibility of death

500 Death

Do you drink too much?

Since not everyone does drink moderately, or less than the maximum intake suggested on pages 192–93, it's a good idea to be aware of the warning signs of alcohol problems. These are:

• A craving for alcohol: being unhappy, edgy and tense without it.

• Drinking to keep B.A.C. at a raised level, in a pattern that becomes more regular, fixed and predictable.

• Family, work and social life taking second place to the fixed drinking pattern and its associated activities.

• Being able to carry on with a B.A.C. level that would incapacitate the ordinary drinker.

• Shakiness, sweating and nausea accompanied by feelings of edginess and tension when the B.A.C. level begins to fall.

• No longer drinking in order to feel better, but in order to avoid feeling worse – to avoid the withdrawal symptoms.

High risk occupations

Certain jobs and lifestyles are associated with an increase in alcohol problems. These are highlighted in the mortality rates for liver cirrhosis, which are considered a reliable indicator of the extent of alcohol dependence. Those at risk include journalists, garage proprietors and doctors, with a cirrhosis death rate of three times the average; members of the armed forces, restaurateurs and insurance brokers, four times; fishermen, seamen and bar staff, six times; and, at the top end of the scale, bar managers and publicans, at 16 times the mortality average.

Occupations and lifestyles associated with a high rate of alcohol dependence include one or more of the following factors: ready access to alcohol; regular social pressure to drink; long-term or frequent separation from normal social or sexual relationships; freedom from supervision; and high stress. If you're in a high-risk occupation or faced with at least one high-risk factor, you may need to make a conscious effort to keep to a moderate level of drinking.

Most alcohol-related problems fall into the following four areas:

• Physical and mental health: brain disorders; disorders of the digestive system such as gastritis and peptic ulcers; fatty liver, hepatitis and cirrhosis; cancers of various kinds; nutritional diseases; disturbances of the metabolism; increased risk of injury, accident or death from the reaction of alcohol with other drugs; emotional disturbance, depression, breakdown and suicide.

• Family and social relationships: family violence and child neglect; debt; separation, desertion and divorce; loss of outside interests and activities; loss of friends; homelessness and destitution.

• Work: unsatisfactory work relationships; bad timekeeping and absenteeism; poor work performance; accidents; lack of promotion; loss of job.

• The law: public drunkenness; motoring offences; theft; violence; sex crimes; murder.

As you drink more heavily, so the range and severity of alcohol-related problems that you suffer from will increase.

Maintaining a daily consumption of 15 or more drinks over a number of years would lead to a serious risk of liver damage. Along the way, you'd almost certainly suffer from other physical, emotional, social and occupational problems, too.

WARNING SIGNS: THE QUESTIONS TO ASK

Can I hold my drink better now than I used to?

Do I ever wake up the morning after unable to remember part of the evening before?

Am I more likely to go to social events if I know that alcohol will be available?

Do I get through my first drink more quickly than I used to?

Do I usually want to drink more than most of the people I'm with?

Do I ever drive my car when I know that I'm over the legal limit?

Am I irritated by comments on my drinking?

Do I ever feel guilty about my drinking?

Do I find that I'm not getting as much enjoyment from my drinking as I used to?

Do I ever regret what I've done or said when I've been drinking?

Do I try to avoid my family and friends when I'm drinking?

Do I spend more on drink than I can really afford?

Do I tend to eat irregularly when I'm drinking?

Do I ever have the shakes in the morning and find that it helps to have a drink?

Have I ever been in trouble with the police because of my drinking?

Have I ever had any work difficulty because of my drinking?

Have I lost any friends because of my drinking?

Has my family life been disrupted at all because of my drinking?

Do I get irritable and edgy if I have to go without alcohol for a few hours?

Have I ever made an effort to cut down on my drinking and not been able to?

If you've answered YES to any of these questions, you may have a drinking problem. You should *almost certainly cut down.*

If you've answered YES to any of these questions, you certainly have a drinking problem. You should probably *stop drinking altogether* and may need specialist help.

How to stop or cut down

If you drink more than the suggested moderate level, you'll benefit physically, socially and financially by cutting down. If you know that you show any signs of dependence or have been in any serious physical, family, work or legal trouble through drink, you should probably stop drinking altogether. As well as answering the questions in the table, above, every drinker should chart his or her drinking behaviour. To do this, write down exactly how much you drink of what, with whom, when and where for a period of a week. This will show you the total of drinks you've had, and in what circumstances.

If you drink too much . . .

The goal to aim for is the moderate level of drinking outlined earlier, or less: not more than 1.8 litres [3 pt] beer or lager, for instance, on any day, on not more than four days a week. This makes a maximum of 24 drinks per week. Even at this level, you'll still increase your vulnerability to misjudgements and accidents if the drinks are consumed too close together.

The strategy for reaching that goal is to cut the overall level gradually, by five drinks each week. But if at present you consume more than 50 drinks in a week, cut down by ten a week until you reach 50, and then by five a week until you reach the moderate weekly level of 24 drinks.

There is more to having a moderate pattern of drinking than just reducing the overall level. Drinking needs to be distributed, so that not too much is drunk at any one time. Your drinking chart will highlight the occasions on which you drink more; these might be on certain days, or at certain times, or with certain people, or in certain places, or in relation to certain events.

To control drinking at these times you'll have to work out strategies, all of which will require preparation and thought. You might have to avoid the event altogether, or arrive late, or leave early, just drink less or not drink at all. Some people, once they've realized how much they're drinking, openly admit to their families, friends and relatives that they've been drinking too much, getting into difficulties, and so want to stop or cut down.

For those who don't wish to come clean, there are many readily accepted reasons for not drinking, or for drinking only a little:

- I'm watching my weight • Money is a bit tight • I'm driving
- I've got a bit of stomach trouble • I'll be drinking later on
- I'm cutting it out at lunchtime/mid-week/on Mondays
- I must cut down since the accident/operation/illness
- I had a bit too much yesterday • I'm in training
- I'm seeing X later, so I'd better not • I've had some already.

Cutting down overall consumption, if it's done gradually and without a great deal of fuss, requires a little planning and record-keeping but is quite manageable for most drinkers.

Outside help

If you want or need to stop altogether, the gradual reduction plan is probably the best method. Some drinkers, however, will need help for physical withdrawal symptoms and other health problems, which any sympathetic family doctor will understand and be able to cope with.

Others, who are severely dependent or severely damaged either physically or socially, may need to stop drinking immediately. Going it alone will probably not be enough. Such drinkers may have to be admitted to a special alcoholism unit for physical and psychological treatment. Alcoholics Anonymous may also help them to stay off alcohol as they become involved in the A.A. system of mutual aid and support. Local councils on alcoholism, social work teams and probation offices, together with advice bureaux and community centres, should all have information on alcohol and its dangers, on how to recognize alcohol problems and on where to go for special help.

Careful drinking

While alcohol has frequently given pleasure, it has also created or contributed to a wide range of serious physical, mental, social and legal problems. Ultimately, individual drinkers have to control their own drinking. Nevertheless, we can all help by:

- Respecting the wishes of the person who chooses to abstain.
- Respecting the wishes of the person who chooses to drink in moderation or to cut down; never insisting on refreshing a drink, refilling a glass or including someone in a round.
- Providing non-alcoholic drinks for those who prefer them, and food with alcohol at all times.
- Recognizing that the host is just as responsible for preventing drunken driving as the guest.

COPING WITH STRESS

The prime objective is to learn how to cope with stress so that you can minimize its potential for damaging health. Obviously this task differs from one person to the next but certain steps must always be taken. The first thing to do is to identify the stress factors themselves and then, having done that, examine your attitude towards them to see whether your response is appropriate. Are you over-reacting? Can the circumstances be altered to reduce stress? A look at your personality type (see page 183) and at your overall vulnerability in terms of stressful events (see page 172) will help you identify some of the factors that are involved.

You have two areas to work in, internal and external. To improve matters internally, it's a question of altering attitudes and habitual responses. To improve things externally involves altering, where possible, those aspects of life that impose stress. The key words in the last sentence are 'where possible' because, as much as anything, it's the ability to accept what can't be changed that enables anyone to stay sane in a world fraught with potential hazards. Once those things over which you as an individual can exert no direct control are removed from the scene, then it's possible, and necessary, to take a sensible look at the problems that remain and that can be solved. These problems may involve feelings of doubt and uncertainty, a long-held feeling of resentment, or hatred, lack of purpose, difficulty in personal relationships, inability to make decisions, or indeed any behaviour pattern that produces unhappiness.

Individual responsibility
Many systems and methods have been evolved that attempt to unravel the confused emotions that prevail increasingly as a result of stress. And although counselling and advice are often necessary, much can be achieved by personal effort. Indeed, in the end, it's up to you to solve your own problems, since the insight therapy and guidance give still needs to be used by you. Above all, the reduction of stress remains a matter of gaining greater insight into your own character, personality and habitual responses. Acceptance of the responsibility for dealing with your problems is a prime requisite for developing awareness and a full personality. For some this means simply adjusting or reorganizing their lifestyle, for others it involves seeking more deeply into spiritual areas and finding purpose and meaning beyond everyday life. Whether you have to do the former or the latter, you'll be in a position to make a start only when you've recognized and come to terms with the need for change and positive effort.

Drugs
The use of drugs to control symptoms should only ever be thought of as a short-term measure. A few days or so, to help overcome a crisis, is justifiable, but beyond that there is the danger that simply masking stress symptoms will lead to more serious problems, as well as the possibility of side effects. Medical research has shown that if any particular symptom of a chronically anxious patient is relieved by drugs, something else crops up to take its place.

Dispelling uncertainty

One of the key causes of stress is uncertainty: it's always easier to take appropriate action after the event. For instance, you lose your job. What do you do? Go out and look for work. Of course, it may not be easy to find work but the immediate question has a simple answer, you know what to do, you can at least try. But if the problem is merely a rumour about jobs being cut back, the uncertainty creates stress; you have sleepless nights, become edgy and argumentative and unable to perform at your best. Ironically the chances of losing the job become even greater.

Having identified the source of stress as uncertainty about the job, the first step towards overcoming it is to think about courses of action, such as contacting other firms or job agencies, and then either discuss them with a sympathetic person or make a firm mental resolve to shelve the problem until there's a chance of more appropriate action. It's important to do one or the other and not just to worry obsessively and speculate endlessly. Taking action immediately reduces stress, and this is true whether the action is going to a job agency or shelving the problem because no appropriate, or further, action is possible for the time being.

To take another example: a swelling appears on a breast, resulting in anxiety, uncertainty and panic. Most such swellings are totally harmless but not knowing the cause can lead to intense stress. The result is a decline in well-being and even more mental turmoil. The answer is to get a diagnosis. Once the enemy is identified, appropriate measures can be started and the stress of uncertainty goes.

Forgiveness therapy

Long-held resentments, grudges and hatreds relating to real or imagined upsets, often years in the past, generate a great deal of stress. One way of releasing the tensions locked up in these emotional cul-de-sacs is by 'forgiveness therapy'. If the very thought of someone results in a marked degree of tension, there's probably a case for forgiveness. In the first place, it's important to realize that what happened lies in the past and nothing can change that. Secondly, you must recognize that by holding on to a negative emotional charge about something that is past you harm only yourself. Whatever the circumstances it's always possible to wipe the slate clean and forgive what has happened. If practical (and it may not be so if, for example, the emotions aroused are directed towards someone long dead), accompany this by an open expression of forgiveness to the person in question, either verbally or in writing, then forgive yourself for your past behaviour. A common reaction to such a suggestion is: 'But I don't want to re-open contact. That relationship is over and done with.' The truth is that the relationship is alive for as long as it continues to hold such emotional power as to make the very idea of contact repugnant. It will be over and done with only when the emotion resulting from the possibility of such contact is one of indifference. And this will happen only when the other party has been forgiven. The degree of tension released by such an action can be truly phenomenal.

Past, present and future

The past is an area in which many people stay trapped emotionally, and it's essential to escape this trap and to concentrate on the present, which is, after all, the only time you're really alive. The future, too, can dominate the present. Since you're as much a product of your expected future as you are of your past, look forward positively – that doesn't mean dwelling on the future but having goals to aim for.

The steps that need to be taken to avoid damage through stress of the 'if only' (past) and 'what if' (future) variety are common-sense ones: living in the present; accepting what can't be changed; forgiving others and yourself for what is past; learning to deal sensibly with real and expected problems; and drawing up realistic goals.

Means to an end

Once you've drawn up your goals, the next step is to plan how to attain them. There's a tendency to expect instant gratification of wants and desires. And if the 'want', whether it's a holiday or a new washing machine, remains unfulfilled, envy, resentment and anger can fill the mind. But if appropriate measures, such as saving, haven't been taken to reach the goal, the all-important means of achieving the end have been neglected. Concentrating on the end and ignoring the means is a common feature of many cases of unfulfilled ambition, which is itself a large stress area.

Taking the stress out of relationships

Relationships require that feelings, needs and desires are expressed to one another in a direct, non-accusative, non-belligerent manner. It does no harm to express emotions strongly, if tensions are building up, but express them in a constructive manner and respect the other person's sensitivities. Remember that nothing and no one makes you angry. Anger is always self-generated; as such, it can be positively used. Bottling it up is harmful because it can be one of the most potent forms of stress.

Equally important, once you've had your say, is being prepared to listen to criticism of yourself without reacting to the fact of criticism. Instead of an angry response, make an attempt at non-critical self-appraisal. Listen to what's being said, evaluate it and then either change your behaviour or explain your reasons for it. Listening to and evaluating what is said will give you insight into how other people see you, and accepting the criticism or explaining calmly why you don't accept it will avoid stressful confrontation. Clarify areas of disagreement so that they're mutually understood. If changes can be made to achieve harmony, make them. If this isn't possible, the best solution to prevent further acrimony is to agree to differ.

It's worth remembering that whenever you behave in a certain way, you add strength to the motivating idea behind your act. If you react angrily to criticism, or fall into a sulky mood in response to real or imagined rejection, for example, this will reinforce your belief that these are the correct responses. By changing the response to a more positive form of behaviour and by repeating it, you'll gradually come to feel that this new response is the correct one.

199

How to reduce stress

1 Work no more than ten hours *daily*.
2 Have at least one and a half days each week free from normal work routine.
3 Allow at least half an hour for each main meal.
4 Eat slowly and chew well.
5 Cultivate the habit of listening to relaxing music.
6 Practise relaxation and/or meditation at least twice (ideally three times) *daily* for no less than 15 minutes each time.
7 Actively cultivate the habit of walking, talking and moving at a slower pace.
8 Smile and respond cheerfully whenever meeting anyone.
9 Plan one 'away from it all' holiday each year.
10 Take ten minutes *daily* (or 20 minutes four times weekly) for physical exercise, some of it preferably outdoors, so you get the added benefit of fresh air and full spectrum light (see page 173).
11 Examine your eating pattern and balance the diet (see pages 129–31 and 138–49).
12 If emotional and/or sexual relationships are distressing you, seek advice.
13 If you're unhappy at work, take stock and look at choices (retraining, new areas of work, job agencies and so on).
14 Cultivate a hobby that's creative rather than competitive (gardening, painting, do-it-yourself) and spend time on it.
15 Have a regular massage or join a yoga class.
16 Concentrate on the present, avoiding the tendency to dwell on past events and future uncertainties.
17 Work and act methodically, that is, finish one task before starting another.
18 Express your feelings openly and without antagonism or hostility.
19 Don't accept, or set yourself, unrealistic deadlines. What can't be done one day can wait until the next.
20 Don't rely on drugs, blaming others or other props in order to cope; accept personal responsibility for your life.

Practical measures

There are practical methods of minimizing the effects of the inevitable stressful episodes of life. A philosophy of living, using intelligently the knowledge of what stress is and what can be done to adjust to it, is the prime necessity, and it should include the 20 basic steps shown above. Don't expect to be able to incorporate all of them into your lifestyle overnight or you're more than likely to fail. Instead regard them as the ideal to aim for. Why not try to work the three that *you* find easiest into your routine this week and proceed from there, adding the other steps in gradually? Pin the list up somewhere where you'll see it so that it becomes automatic to check on your progress every day.

Making decisions

Although there's no way of anticipating all possibilities, basic planning is a good first step towards sound decision-making and so reducing the stress that this process often entails. Start by writing down the nature of the problem and defining the choices that appear to exist. Don't forget one important choice, which is sometimes overlooked: the positive decision to do nothing. Usually only a limited number of choices exist, so write down the merits and demerits of these. Having an ideal end-result in mind helps, so write this down as well. Most decisions are based on linear thinking – starting at one end and working towards a desired objective at the other, and this is often the best way of dealing with everyday problems. However, if, after you've defined your problem and all the reasonable options open to you, no solution is obvious, spend a little time doing some lateral thinking, looking for unusual solutions. You'll probably find in the end that you'll have to make a compromise because there's seldom an ideal answer if a decision has been creating anxiety.

Take, for example, the case of a widow who lives alone and isn't well enough to take care of herself. She has two married children who live in different places. Both want her to go and live with or near them. She believes that whichever she chooses the other will feel slighted. What should she do? She could stay where she is, or go to one or other of her children. Compromise solutions would be to spend time with each or to choose an alternative companion with whom to share her own home. There's no ideal solution, especially if she's uncertain whether her children genuinely want her to live with them, but it's essential to make a decision, to make the most desirable – or at any rate the least undesirable – choice. It's the initial indecision that creates the stress; once the decision is made, stress is greatly reduced. It's important, too, to be positive about the decision once you've taken it, while bearing in mind that there's always room for modification if, for whatever reason, it doesn't turn out to be as successful as you'd originally hoped it would be.

Habits

Everyone lives their lives by habit to some extent. The question to ask yourself with regard to stress is: Are your habits likely to reduce or create it? As discussed earlier, it's easier to change yourself, and your habits, than it is to change the rest of the world. Altering your personal habits so that you eat better, sleep better and exercise more will pay real dividends in terms of reduced stress, improved health and a heightened sense of well-being. It's worth noting here the role that exercise plays in stress reduction and improved health. Many people take no exercise at all, yet the body was designed for activity. As the circulation is stimulated by exercise, the presence of lactic acid, which not only fatigues the body and dulls the brain but heightens anxiety, is reduced, while the production of adrenalin and noradrenalin, which can be linked with a general feeling of happiness and alertness, is increased. Although jogging round the block, or taking any form of exercise for that matter, won't solve all your problems, it will

201

have an invigorating effect on both the mind and the body, helping to banish lethargy and boredom and even alleviate depression. It can also provide an outlet for aggression (this is particularly true of competitive sports) and pent-up emotions.

Eating, sleeping and exercise habits are easily recognizable but there are other, more subtle habits that can affect your ability to cope with stress. You're probably not even aware of them. For instance, are you in the habit of looking serious, unsmiling and severe? It's just as easy to look unworried and to smile. The strange fact is that your emotions will respond to the way you look, just as much as the other way round. What is the image you have of yourself? Does this correspond to the image others have of you? If there's a lack of harmony in the environment, whether at work or home, you may be projecting an unhappy, stress-inducing image. On the other hand, a friendly word, a smile, active interest in others, tolerance and praise rather than criticism will lead to a feedback of warmth and happiness – which reduces stress enormously. The changes in thinking and behaviour that this involves take real effort but the results that they bring are well worth it.

A positive choice

In summation it's worth repeating that you can choose to be happy and relaxed or tense and unhappy, either by altering circumstances, where feasible, or by altering your attitudes and behaviour towards them. If you do the following:
• take a close look at avoidable stress factors and consider ways of eliminating them
• make an attempt to increase your self-awareness and to understand yourself and others
• take steps to balance your diet properly, as well as taking the other practical measures outlined on page 200, including regular exercise sessions and practising a relaxation technique, yoga or meditation as frequently as you can
then you will be able to give an honest 'yes' to most of the following questions:
1 Do you feel relaxed and happy?
2 Do you feel well?
3 Are you sleeping well and waking refreshed?
4 Do you like most people?
5 Have you confidence in the future?
6 Is life enjoyable?
7 Do you feel satisfied with your appearance?
8 Have you a satisfactory emotional and/or sexual relationship?
If you answered 'yes' to most of these, you are in a secure emotional state and should guard this by avoiding the pitfalls already outlined. If your answer was 'no' to most of the questions, use this book as a guide, take professional advice and, above all, have confidence that, if you set your mind to it and try, you can achieve physical and emotional well-being.

Biofeedback

This technique represents a breakthrough in understanding our ability to manipulate body functions and so influence health, both physical and mental. In particular, it offers an effective method of learning to control the harmful consequences of stress without recourse to drugs, but it has also proved successful in controlling a variety of complaints, from ulcers to abnormal heart rhythms.

How it works

As the name suggests, it's based on feeding back, by means of sound or visual display, information about body processes that are generally outside voluntary control. The essential feature of the technique is that the person using a biofeedback machine learns, by trial and error and by repetition, what it is that has to be done by the mind to control a particular physical function. The equipment can be used to help a person control heart rate, blood pressure, the activity of the sweat glands (which is higher when you're anxious) and, as shown below, muscle tension and types of brain rhythms.

Biofeedback machines are easily obtainable for home use, but it must be emphasized that no biofeedback method should be used without supervision, if you're attempting to improve an existing health problem. For the purposes of relaxation, results to date suggest that the best way to use biofeedback is in conjunction with meditation or relaxation techniques. It's not certain whether in the long term the results can be carried over into everyday life without the aid of the equipment, nor is it certain that by learning to control one symptom of stress, such as high blood pressure, it's possible to achieve overall relaxation. For the time being, biofeedback is best regarded as a useful aid rather than a complete answer to reducing stress.

This machine measures both muscle tension and the electrical rhythms of the brain: one or other is selected by the brain rhythm/muscle tension switch. Electrodes placed anywhere on the skin's surface pick up the small electrical signals caused by muscle activity, allowing you to monitor physical tension. Brain rhythms are measured by an electrode behind each ear and one at the back of the head; the reading is taken from the side of the brain selected by the changeover control. The brain-wave frequency selector measures each of the brain rhythms – alpha, the relaxed waking frequency; beta, the active waking frequency; theta, the dreaming rhythm; and delta, the non-dreaming, deep sleep waves. The information is registered by the needle on the panel and by an audible tone fed through an earphone. Muscle tension is usually measured by a rising tone, alpha brain-waves with an on/off one. For both, the baseline selector sets the level at which the machine begins to register.

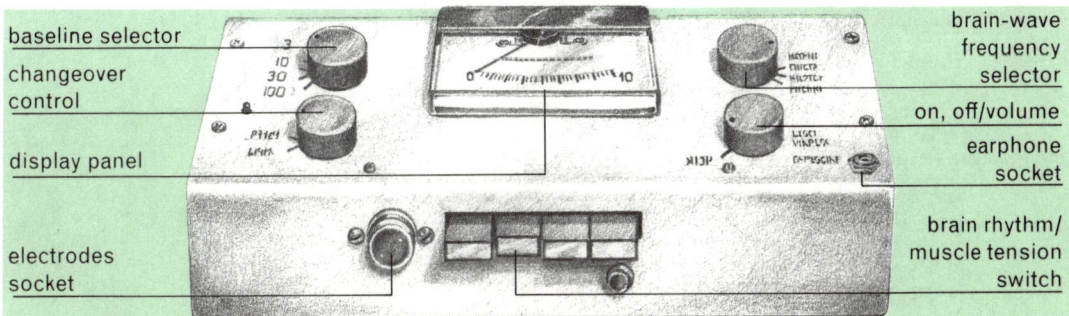

baseline selector

changeover control

display panel

electrodes socket

brain-wave frequency selector

on, off/volume

earphone socket

brain rhythm/muscle tension switch

Sleep and stress

Sleep and stress make poor bedfellows. Stress often leads to insomnia while insomnia, in turn, can be the cause of stress and a vicious circle is quickly drawn.

When stress disturbs sleep – and this is recognized as one of the most striking symptoms of a stress condition – the disruption can take a variety of forms: difficulty in getting to sleep; fitful, disturbed sleep; waking up early, unable to fall asleep again. Even the mildest cases of insomnia can increase the stress level.

The value of sleep

Sleep is vital to health and probably life itself. Its disruption can cause: deterioration in perception; slower, more erratic reaction time to stimuli; lower energy level; lapses of memory; increased pain sensitivity; and a tendency towards irritability and depression.

There are two main kinds of sleep: deep, and dreaming, lighter sleep. In the deep stage vital hormones are produced from the pituitary gland, which have a restorative effect on the body. Consequently, if you're woken up during this phase, you'll recall almost nothing of what happens and will behave in a zombie-like way. Dreaming is considered important not only because it helps consolidate new information in the memory, but because it frees the unconscious and relieves tension built up by repression. Distressing symptoms, such as confusion and increasing difficulty in performing simple tasks, have resulted from dreams being constantly disturbed experimentally. Poor sleepers spend less time in both the deep phase and in dreaming sleep, and more in the less valuable, lightest stages.

In industrialized societies a variety of factors work against the

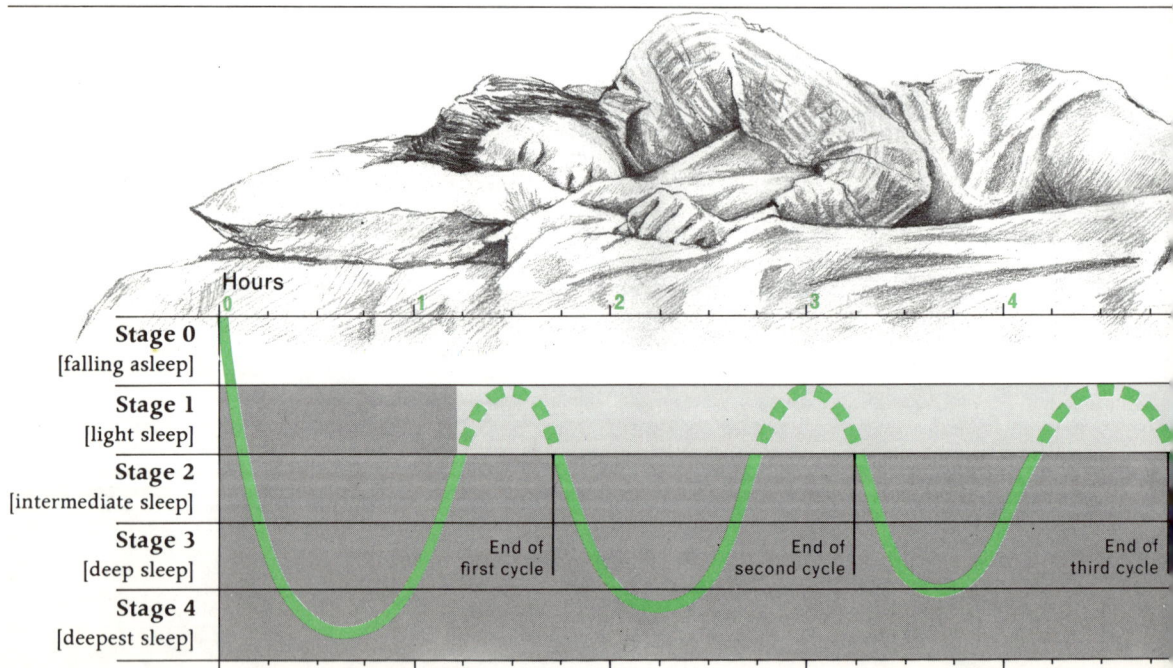

Hours

Stage 0 [falling asleep]				
Stage 1 [light sleep]				
Stage 2 [intermediate sleep]				
Stage 3 [deep sleep]	End of first cycle	End of second cycle		End of third cycle
Stage 4 [deepest sleep]				

pattern of sleep that nature demands. There is, for example, the pressure of conformity. We wake up and get up at times determined by outside schedules and not by the body's needs. The full sleep cycle is not always completed. If there are additional stress factors – awkward journeys to work, difficult relationships, financial anxieties and so on – the picture begins to look ominous. Together with an all too common tendency to snatch meals in the form of snacks of poor value, too little exercise, and too many breaks in the natural pattern of sleep by burning the midnight oil, this sort of stress readily sets the scene for insomnia.

Sleeping tablets

At this stage many people turn to medication for help but the results are less than satisfactory. The fact is that when sleeping pills do work they don't induce normal sleep but simply a knock-out effect, and being unconscious is not the same as being asleep. They reduce the amount of time spent dreaming, as well as the intensity of dreams.

Sleeping tablets can also have a number of side effects including indigestion, respiratory ailments, loss of appetite, skin rashes, increased blood pressure, kidney and liver dysfunction, lowered resistance to infection, mental confusion and circulatory problems. Apart from this, if not technically addictive, as are barbiturates, all sleeping tablets with a sleep-inducing effect that is rapidly lost create a dependency. Since all such drugs become less effective as the body develops a tolerance to them (within three or four weeks at the most), this dependency is the rule rather than the exception. Lastly, the greatest irony of all is that withdrawal results in worse insomnia.

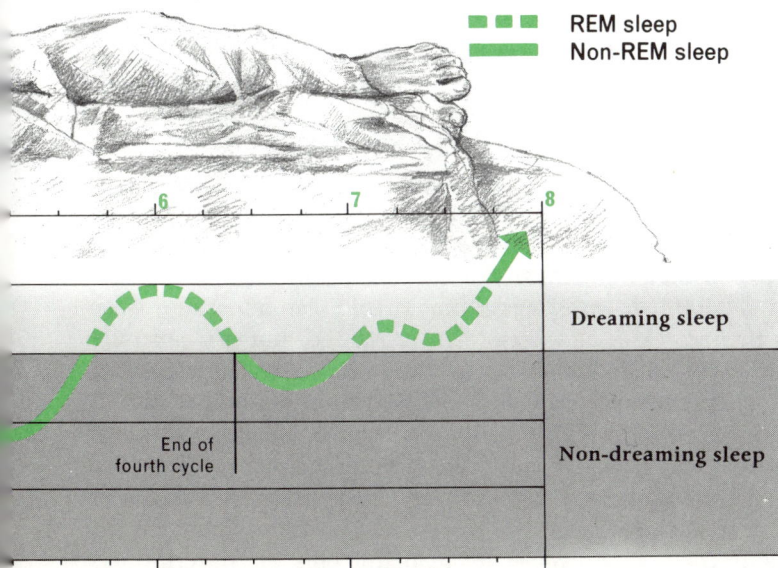

- - - REM sleep
——— Non-REM sleep

6   7   8

Dreaming sleep

End of fourth cycle

Non-dreaming sleep

Sleep begins with a borderline state between waking and sleeping. The mind wanders and awareness is dull; there's a general decrease in muscular tension. Gradually, body functions slow right down and sleep becomes deeper until the deepest stage is reached. This is followed by a lighter, dreaming phase, in which the closed eyes move rapidly – hence the name REM, rapid eye movement, given to this phase. Fingers and toes often twitch during this phase, too.

The whole cycle from dropping off to sleep to the end of the first dreaming phase takes less than two hours. The deep and dreaming cycle is repeated four or five times in an average night's sleep, with the deepest sleep in the first few hours of the night and dreaming phases dominating in the morning.

How to combat insomnia

With sleeping pills discredited, the question remains: what can provide the answer to insomnia? There are a number of possibilities that are worth considering.

The first concerns your pre-sleep pattern, much of which is established from the earliest years. Choice of bed, as well as what you do before going to sleep, is all part of this. Whether the ritual consists of taking a bath, reading, making love, praying or even the way you lie in bed, any variation in it can disturb sleep, so it pays to look at the pre-sleep pattern that existed before the onset of insomnia. Obvious causes of a change in the sleeping pattern can often be identified in this way and the usual pattern of preparation for sleep re-established.

If the change in the sleep pattern is to waking in the early hours, it often helps to get up rather than lie and worry. If personal circumstances permit, take a midday nap either after or instead of a meal. This won't detract from the chance of sleeping well that night but, by helping to restore relaxation, will enhance it. Where an afternoon nap isn't possible, try relaxation exercises, autogenics and/or meditation; turn to the How to relax section, pages 207–40 for a variety of self-help methods. If the problem persists, a depressive illness may be responsible, so seek medical advice.

Sex, or the lack of it, is a major area of stress that may lead to insomnia, and advice from special counsellors may be necessary. Some such experts now suggest masturbation for those who live alone, but this meets with strong resistance in many people. Whatever the problem, individual counselling is recommended; consult a medical advisor to arrange for this.

Exercise and nutrition also play a part in re-establishing normal sleep patterns. Try to ensure that you take adequate exercise, but not just before going to bed, unless this is part of the normal pre-sleep ritual. Aim for a well-balanced diet that includes around 45g of protein a day. Don't drink tea or coffee just before going to bed as the caffeine in them acts as a stimulant; instead try a herbal tea (see page 137) or have hot milk. Some insomniacs have been found to have low blood sugar; this condition, hypoglycaemia, can be caused by eating too much food containing highly refined sugar, so try cutting down. Some researchers have also found insomniacs to have low levels of nicotinic acid, vitamins B_6 and B_{12}, zinc, calcium, magnesium and manganese, all of which indicate an inadequate diet. The general advice is to consult a nutritionally orientated doctor.

Lack of tryptophan, an essential amino acid, can also cause sleep problems (in rare cases an excess can do so, too, but it's generally neutralized in a healthy body). One of the proteins, and so contained in protein-rich foods, tryptophan should be supplied by the diet. It helps produce serotonin in the body, a substance essential for sleep. Insomniacs should try a 1g dose, 20 minutes before going to bed (don't persist indefinitely if it doesn't help). Tryptophan is available from health food stores as part of sleep-assisting compounds but it's expensive. In the U.K., however, it's available only on prescription.

HOW TO RELAX

Relaxing thoroughly can be a much harder task than eating or exercising properly. It may be difficult for you to acknowledge to yourself the whole basis of relaxation – letting go and allowing your body's restorative side to take over. You may spend most of your life in situations where drive is essential, but remember that you need regular periods of rest as well, or sooner or later you'll react with one or more of the symptoms of stress. Learn to be in control of your body rather than the other way round: experiment with the range of relaxation techniques outlined here to find the methods that appeal most and work best for you. Even a technique that's specifically designed to relax your muscles has a calming effect on your mind and one that helps you to become less anxious will also ease physical tension. You may find that some methods are particularly useful for coping with periods of great stress, whereas others encourage you to develop, in general, a calmer and more equable approach to life.

The range of methods

Relaxation techniques will help you to unlearn the habits of tension and to replace them gradually with beneficial ones. The routine on pages 208–09 shows you how to counter the usual muscular responses to stress with the opposite action and takes you through the basic steps needed to relax your whole body. After some practice, you'll be able to trigger off a chain of relaxation responses with one simple movement, such as pulling down your shoulders. The section on page 211 explains the effects of one common symptom of tension, inhibited breathing, and offers some advice on coping with it.

Most forms of exercise help to ease strain by giving your body a chance to stretch out tense muscles. Yoga (see pages 214–20) is particularly useful as it not only includes poses that are specifically intended to help you relax but as, eventually, each pose is held for a few minutes, it also encourages you to slow your pace. The exercises on page 210 focus on relaxing the back of the neck and shoulders, an area that's particularly prone to accumulate tension, while those on pages 212–13 are designed to reduce the stress and minimize the discomfort of long journeys.

Massage has been used to heal, relieve pain and give pleasure by many people from the ancient Hindus to the classical Greeks and Romans. Several different forms have developed. The Swedish massage on pages 221–29 and the Oriental system on pages 230–35 have different roots and so involve different techniques, but they both help to release accumulated tensions from the muscles by direct manipulation. Water therapy (see pages 236–37) is another way of directly tackling the physical effects of stress, through baths, saunas and wrapping treatments.

There are also methods that induce physical and mental relaxation by creating a peaceful state of mind (see pages 238–40): meditation, which helps you to develop inner calm and stability and also encourages you to relax physically; and autogenics, in which regular practice of self-suggestion exercises brings relaxation.

207

Relaxing your muscles

Follow this sequence of direct physical orders (in bold type) to relax each part of your body. Read the instructions, or tape them, before you start. It may take a little while to get the best response, so practise the sequence regularly. It's probably easiest to let go completely lying down, but gradually you'll be able to apply the technique anywhere, any time.

Lie facing up on the floor or on a bed. If this makes your lower back uncomfortable, place a cushion or pillow under your thighs; or lie on your side, adapting the instructions as appropriate – this is a good position for late pregnancy. Rest your hands on your pelvis or on the floor beside you.

1 Check that the back of the neck is long by tucking in the chin. Place a cushion or pillow under your head if necessary.

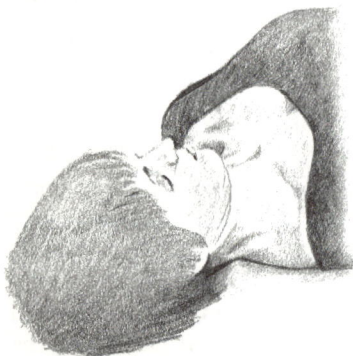

2 Press your head and elbows into the floor. As your upper back lifts off the floor slightly, you can easily **pull your shoulders down away from your ears.** Replace your upper back on the floor.

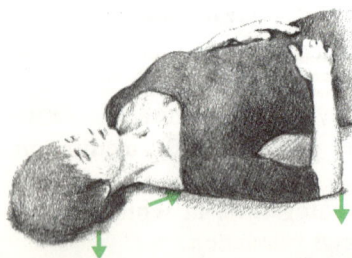

3 Think about the feeling of ease and freedom in your neck after lengthening it fully. If there is still a feeling of tightness, **roll your head gently from side to side**, keeping it fully supported on the floor, and start again.

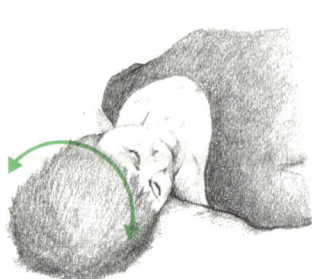

4 Push your elbows outwards, without lifting them up; as you're trying to let go, allow their weight to be supported. A common sign of tension is to hold the arms close in to the body. To induce the opposite, relaxed, body reaction, perform the opposite action by pushing your arms away from you.

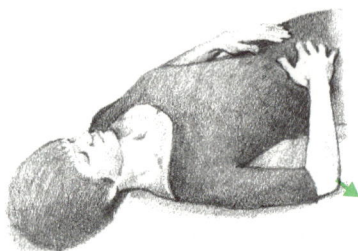

5 Stretch the fingers and let them fall back on to the support. You may tend to clench your hands unnecessarily in everyday life: notice how it feels to have the fingers lengthened instead.

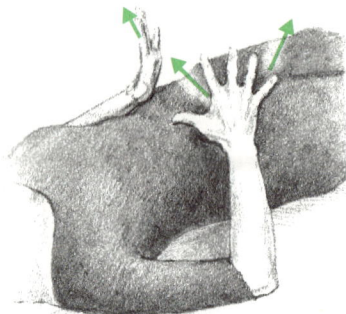

6 Press your whole trunk into the floor, in effect doing a small pelvic tilt and lengthening out the lower back (see exercise 8, page 33).

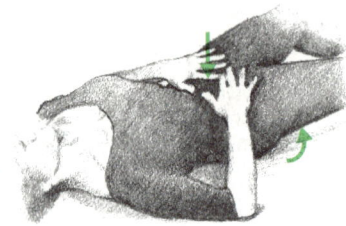

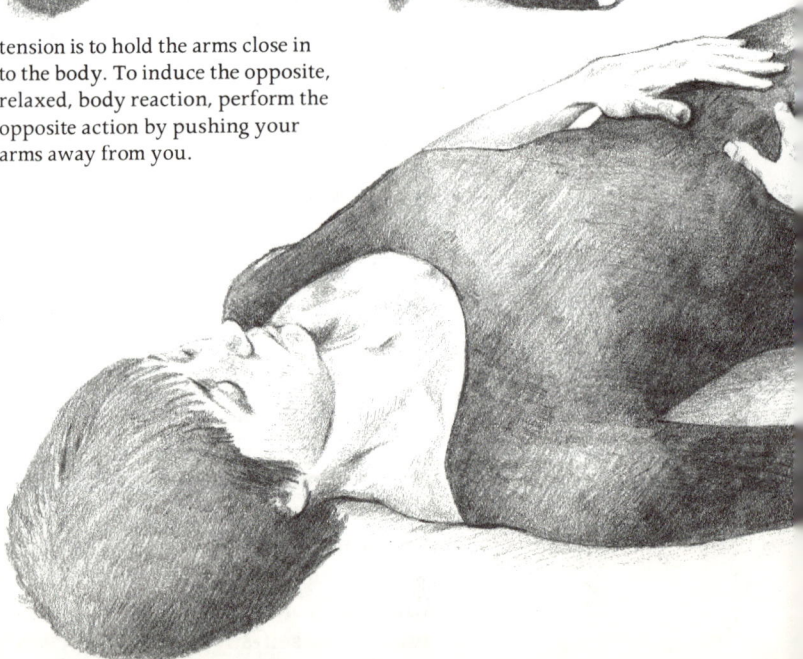

7 Bend the knees, pressing the heels into the floor to help you with your pelvic tilt if the movement doesn't come easily at first.

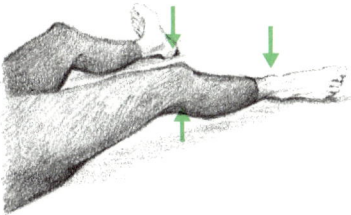

The two natural curves at the back of the neck and waist will be slightly off the floor but require no effort to keep them there. Realize that the trunk is fully supported and that you no longer have to hold it up, but can let go completely. It may not be easy to let go if you suffer from backache, as it's natural to hug any sensitive area. But the moment of unpleasantness as you let go is followed by great ease as the tense muscles release and the blood flows into the sore area to do its healing work.

8 Your thighs will tend to turn out naturally with the pelvic tilt, but at first you may need to do this consciously. **Turn the legs out** so the knees face away from each other. Wiggle the knees about gently if necessary until they feel totally at ease.

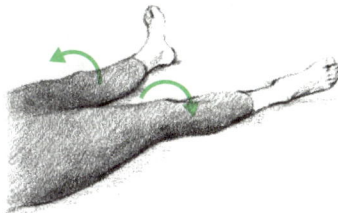

9 Let the feet be loose at the end of the ankles. At first, two small movements may help the feeling of complete ease in the feet. Gently push the heels away from you (a) and, even more gently, push the toes away from you (b).

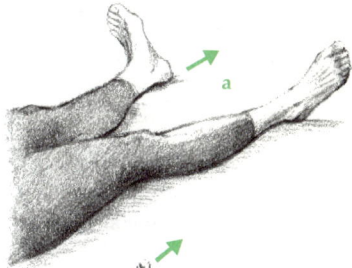

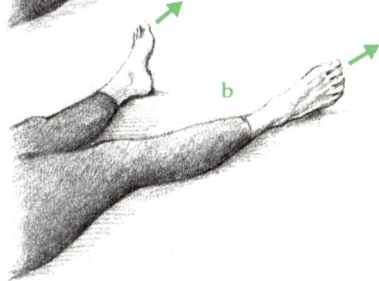

10 Take a good deep breath and let it out in a long deep sigh. Be aware of the ribs working well, as they should for normal breathing, so the breath gets down into the body and isn't stopped half way in the upper chest.

Relaxing the face
Shut your eyes, if you haven't already done so, by gently lowering the top lids without any squeezing or puckering of the skin.

Make sure that your lips aren't pursed, but are soft and lightly touching each other. The jaws should be separated. If they aren't, drag the lower jaw down away from the top one, like a tiny yawn inside the closed mouth, and let go so that the lower jaw finds its own level. If the tongue is on the roof of the mouth, pull it off and let it hang loosely inside the mouth so the tip lies behind the lower front teeth. The throat is now able to relax completely.

Feel the whole face opening outwards from its centre, like a flower opening out. Be aware of space between the eyebrows and of the skin on the forehead releasing up through the hairline. Try stroking your forehead up through the hair before you start, to get the feel of this.

You can now allow your body to lie in peace and tranquillity, not being held still but resting still because you have let go. Gradually the mind can begin to let go too.

Easing tension in your neck and shoulders

Tension collects easily in this area: the head itself weighs 4.5–6.7 kg [10–15 lb], so after a trying day when your shoulders tend to hunch up, it's not surprising if headaches and aches and pains in the neck and back develop. Be careful to work the neck gently and slowly, never pulling or jerking it. Avoid circling the head round in one movement as this grinds down the vertebrae; if you have any neck problems, consult a doctor before starting.

2 A squeeze to release tension between the shoulder blades, useful after working with your arms forwards. Clasp your hands behind you, fingers interlocking. Bending the elbows, press the upper arms in, squeezing the shoulder blades together. Repeat several times. *Bonus: opens the chest, encouraging good breathing.*

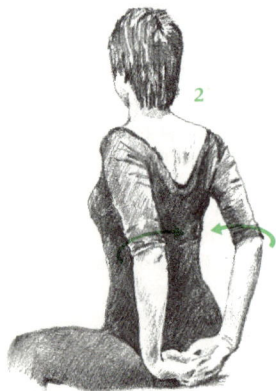

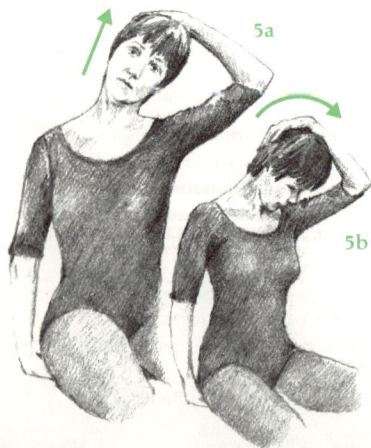

1 To strengthen the upper back and release tension. Lift your shoulders up to your ears (a). Notice how it feels as you raise them deliberately. Pull your shoulders back (b), feeling a squeeze in the upper back.

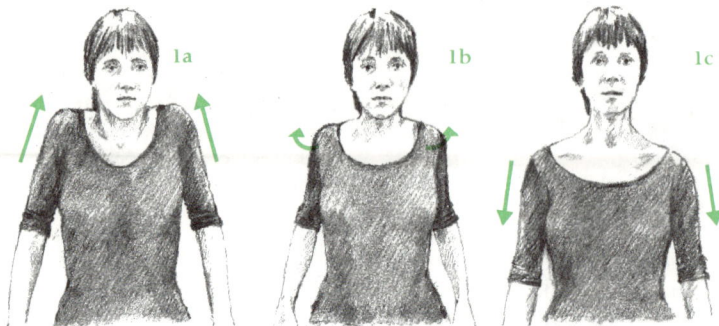

Most important, pull the shoulders down as far as possible (c). Do this as often as you can or whenever your shoulders are raised. Repeat the up, back and down movements several times.

3 To stretch the back of the neck and the spine to ease tension. Sit with your hands on your thighs and legs uncrossed. Drawing the chin in, lower your head slowly forwards (a). When this becomes easy add the weight of your arms. Clasp your hands behind the top of your head and let the elbows fall forwards, but don't pull with them. Draw in your chin, lowering the head until you feel a stretch (b). As this subsides, lower the head further, letting your back round. Hold, breathing well; slowly lift the head.

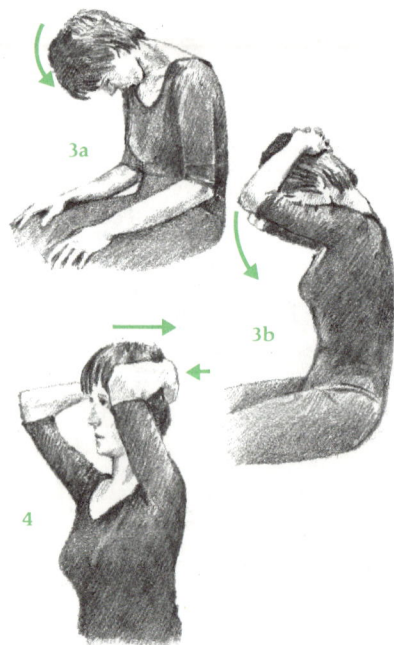

4 To strengthen the muscles at the back of the neck. Clasp your hands behind your head and draw your chin in. Pressing your head back, pull forwards with your hands. Stop, holding your arms in position. Repeat up to six times.

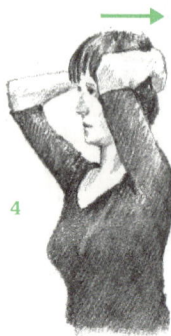

5 To stretch the sides of the neck. Sit with your right hand tucked under your thigh to anchor the right shoulder. Draw in your chin and tilt your head to the left until you feel a gentle stretch on the right of the neck. If this is easy, add the weight of your left hand: do not pull, just rest it across your head (a). Hold for a while and slowly lift the head. Repeat to the right.

Tuck your right arm under you at the back of the chair. Draw in your chin and lower your head diagonally to the left until you feel a stretch from your right shoulder to the base of your skull. Place your left hand diagonally across your head for extra weight if you want more of a stretch (b). Hold for a while; raise your head slowly and repeat to the other side.

210

Breathing

It's possible to survive for weeks without food and days without liquid, but without breathing you can last only a matter of minutes. For this reason, breathing is carefully controlled by a special centre in the lower brain, which automatically regulates the intake of oxygen and the blowing out of carbon dioxide. If you interfere with this fine balancing mechanism – by trying too much deep breathing without adequate physical preparation, for instance – you may become dizzy and eventually faint, a safety mechanism that allows the automatic centre in the brain to regain control.

Posture and exercise

Almost every form of exercise increases the demand on the lungs for oxygen, so that any exercise practised regularly helps to open out the chest area and encourage deeper, stronger breathing. Carefully graded aerobic training (see pages 67–75) is specifically designed to increase your lung capacity. When possible, during exercise, try to breathe through your nose, not your mouth, as the nasal passages filter the air, purifying, warming and moistening it.

Good posture (see pages 12–15) is also essential for good breathing, as your ribs need space to move up and outwards as you breathe in, and down and inwards as you breathe out. If you slouch regularly, your ribs are likely to give up the struggle to move as they were designed to, because of the heavy weight bearing down on them from above. Instead of filling your lungs fully, you use your upper chest only, so your breathing becomes shallow and inadequate. This upper-chest breathing is designed for use in emergencies, when the muscles have used up their supply of oxygen and you need to pant to get as much air into your body as quickly as possible to oxygenate the blood. If you've been running, for example, this happens automatically. However, if you habitually breathe in this way, it sets the body into a permanent alert, which is a state of great stress (see pages 175–77). This develops into a vicious circle as, when you're anxious, you tend to hold your breath.

Breathing for relaxation

Just as anxiety can affect breathing, so good breathing is an important way of learning to control stress and nervousness. Train yourself to keep breathing evenly: concentrate on exhaling, and the inhalation will look after itself. When you're feeling anxious, try the old theatrical trick of taking a few deep breaths to control your nerves. Straighten up your head and shoulders, expand your ribs as you inhale, and exhale slowly – the effect is immediately calming. Practising yoga (see pages 214–20) is particularly useful for developing control, as breathing well in an awkward pose trains you to keep breathing evenly in any difficult situation; singing is also excellent training. Be aware of your normal breathing every once in a while, and if you find it's stilted, try to even it out with a leisurely inhalation, pause, exhalation, pause sequence, rather like the ebb and flow of gentle waves lapping the seashore. If you suffer from asthma or bronchitis, see page 83 for exercises to help you breathe more easily.

211

Are you travelling comfortably?

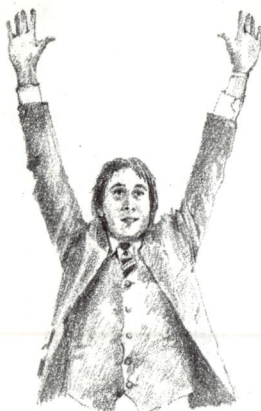

A really good stretch and some deep breaths every so often can help to prevent stiffness.

To make the best of your journey, use your seat. Sit well back and let your body be completely supported by it, sink into it deliberately. If you have a headrest or armrests, relax into them. This is difficult if the chair's badly designed for you, which is especially likely if you're very tall or short: see pages 20–21 for advice on how to adapt your seat to give you better support.

Sitting with your weight unevenly distributed, your legs or arms crossed or your spine slumped puts extra strain on your body and tends to lead to aches and pains, so sit with your body well balanced and lengthen your spine as much as possible (see pages 12–15). If you're anxious or worried, tension at the back of the neck and around the shoulders may make your back arch and your shoulders lift, straining the muscles and affecting your breathing. Remember not to hold your breath and practise a relaxation technique to help you to let go: the routine on pages 208–09 can be done in a seat.

These exercises show how to make the maximum use of limited space to relieve stiff and cramped muscles and will help you to arrive feeling as fresh as possible, whether travelling by plane, train, car or boat. Practise them in any sequence, holding the positions as long as feels comfortable and repeating each exercise as often as you like: aim for about five repetitions. They're designed for exercising in a seat, but some can also be done standing, leaning back or lying down. You may also like to adapt some of the exercises on pages 26–29, 32–45 and 210 for use when you're travelling.

1 If you have weak knees, this exercise is especially helpful, as it strengthens the quadriceps muscles which enclose the knee-caps. Sit with your legs straight out in front of you. Straighten them as strongly as you can, pushing away with the heels and lifting the toes in towards you. Hold for a count of ten if possible and then stop. If this is difficult, work up to ten gradually.

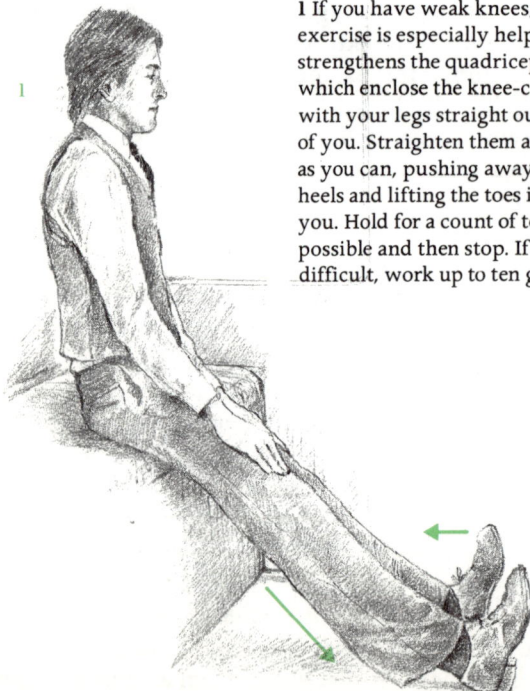

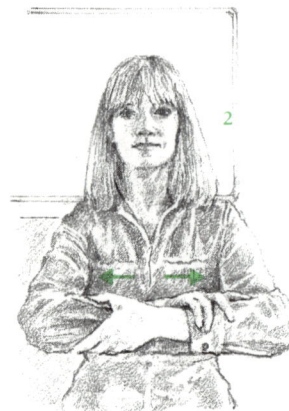

2 To stimulate circulation in the chest and arm muscles. Lift your arms to chest level and clasp each hand round the opposite wrist, holding your elbows up. Push your hands slowly up your arms, as if pushing back tight sleeves. Release when you reach the elbows. Repeat two or three times with your arms at waist level and at eye level.

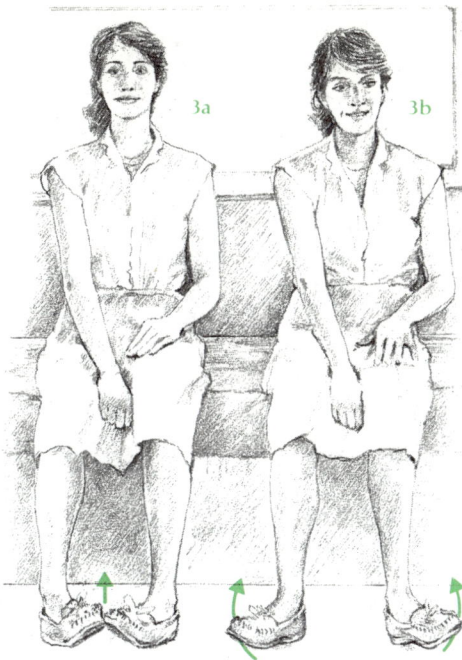

3a 3b

You may like to try exercise 1 on page 210 and exercise 3 on page 28, which are also helpful when you're travelling.

3 To bring circulation to the calves and feet and strengthen the ankles. Put a fist between your knees and hold it there through the exercise. Keeping your heels on the floor, turn your toes in, and lift the big toes up towards the insides of your knees (a). Brush your feet along the floor, turn them out and lift the little toes up towards the outsides of your knees (b). Finish with a few repetitions of the outward movement only, releasing your feet to the floor between each lift.

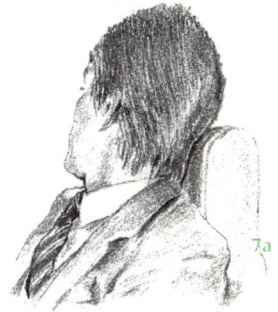

7a

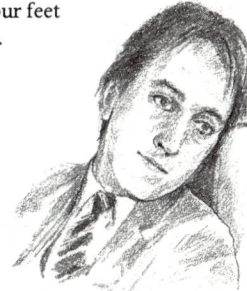

7b

4 To prevent stiffness in the legs and aid circulation; this is a helpful exercise for flabby inner thighs. Sitting down, clench one hand between your knees, as in 3. Press your thighs inwards strongly.

5 This twist helps to prevent stiffness, as well as keeping your spine flexible. Sit forwards so the back of your seat doesn't get in the way. Lengthen your spine and turn from the waist as far as you can to the right, looking behind you. Repeat to the left.

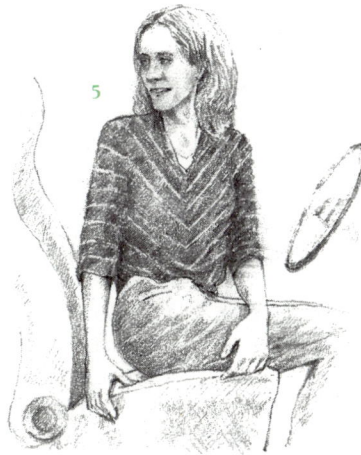

5

7 The spine, particularly at the neck, is beautifully designed to turn, so do this regularly to keep it flexible. Sit well back into the seat with your head supported, preferably by a headrest. Slowly turn your head as much as possible, to the right (a) and the left (b).

8 This helps to mobilize the thumb joints. Rest the outer edges of your hands on your thighs and rotate both thumbs in as wide a circle as possible. Repeat, circling in the opposite direction.

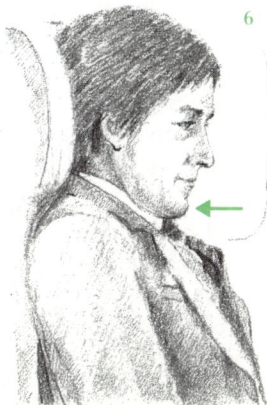

6

6 This exercise strengthens the muscles that support the head and increases the circulation to them. It also encourages full use of a headrest, allowing the head to sink into it and stay supported and at ease. Sit well back so your spine and head are supported and upright. Tuck your chin into the neck and press your head back into the headrest; hold for a few moments.

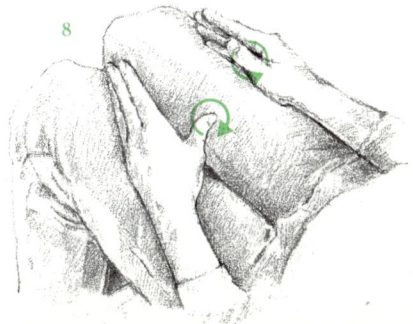

8

213

Yoga

Yoga is a practical holistic philosophy designed to bring a profound state of well-being to body, mind and spirit. It has roots dating back about 5,000 years and was systematized in the 2nd century BC by an Indian sage named Patanjali, who enumerated its eight stages or 'limbs': *nama* and *niyama*, the ethical precepts; *asana,* the practice of physical postures; *pranayama*, control of the breath; *pratyahara*, the development of mental calm and balance; and *dharana, dhyana* and *samadhi* – concentration, meditation and joy. Real yoga, or union, comes with the integration of all these aspects.

The branch that has become most widely known is hatha yoga, the physical exercises, or asanas. Practising these poses not only brings strength, flexibility and grace but also benefits most of the glands, organs and muscles of the body; after a session, you should feel both alert and relaxed. Everyone finds some poses easier than others, but the aim is to perform them all equally well.

The poses on the following pages are based on the work of Sri B.K.S. Iyengar, a modern authority and author of the essential book, *Light on Yoga*. Course One is a brief, basic routine, suitable for beginners. Course Two is for those who have been doing yoga for some time and want to expand their routine. Course Three is harder and takes longer, so you may have time for it only on days when you want a thorough work-out. Courses Two and Three each include poses from the course before: the instructions in italic refer back to asanas already described. However, this selection is intended only as reference for practice between classes. If you want to learn yoga, it's essential to have personal supervision from a teacher, who can help you to overcome any problems, drawing from the whole range of asanas. It's particularly important not to start on your own if you're pregnant, or have backache or heart problems, or any long-standing complaint.

Bear these points in mind when practising:
• Wear loose clothing that allows you to stretch and move freely, and practise in bare feet so you don't slip.
• Try working on a blanket for comfort when sitting or lying down.
• Don't work on a full stomach.
• Breathe through the nose and don't hold your breath in a pose.
• Hold each posture only as long as it's comfortable – a few seconds may be long enough at first. It's better to do an asana intelligently than to strain to do it fully.
• In standing poses where one foot is turned in, the other out, turn the first foot only slightly in, the second out at 90° and make sure that the heel of the second foot is in line with the instep of the first.
• Try to practise a little every day. If you're pressed for time, just do two or three poses that you find more difficult. Ideally, each practice should always include two or three standing poses; both forward and back bends (more forward than back, if there's an imbalance); a twisting exercise; more shoulderstand (9) than headstand (18), if the headstand is done; and finally savasana (11).

COURSE ONE

Children often enjoy yoga, but they should never be pushed into it – let it be a game that they can start and stop whenever they like. The poses that are most fun for them are shown by a child. Adults of any age can start yoga: being fairly gentle, it's an especially good form of exercise for the elderly.

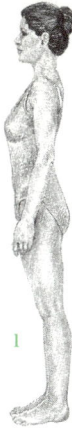

1 Tadasana
The basic standing pose to develop correct posture. Stand with feet touching, spreading your toes to give firm support. Lift your knees, contract your buttocks and stretch up from the pubis, feeling your abdomen flatten. Elongate the whole spine, including the neck. Open the chest and drop your shoulders.

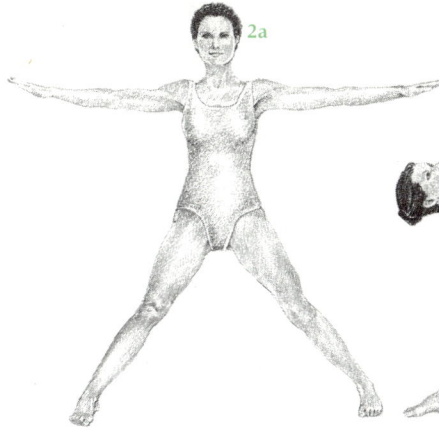

2 Trikonasana
Strengthens the legs and back and makes the legs and hips more supple; helpful for backache. From tadasana take feet 1 m [3–3½ ft] apart and stretch arms out at shoulder level, palms down (a). Turn left foot in, right foot out. On an exhalation, stretch from the hip and take your right hand down to hold your right leg or touch the floor; raise your left arm vertically and look up at your left thumb (b). Lift your knees and stretch your arms and spine fully. Inhale as you come up. Repeat on the other side.

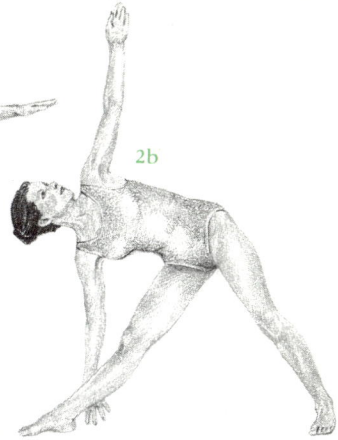

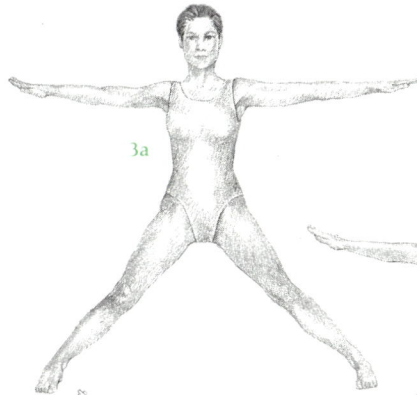

3 Utthita parsvakonasana
Opens and develops the chest, helps to slim the waist and hips and to settle digestion and excretion; relieves sciatica and arthritis. From tadasana, take feet 1.3 m [4–4½ ft] apart. Stretch arms out at shoulder level, palms down (a). Turn left foot in, right foot out. On an exhalation, bend your right knee to make a right angle, with your thigh parallel to the floor, your calf vertical (b). Stretch your trunk on to your right thigh, putting your right hand by your right foot. Extend the left arm over your head and look up, stretching the back of your body from left heel to fingertips and keeping your head, chest and hips on one plane (c). Inhale as you come up. Repeat on the other side.

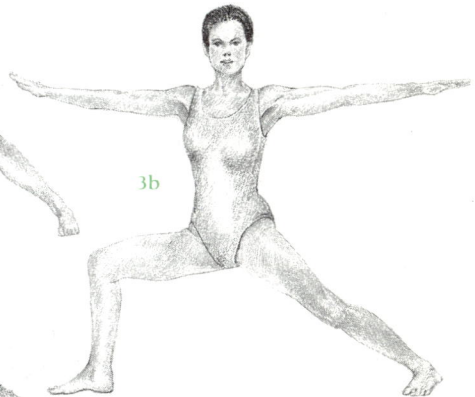

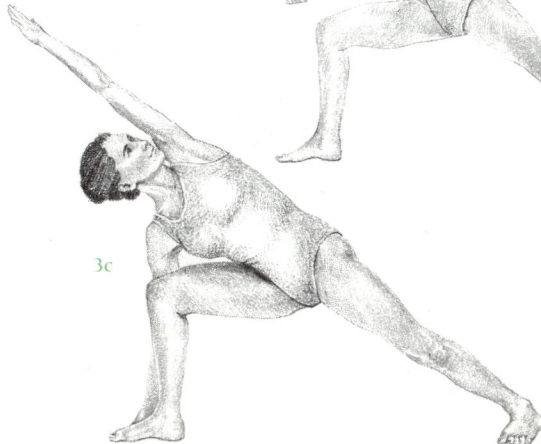

215

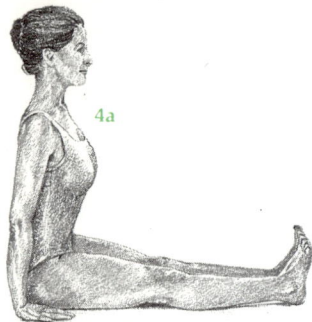

4 Paschimottanasana
Tones the abdominal organs, calms the heart and mind. Sit with legs straight out in front, feet flexed, hands by hips and stretch your spine and neck up, holding your shoulders down (a). On an exhalation, extend your spine forwards, keeping your back concave and your head up. Hold your toes (b) or, if you can't, a towel or belt looped around your feet. Breathe out and lower your chest on to your thighs, if you can do so with a straight back (c). Inhale as you come up.

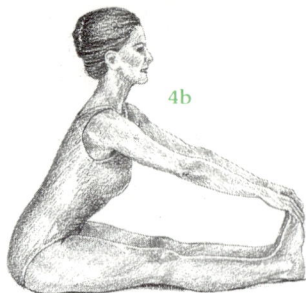

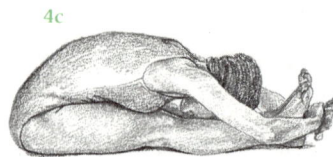

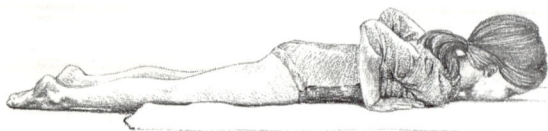

5 Bhujangasana
Strengthens the spine and opens the chest. Lie facing down, legs and feet stretched out together, palms down at chest level (a). On an inhalation, lift up, pushing with your hands, and lengthen the spine upwards while you take two breaths (b). Breathe in and roll your head back, contracting the buttocks and tightening the thighs as you stretch the legs strongly (c). Breathe out as you lower to the floor. Repeat up to three times.

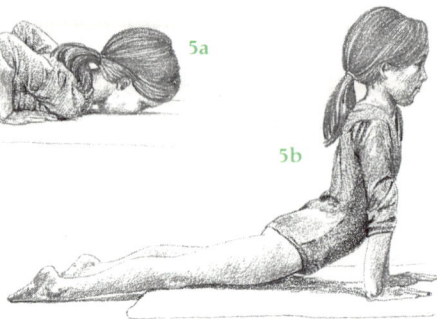

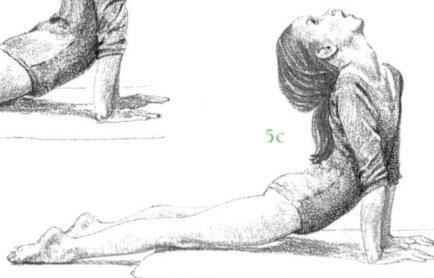

6 Bharadvajasana
Relieves stiffness in the lower back and eases arthritic pain in the hips and shoulders. Sit with a straight back (a), as in paschimottanasana. Bending your knees, swing your feet back to your left hip. Keeping both buttocks on the floor, turn to the right. Try to bring your chest in line with your thigh, but don't let your lower back curve forwards. Pull in your waist and abdomen, stretching from pubis to chest. Tuck your left hand under your right knee. Put your right hand behind you to help you stretch up or, if your lower back is straight, exhale, and take your right hand behind you to clasp your left elbow (b). Repeat on the other side.

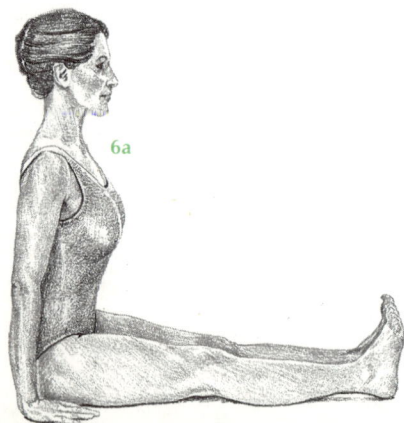

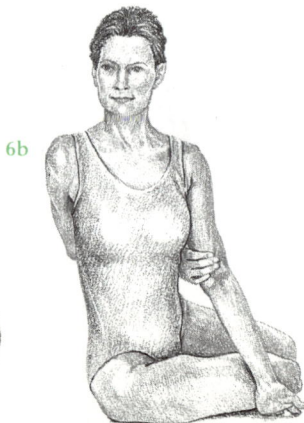

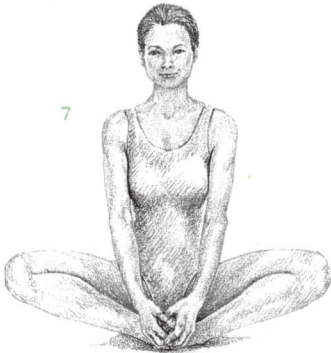

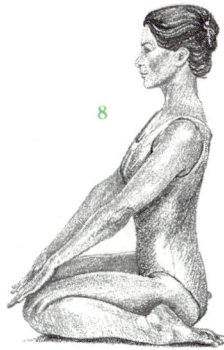

9 Salamba sarvangasana

Women should avoid this when menstruating. Brings all the functions of the body into balance; restores energy. Place a folded blanket on the floor and lie facing up with your shoulders and elbows on it. Bend your knees up to your chest and, exhaling, roll up on to your shoulders, supporting your upper back with your hands (a). Stretch the spine up and straighten your legs. Your body should be vertical, your chest touching your chin (b). Aim eventually to hold this pose for ten minutes. Exhale as you come down.

7 Baddha konasana

Helpful for urinary or menstrual difficulties; relieves sciatic pains. Sit with knees bent and bring the soles of your feet together. Keeping your back straight, draw your feet in towards you, lowering your knees as far as possible.

8 Virasana

Eases rheumatic pains in the knees, corrects flat feet. Kneel on the floor with knees together and feet apart, toes pointing back, hands on your knees. Try to lower your buttocks to the floor. Sit on a cushion if your knees are stiff.

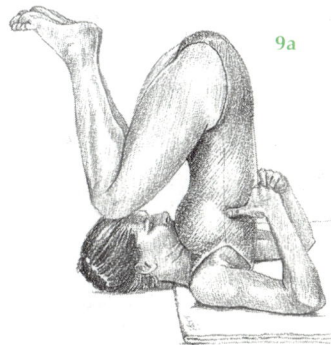

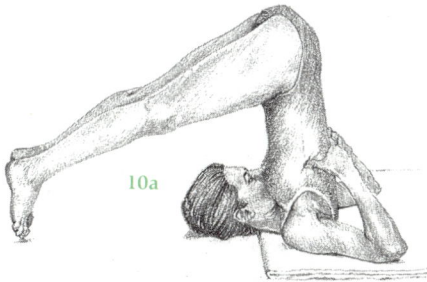

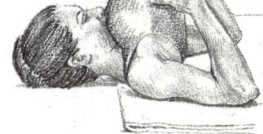

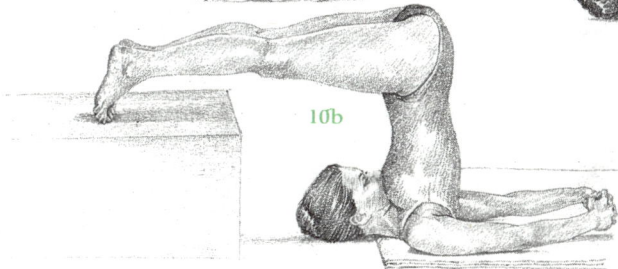

10 Halasana

Women should avoid this when menstruating. Benefits as in 9; also gives a relaxing stretch in the thighs. From sarvangasana, lower your legs over your head, until your toes touch the floor (a); don't let your spine sag. Rest your feet on a box or chair if you are a beginner or have a stiff back (b). Once in the pose, straighten your arms back, as in (b). Aim eventually to hold this pose for ten minutes.

11 Savasana

Quietens the mind and refreshes the body, especially the nerves. Lie on your back. If your neck and shoulders are stiff, rest your head on a book or put a cushion under your head and shoulders. Drop your

shoulders, stretch your legs, and take your arms a little away from your trunk, palms up. Keep your body even. Close your eyes, relax every part of your body and let your breathing become quiet. Stay in the pose for about ten minutes.

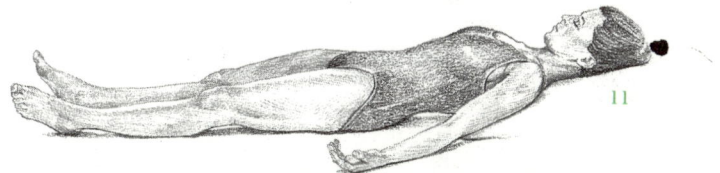

COURSE TWO

Begin with poses 1, 2 and 3 from Course One.

12 Janu sirsasana

Tones the abdominal organs and aids digestion. Sit with legs straight out in front. Bend your right leg, letting the knee fall outwards and moving it to the right so the foot doesn't touch the left leg; keep the left foot flexed. Put your right wrist on your right knee, your left hand behind you, and lift the spine up straight (a). On an exhalation, bend forwards to clasp your left foot with both hands, if you can do so with a straight back (b); otherwise hold (a). Repeat on the other side.
Now do pose 4 from Course One.

13 Navasana

Helpful for a bloated feeling in the abdomen and gastric complaints, benefits kidneys and trims the waist. Sitting down, bend your legs up to your chest and lean back. On an exhalation, straighten your legs up in front of you; aim to raise your feet higher than your head. Stretch your arms out in front, parallel to the floor, palms facing each other. Keep your weight on your buttocks, not on the base of your spine. Exhale as you come down.
Now do pose 5 from Course One.

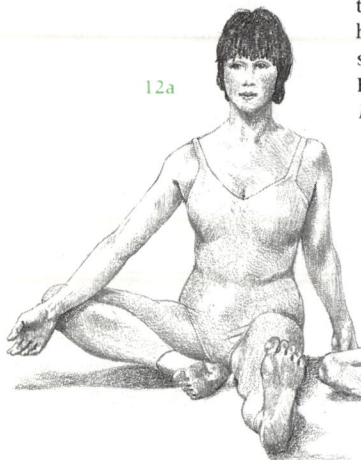

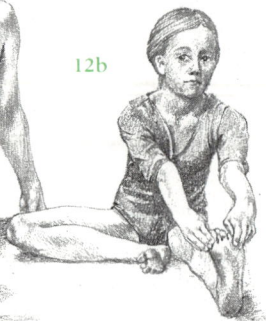

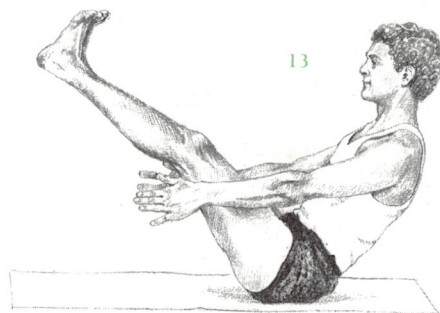

14 Ustrasana

Stretches and tones the back; helps to correct rounded shoulders and a hunched back. Kneel down and push the heels of your hands into your lower back, fingers pointing out (a). On an exhalation, lower your left hand to your left foot and your right hand to your right foot. Lift your hips up, pushing your thighs up until they are vertical, and let your head roll back (b).

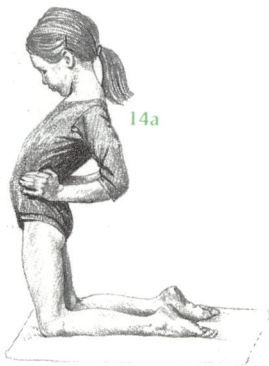

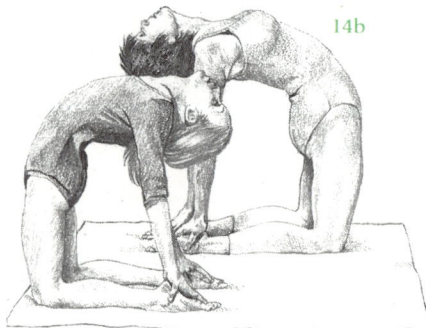

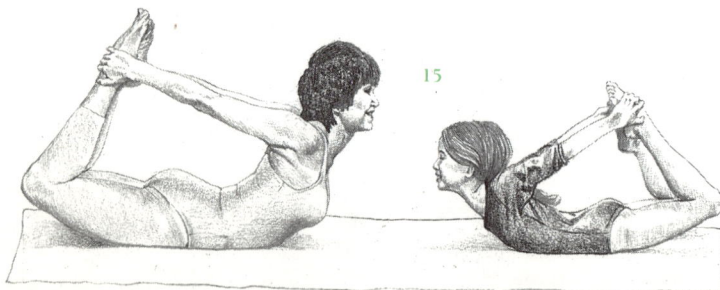

15 Dhanurasana

Stretches and mobilizes the spine, tones the abdominal organs. Lie facing down, bend your knees and hold your left ankle with your left hand, your right ankle with your right hand. On an exhalation, lift your chest and thighs up as far as possible, looking up. Hold, pulling upwards. Exhale as you release.

16 Mandukasana

Relaxes all the abdominal organs and opens the chest. Kneel down, sitting on your heels and, keeping your big toes touching, take your knees wide apart. On an exhalation, bend from the hips and stretch your arms forwards on the floor, holding your buttocks down on your feet. Try to lower your abdomen to the floor. *Now do poses 6, 7, 8, 9 and 10 from Course One.*

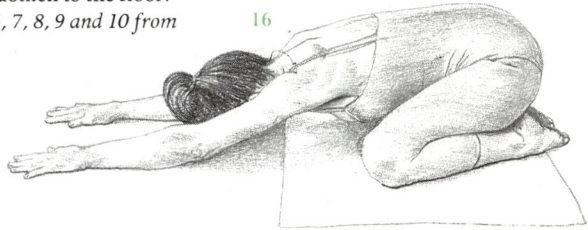

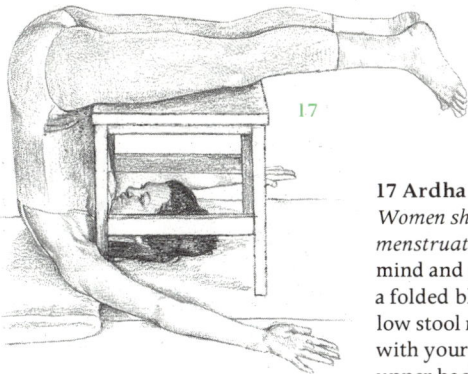

17 Ardha halasana

Women should avoid this when menstruating. Relaxes the body and mind and stretches the back. Place a folded blanket on the floor and a low stool next to it. Lie facing up, with your shoulders, elbows and upper back on the blanket, your head on the floor under the stool. Bend your legs; on an exhalation, lift your back up and lower your thighs on to the stool, your hips touching the edge. Straighten your legs and arms out. Aim to hold the pose for about ten minutes. *Now do pose 11 from Course One.*

COURSE THREE

18 Sirsasana

Women should avoid this when menstruating. This brings fresh blood to the brain, vigour to the lungs and balance to the body and mind. Practise this only when you can do all the other asanas easily; damage can result from doing it incorrectly. Place a folded blanket on the floor and kneel beside it. Place your elbows on it, no more than shoulderwidth apart. Interlace the fingers firmly. Rest the crown of your head on the floor against your cupped hands. Straighten your legs and walk your toes in towards your head. Hold for a few moments, making sure your back is extended (a). Breathing out, bend your knees, lifting your feet and bringing your knees in to your chest (b). If this is hard, gently jump one leg up at a time. When you feel stable, gradually straighten your legs until your body is vertical (c). At first, it may help to practise this with your back a little way from a wall to prevent you falling back. Aim eventually to hold this pose for ten minutes. Exhale as you come down.

Now do poses 1, 2 and 3 from Course One; pose 12 from Course Two.

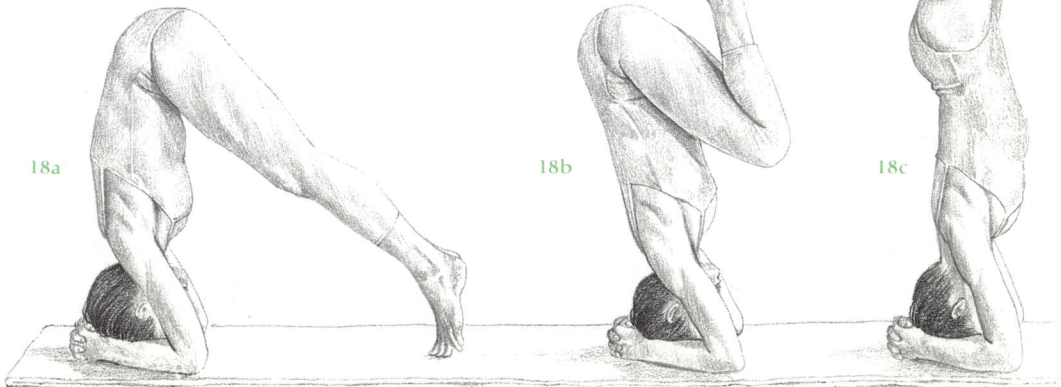

19 Triangamukhaikapada paschimottanasana

Helps to cure flat feet, relieves sprains in the ankles and knees and tones the abdominal organs. Sit with legs straight out in front, feet flexed. Bend the right leg up behind you, sitting up straight on both buttocks (a). If this is easy, exhale and bend from the hips over the left leg, stretching both arms forwards (b). Inhale as you come up and repeat to the other side.
Now do pose 4 from Course One.

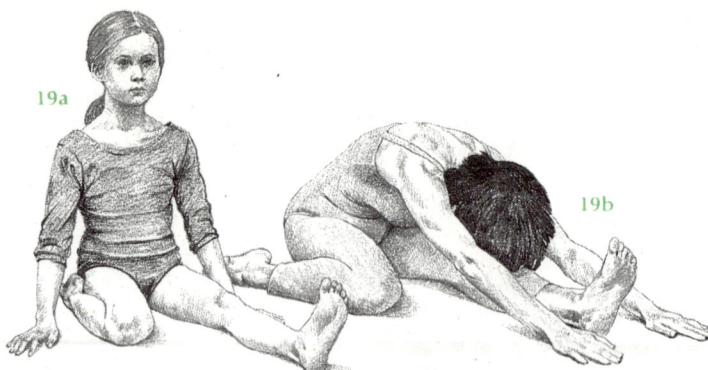

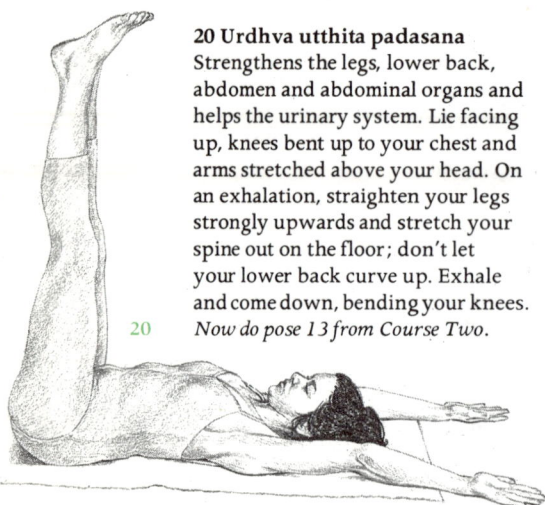

20 Urdhva utthita padasana

Strengthens the legs, lower back, abdomen and abdominal organs and helps the urinary system. Lie facing up, knees bent up to your chest and arms stretched above your head. On an exhalation, straighten your legs strongly upwards and stretch your spine out on the floor; don't let your lower back curve up. Exhale and come down, bending your knees.
Now do pose 13 from Course Two.

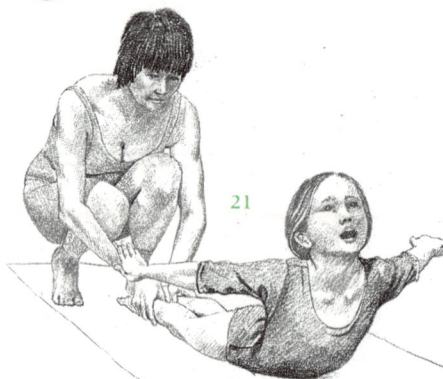

21 Salabhasana

Aids the digestive and urinary systems, mobilizes the spine and relieves pain in the lower back. Lie facing down, arms outstretched at shoulder level. Ask a partner to hold your feet down firmly. On an exhalation, lift your chest up as high as you can; hold, trying to lift further.

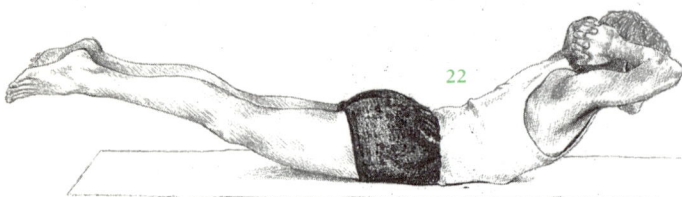

22 Makarasana

Benefits the digestive and urinary systems and strengthens the back, relieving pains in the lumbar area. Lie face down, hands clasped behind your head. On an exhalation, raise your legs and chest up as high as you can, keeping your legs straight.
Now do pose 5 from Course One; poses 14, 15 and 16 from Course Two; poses 6, 7, 8, 9 and 10 from Course One; pose 17 from Course Two.

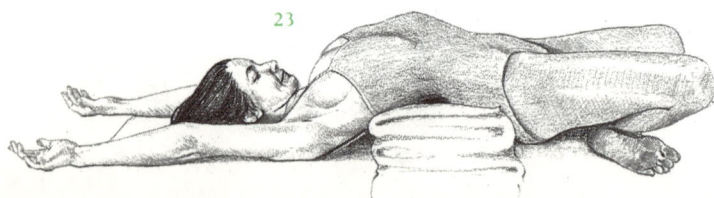

23 Supta sukhasana

Relaxes all the internal organs, quietens the nerves, improves breathing and develops the shoulders. Sit with your legs crossed, with a large cushion or several folded blankets behind you. Let your knees fall apart and wriggle each foot under the opposite shin as far as possible. Lie back over the cushion or blankets so they support your trunk, stretching your arms over your head and keeping your buttocks on the ground. Repeat, crossing your legs the other way.
Now do pose 11 from Course One.

Swedish massage

The value of a caring touch, both given and received, is enormous. Touching should be an instinctive way of giving comfort and reassurance, but because of cultural taboos, it's a pleasure often denied. Part of the health-giving potential of massage is the contact it gives, but it also has many other benefits for the recipient.

The massage on pages 222–29 is based on the work of Peter Henrik Ling, a 19th-century Swedish fencer and gymnast who blended European and Oriental practices, creating a system that covers the whole body with a variety of strokes, some deep, some superficial. Its most obvious function is to relax the person being massaged, but it also brings several other benefits. Friction from the masseur's hands generates heat and so increases perspiration, helping the body rid itself of waste products. Pressure encourages the flow of fluid between the lymph glands, improving the body's natural immunity to infection; it also hastens the flow of blood back to the heart from veins close to the skin which, together with the increased flow of lymph, helps to remove the waste products accumulated in the muscles. Tissues near the surface are stretched directly so muscles that are bunched and shortened (by overuse, bad posture, tension and so on) are helped to return to normal; as the muscles relax, blood flows in, bringing fresh oxygen and nutrients and carrying away toxic wastes.

Whether it's intended as therapy or as a means of relaxation, however, there are some things that massage can't do. It's impossible to lose weight or 'tone up' muscles by being massaged. Massage can never act as a substitute for proper diet and exercise, although it can complement them by creating a sense of well-being and by encouraging a return to normal muscle and tissue metabolism.

Don't attempt a massage on anyone with a high fever or when there's a possibility of dislodging a thrombus, or blood clot, in the veins. Avoid working over varicose veins, recent injuries or areas of active skin disease. There's a danger that an inexperienced person might damage the internal organs while massaging the abdomen, so it's best left out of this basic home massage. If you're in any doubt, or need treatment for a specific problem, seek professional advice.

Before you start Home massage should be both enjoyable and relaxing, so make the room as comfortable as possible. Keep the lighting soft and, as your partner should wear no clothes or only underwear for a body massage, make sure that the room is warm and cover the parts that you're not massaging. It's easiest to reach each area without straining if your partner lies on a large table covered with a blanket, but if necessary you can spread some blankets on the floor. Don't use a bed, as most of the pressure is absorbed by the mattress, not the body.

You may like to use a lubricant, such as hand cream, baby, mineral or even vegetable oil. This helps to avoid uncomfortable friction: if you don't use one, make sure your hands aren't moist, as this prevents them from moving smoothly. Choose a lubricant that doesn't irritate your partner's skin and don't use too much, as your hands may slip and slide. Aromatherapists lay special emphasis on the lubricant, and massage with essential plant oils for specific effects.

Minimize the distractions, and the conversation, so you can both concentrate on the massage. If your hair is long, tie it back, and remove your watch and any jewellery that might irritate your partner. Make sure that your fingernails are short, so they can't dig into the flesh, and roll back your sleeves if they're loose. You may want to use only a part of the massage on pages 224–27 – for example, a few minutes' work on the shoulders when your partner has had a hard day – but if you want to do the whole massage, allow at least an hour.

Be aware of tension in your body before beginning. If you're not relaxed, you have to work through your own muscle tension, as well as your partner's. Learn to recognize tension with this exercise: let one arm hang by your side and feel the texture of the muscles; then stretch it out in front, clenching your fist, and notice the difference in texture. If you are tense, try the relaxation technique on pages 208–09 before you begin and remember to breathe evenly as you work.

Basic techniques

The art of massage lies in deciding which part of the hand to use and how much pressure to apply. It's also important to establish a smooth rhythm and to flow evenly from one movement to the next. The techniques that you'll need in the massage are described below and opposite – they're given in bold type where they occur in the instructions on pages 224–29. At first, follow the directions closely – a good place to try them out is on your partner's back – but as you practise, you'll naturally evolve your own style.

STROKING

Deep stroking *right*
Use this at the start of a massage to distribute any lubricant evenly and encourage relaxation; you can also use it between other strokes to soothe and give the tissues a rest from deep work. Run your hands smoothly over the skin, curving them over the body's contours and giving a deep stroke, mainly from the palms. This encourages the flow of lymph and of blood returning to the heart, so the massage must be towards the heart when working on the arms or legs. Apply pressure only as your hands move away from you, but maintain contact in both directions. When working over a small area, you can use just your thumbs or fingers.

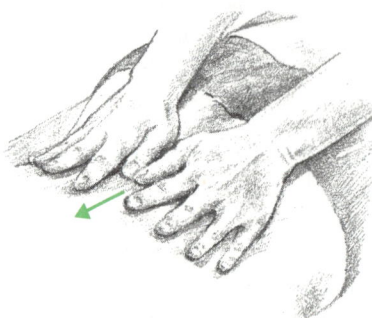

Superficial stroking *right*
The reflex reaction of the nerves to this movement should result in relaxation. Glide your fingers or fingertips very lightly along the skin. Use each hand alternately, the second beginning a sweep just as the first finishes, so you build up a

flowing rhythm; keep the motion slow to help your partner relax. It doesn't matter which direction you move in, as long as you're consistent. This is a particularly relaxing movement at the end of a massage, but don't use it for more than a few minutes, or it may become irritating.

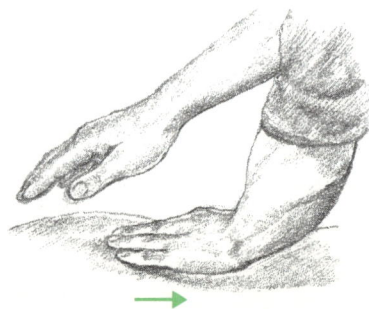

KNEADING MOVEMENTS

The benefit of these is the stimulation of the blood supply. Gently lift, wring and squeeze the muscles – the only gliding motion is when your hands move from area to area. You should use both hands alternately but you may be able to use only one over a small area. Make each movement slow, gentle and rhythmic, and as deep as can comfortably be tolerated. Don't work too long in one place in case you bruise the skin, and don't pinch.

Kneading *below*

Rest the heels of your hands and your thumbs on your partner's body and mould your fingers, held together, round a muscle mass. Roll the flesh under each hand with the outer edge of the hand and wrist.

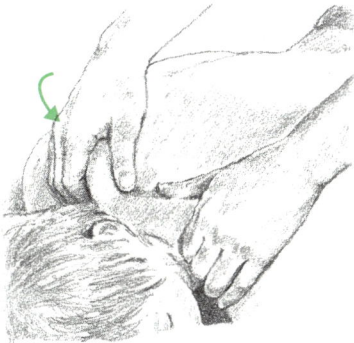

Picking up *below*

Begin with your hands in the same position as for kneading, but bring the muscle mass towards the thumb and heel of each hand with your fingers. Lift the flesh up, away from the bone, and squeeze it gently at the end of the movement.

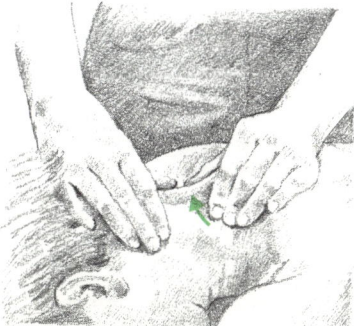

Skin rolling *below*

Rolling, in particular, helps to promote a good blood supply to the skin. Grasp some tissue between the thumb and fingers of each hand, so a ridge of flesh is raised, and move each thumb in towards the fingers, creating corrugations in front and smoothing the skin behind as it moves. Take great care as this can be uncomfortable and it's easy to bruise your partner if you're over-enthusiastic.

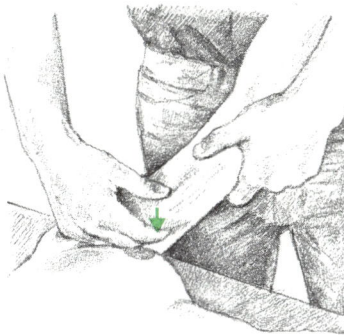

FRICTIONS *below*

Use this spot action for areas where deep tissues need to be worked on: for example, where the tissue feels tense, stringy or knotty, or where it feels tender to your partner. Press down with the pads of one or more fingers, your thumb or the heel of your hand and give a deep, even, circular massage for about three seconds. You can repeat the movement but don't work on the same place for longer than your partner can comfortably tolerate. Using both hands, one on top of the other, gives extra reinforcement on large muscle masses, such as the buttocks.

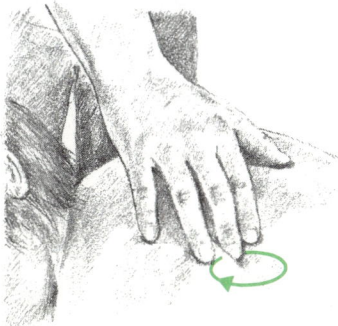

PERCUSSION

All the movements in this group – hacking, cupping, slapping, beating, tapping and pincement – are stimulating, not relaxing, and so are more appropriate for a remedial massage given by a skilled practitioner. There are times, however, when stimulation is helpful in a home massage so hacking and tapping are included.

Hacking *below*

Start with relaxed hands and wrists, fingers loosely together, hands parallel and palms facing, and drop each hand alternately down on to the skin. It's not a chopping action – curl your outer three fingers under as your hands meet the flesh. Make the movements quick and brief, trying to keep your timing even, so you don't develop an unbalanced rhythm. You may like to practise this on a soft cushion or pillow.

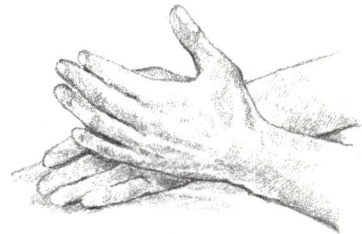

Tapping *below*

Using the index and middle fingers of both hands, tap briskly and rapidly over the skin, as if tapping on a table.

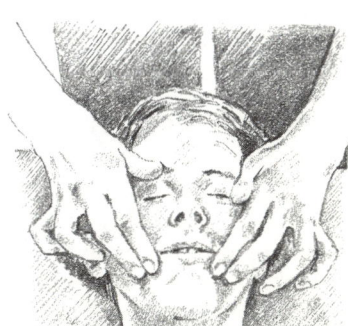

223

Head to toes massage

FACE AND FRONT OF THE NECK

1 Stand behind your partner's head. Rest the pads of your thumbs just above the inner corner of each eyebrow. **Stroke deeply** with each thumb out to the side towards the temple. Repeat, moving your thumbs further up away from the eyebrows with every stroke, until you reach the hairline. One sign that your partner is relaxed by this stroke is an open mouth, showing a release of tension from the jaw.

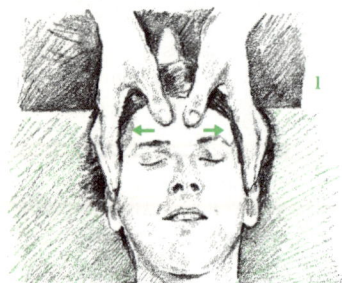

2 With great care, repeat the movement immediately below the eyebrows, **stroking deeply** along the rim of the bone to the outer edges of the eyes. Repeat once.

3 Cup your hands round your partner's chin and give **deep strokes** below the jaw, some to the ears and others continuing in front of the ears up to the temples.

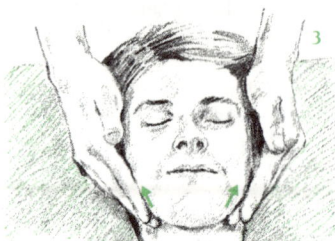

4 Turn your partner's head to the left, supporting it with your left hand, and give **frictions** to the area round the hinge of the jaw with your right thumb or fingers.

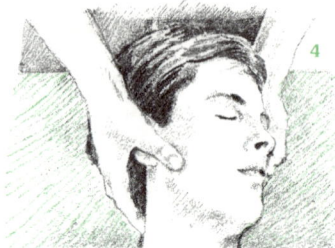

5 Give **deep strokes** from the jaw to the collarbone with your thumb, working on the fleshy parts at the side of the neck.

6 Give **frictions** round the hinge of the jaw with your thumb or fingers.

7 Finish working on the neck with a few more **deep strokes**. Turn your partner's head and repeat stages 4, 5, 6 and 7 on the left of the neck.

8 With an index finger on either side of the bridge of the nose, **stroke deeply** down the nose. Repeat twice, moving out from the nose.

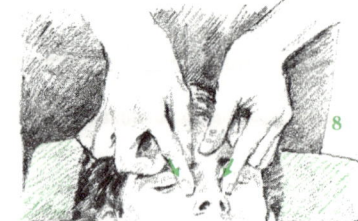

9 **Tap** over the cheeks, chin, sides of the face and round the mouth.

10 Finish with a repeat of 1.

ARMS

1 Stand by your partner's left arm and firmly but gently hold the wrist in your left hand. With your right hand, **stroke deeply** from the wrist to the shoulder, moulding your hand to the contours of the arm. Repeat five times, changing hands so you cover both sides of the arm.

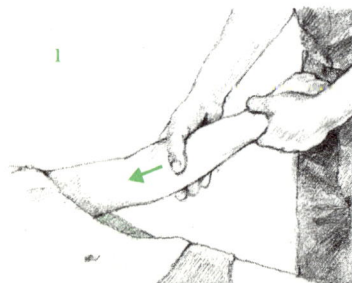

2 Grip your partner's hand under your left arm and use your forearm to help keep it in place. **Knead** the muscles of the upper arm with both hands (below), working on the inside from underarm to elbow and the outside from elbow to shoulder. Knead the muscle mass at the top of the arm thoroughly, taking handfuls of skin and muscle between the fingers and thumbs. Repeat the same sequence with **picking up**.

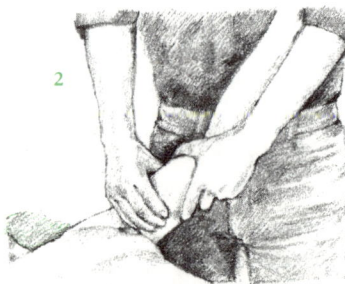

3 Letting your partner's arm rest on the table, palm up, **knead** the muscles of the forearm, working from elbow to wrist along the fleshy part. **Pick up** over the same area.

4 Repeat the deep stroking, as in 1, making three full strokes.

5 Using your thumb or fingers, give **frictions** where needed. Pay particular attention to the shoulder and the crease of the elbow.

6 Rolling is excellent for getting the circulation going, especially on the upper arm, which tends to become flabby, losing its smooth skin texture. With your partner's hand under your arm, as in 2, **roll** the length of both the inside and outside of the upper arm.

7 Work over the fleshy areas of the arm with **hacking**.

8 Finish with a repeat of 1, making three strokes, either deep or superficial, as you prefer.
Walk round and repeat 1 to 8 on the right arm.

HANDS

1 Stand at your partner's right side and support the right hand and wrist, palm up, in both your hands. Give thumb **frictions** to the wrist, paying particular attention to any tendons that feel very tight. Work over the palm with frictions, releasing any tension you feel.

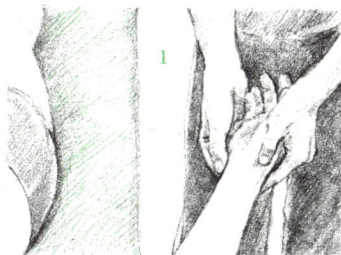

2 Support your partner's hand at the wrist with your left hand. Place the length of your right thumb along the base of the palm, letting your fingers cradle the back of the hand. Starting at the outer edge of the hand, make **deep strokes** with your thumb from wrist to fingertips. Finish the stroke in the air at the end of the fingertips to give your partner a floating, relaxing feeling. With each stroke move your thumb further in towards the index finger.

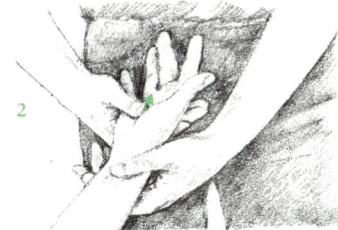

3 Turn your partner's hand over and, supporting the palm, give thumb **frictions** to the back of the wrist and from wrist to fingers, working between the bones.

4 Holding your partner's hand in both of yours, take hold of the base of a finger between your thumb and fingers. Pull firmly and slowly up its length, continuing a little way beyond the fingertips. Before you reach the end of the first finger, begin pulling another with your other hand and repeat with all the fingers and the thumb, releasing only one at a time so your partner's hand is always supported.
Walk round and repeat 1 to 4 on the left hand.

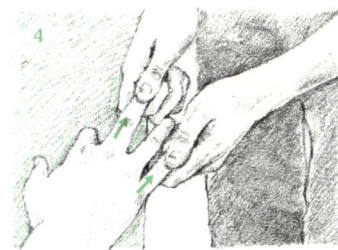

LEGS – FRONT

1 Stand at your partner's feet, or slightly to the side if you're not tall enough to reach from ankle to thigh in one easy movement. Clasp your partner's left ankle with both hands, so your thumbs overlap, and **stroke deeply** up the length of the leg. Repeat five times.

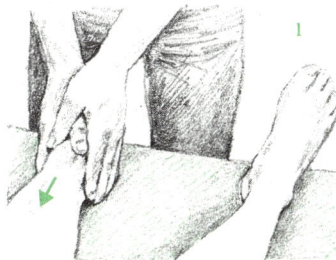

2 Move round to your partner's left side and, using both hands, **knead** the thigh muscles. Work along the outside from hip to knee and the inside from knee to groin. Knead the middle of the thigh, with one hand on each side of the leg or with both hands working on the centre. Repeat with **picking up**. Squeeze and wring gently (as shown) where you can pick up enough tissue.

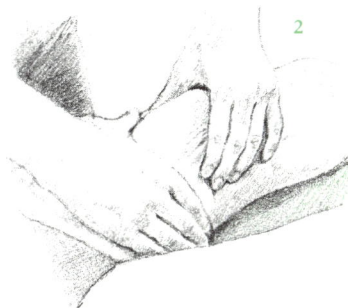

3 Repeat deep stroking, as in 1, for three strokes.

4 With the thumb or fingers of one or both hands, give **frictions** where necessary: working round the knee-cap is often helpful as there are many tendons that may have become tight and stringy.

5 Circulation in the thighs is often sluggish and fat tends to accumulate on the outer thighs, changing the skin texture, so rolling is useful here. Use both hands over this large area. **Roll** systematically from hip to knee on the outside, from knee to groin on the inside and from groin to knee on the centre.

6 Work over the whole thigh with **hacking**; avoid the shin, as it's too bony.

7 Repeat deep stroking, as in 1, for three strokes.

8 Bend up your partner's left leg so the foot rests firmly on the table or couch. Sit on the edge of the table or couch by the leg, with your left hand holding the knee steady. With your right hand, grasp the calf muscle close to the ankle and move it sideways, to your right. Repeat, working up the calf.

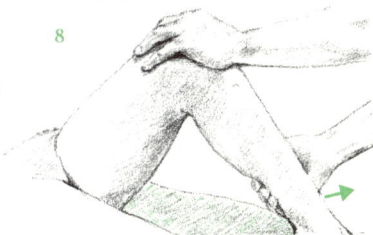

9 Finish with three full strokes, as in 1 – these can be deep or superficial as preferred.
Walk round and repeat 1 to 9 on the right leg.

▷

FEET

1 Stand at the end of the table and cradle your partner's left foot with both hands, one over the ankle and the other under the heel. Make **deep strokes** with both hands along the length of the foot to the ends of the toes. Repeat five times.

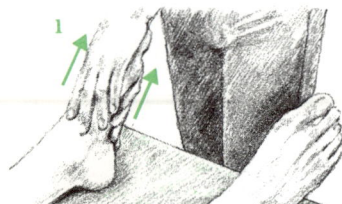

2 Supporting the foot with both hands, give thumb **frictions** round the inner and outer ankle bones and to the top of the foot, working from ankle to toes between the bones.

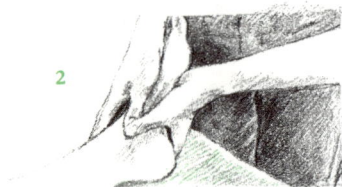

3 Place both thumbs on top of the foot, near the middle of the toes, and let your fingers curl round the sole. Apply pressure and **stroke deeply** with your thumbs out to the sides of the foot. With each stroke, move a little further towards the ankle until the whole foot has been transversely stretched.

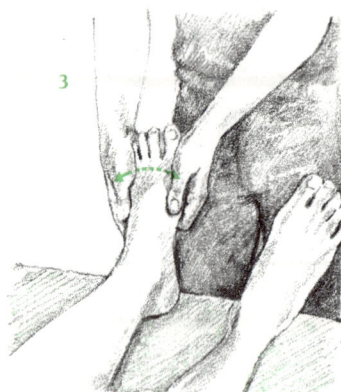

4 Support the foot at the heel with your left hand. Work on the sole, giving **frictions** with your right thumb from heel to toes and from the outer to the inner edges of the foot.

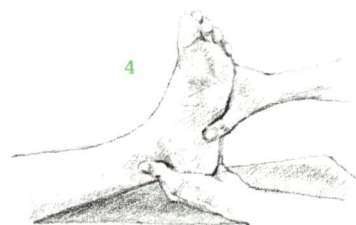

5 Holding your right hand over the ankle for support, **stroke deeply** up the sole from heel to toes, with the base of your left palm covering the width of the foot. Repeat twice.

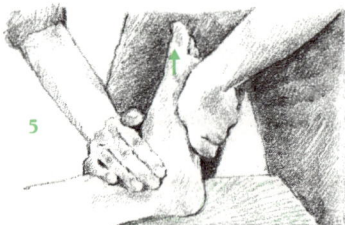

6 Firmly and slowly, pull each toe between your thumb and forefinger, working on all five toes, using alternate hands, as with the fingers (see page 225).
Repeat 1 to 6 on the right foot.

LEGS – BACK

1 Ask your partner to turn over, and stand at the left foot or left side. Cross your thumbs over the back of the left ankle and give six **deep strokes** up the leg.

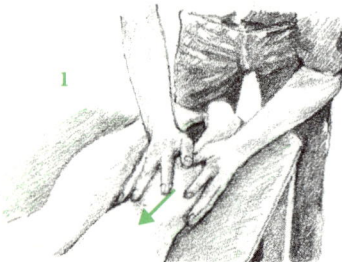

2 Stand by your partner's left thigh and **knead** the thigh muscles with both hands (as shown). Work on the outside from hip to knee, the inside from knee to groin and the middle from the top of the leg to the knee. Repeat the same sequence with **picking up.**

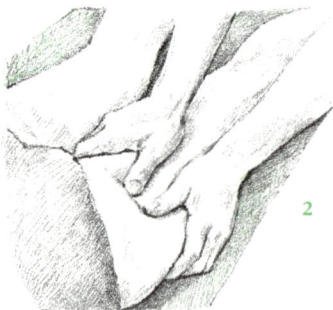

3 Massage the fleshy parts of the calf with **kneading** and **picking up.** Work with both hands from ankle to knee on the inside and from the knee to ankle on the outside.

4 Repeat deep stroking, as in 1, for three strokes.

5 Give **frictions** with your thumb or fingers where appropriate, concentrating on the crease of the knee and the Achilles tendon.

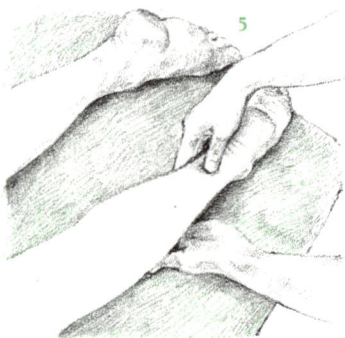

6 **Roll** the whole thigh and calf, following the same sequence as for kneading and picking up.

7 Work thoroughly over the thigh and calf with **hacking**.

8 Finish with three full strokes, as in 1 – these can be deep or superficial as preferred.
Walk round and repeat 1 to 8 on the right leg.

BACK, NECK AND SHOULDERS

1 Your partner's arms should be at the sides or bent above the head. Stand close to one side at about waist level. Put both hands flat on the small of the back, thumbs on either side of the spine. Make two **deep strokes** close to the spine in a straight line up to the neck, moving slightly out to the shoulders at the top (a).

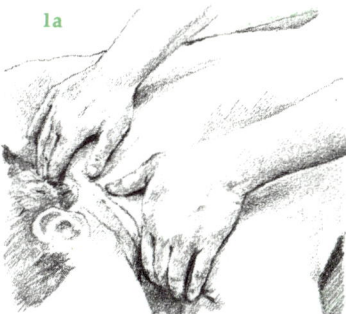
1a

Repeat twice, moving your hands a little way from the spine each time; finish both strokes at the underarms instead of the shoulders (b).

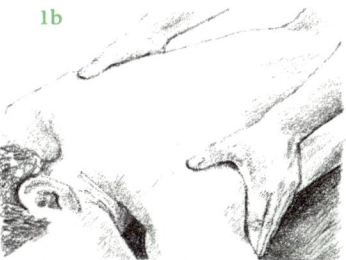
1b

2 **Knead** the top of the back and the shoulders, using both hands on the same shoulder or one hand on each. Work thoroughly over the area including the muscle mass at the top of the arm (below). Follow with **picking up** over the same area.

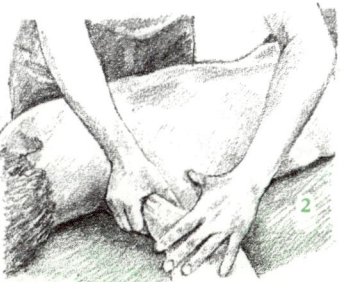
2

3 Give **frictions** with your thumbs or fingers wherever necessary: usually around the shoulder blades, top of the back and shoulders.

4 Place one hand flat on your partner's back, with the heel of your hand just beyond the spine on the side opposite you, and reinforce it with the other hand. Pressing down, **stroke deeply** outwards from the spine. Repeat, until you've transversely stretched the length of the back from buttock to underarm, working carefully over the shoulder blade as the muscle mass is smaller in this area.

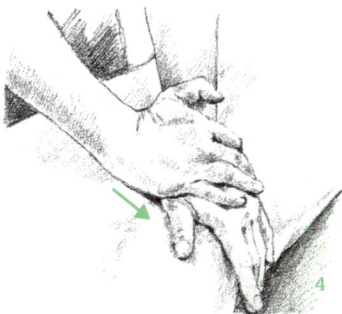
4

5 With one hand flat on top of the other, give **frictions** with the heel of your hand to the buttock furthest from you. Work over the buttock with large, circular movements. Both hands are used as the muscle mass is large and, although tension collects here, it's hard to detect.
Walk round and repeat stages 4 and 5 on the other side.

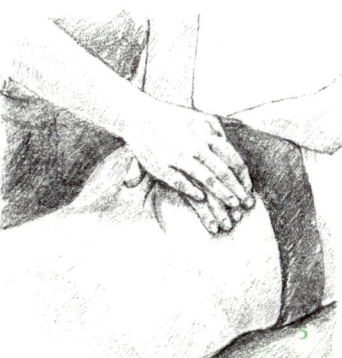
5

6 Repeat the sequence of deep stroking, as in 1.

7 Work over the back and shoulders with **hacking**, concentrating on muscled or fatty areas, but avoid the lower ribs, as you might hurt the kidneys.

8 With a thumb on either side of the spine at the base of the neck, make **deep strokes** to the top of the neck, moving further to the sides of the neck with each stroke.

9 **Knead** (below) and **pick up** over the length of the neck, using both hands, one above the other.

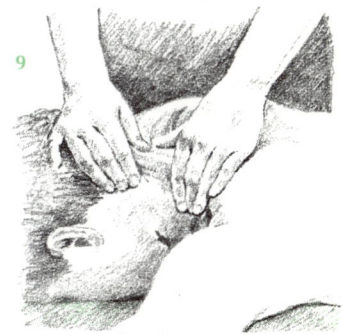
9

10 Rest one hand on your partner's head and, with the other, give thumb **frictions** wherever needed, paying particular attention to the area just under the base of the skull.

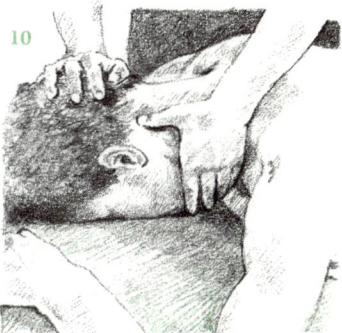
10

11 Give **deep strokes** with your fingers down the neck from the base of the skull, moulding your hands to the shoulders at the end of each stroke.

12 Finish with a few **superficial strokes** along the spine – keep the strokes in the same direction.

Self-massage

It's more difficult to relax fully when massaging yourself than when being massaged, as some of your muscles are always tensed. However, if you're on your own, self-massage can certainly help to ease tension; it's particularly useful for relieving aches and pains accumulated during the day, from headaches to tired feet. The selection of simple and effective strokes below can be done in any sequence; you can also add any movements from the body massage that you enjoy and can adapt. It's easier to work directly on your skin, but there's no need to take off all your clothes – just change out of anything bulky or constricting. Massage yourself while reading, watching television or having a bath, and if you moisturize your skin, try incorporating the strokes as you apply the lotion. Let massage add some luxury to your life – it's free and a little pampering goes a long way.

FACE

1 Sit with your elbows comfortably supported and put the palms of your hands side by side over your eyes. This helps you to focus on yourself. After a few moments, move your hands up to your forehead. Using the heels of both hands, **stroke deeply** across your brow from the centre out to the sides. Repeat, working up to the hairline.

2 Temple circling is also very relaxing. Using one or two fingertips on each side, gently give **frictions** beyond the outer edge of each eye and just above it.

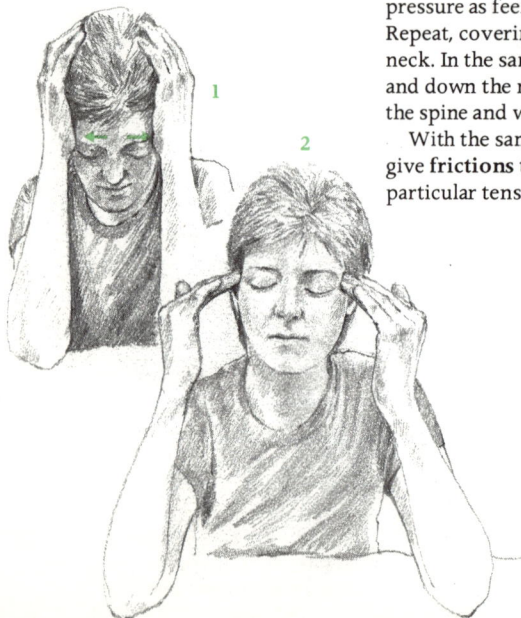

NECK

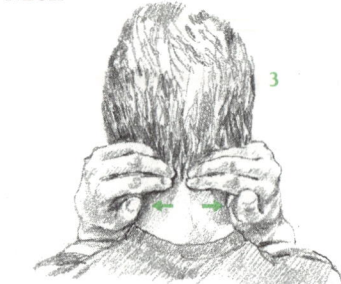

3 Place the middle three fingers of each hand on either side of the spine and give **deep strokes** outwards with your fingertips, using as much pressure as feels comfortable. Repeat, covering the length of the neck. In the same way, stroke up and down the neck, starting next to the spine and working out.

With the same three fingertips, give **frictions** to any areas of particular tension.

ARMS/SHOULDERS

4 Sit with your left arm supported by a cushion or pillow. Slowly and gently **knead** the arm and shoulder with your right hand, grasping as big a mass as possible and making large circular motions.

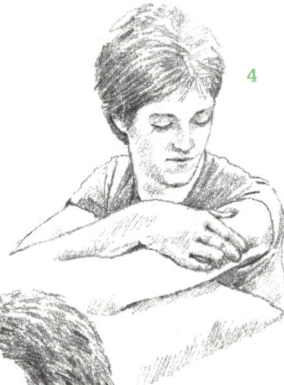

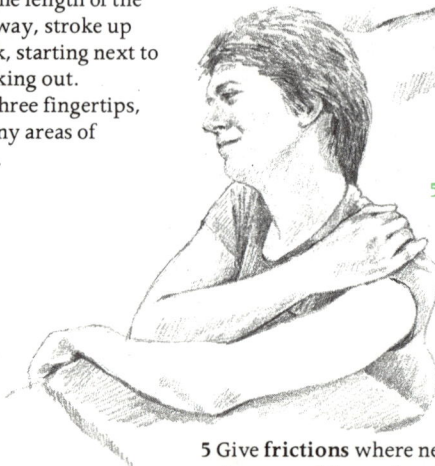

5 Give **frictions** where necessary, using several fingertips, if possible, to give a less concentrated, more relaxing sensation.
Repeat 4 and 5 on the right arm.

BACK

6 Place your hands on either side of the spine, with your wrists uppermost, and make **deep strokes** out to the sides; press with the whole hand or just the palm. Repeat, working up the spine. With your hands in the same position, stroke in the same way, from the base of the spine up as far as possible.

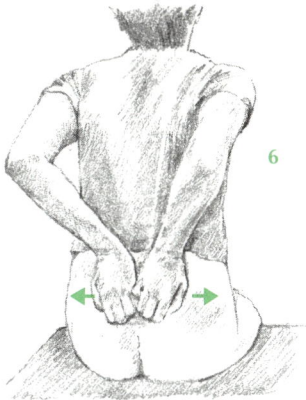

HANDS

7 Cradling the back of your left hand, give **frictions** to the wrist and palm with your right thumb.

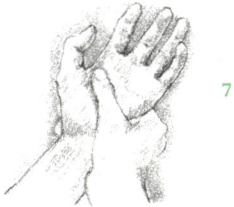

8 Clasp the back of your left hand, with the heel of your right hand near the base of the thumb. **Stroke deeply** with your right hand across to the outer edge of the left hand. Repeat, starting a little further up from the wrist with each stroke until you reach the knuckles.

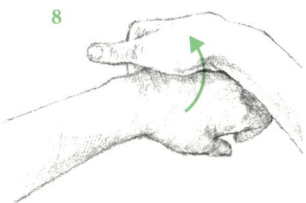

9 Give **frictions** with the thumb to the back of the left hand, working across the wrist and between the bones from wrist to knuckles.
Repeat 7 to 9 on your right hand.

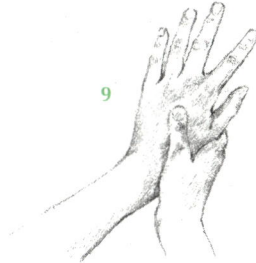

LEGS

10 The easiest part of the leg to massage yourself is the lower leg. Sit on the floor and bend your left leg, resting the foot firmly on the floor. Put both hands, fingers pointing down, in the centre of the calf and move each hand out to the side, **stroking deeply** with the whole of each hand but mainly with the heel. Work up the length of the calf in the same way.

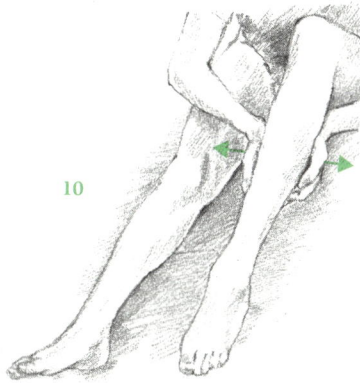

11 Give **frictions** with your thumbs or fingers where necessary – pay particular attention to the Achilles tendon.
Repeat 10 and 11 on the right calf.

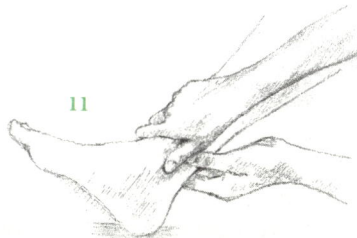

FEET

12 Rest your left ankle over your right knee. Using one hand to hold the left foot, give **frictions** with your right thumb along the sole.

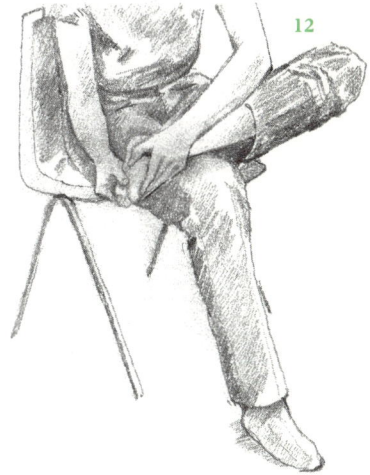

13 With your left hand over the ankle to give support, give **deep strokes** with the heel of your right hand to the left sole from heel to toes (a).

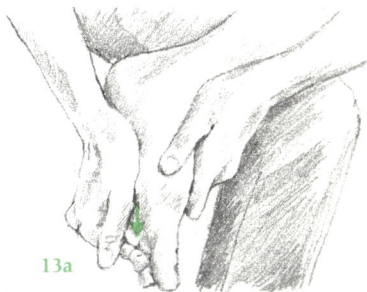

When you reach the toes, clasp them and pull them upwards (b); this stretches the muscles, ligaments and tendons.
Repeat 12 and 13 on the right foot.

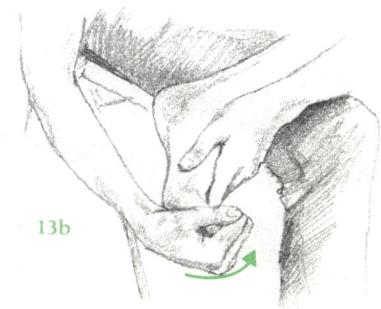

229

Oriental massage

Although Oriental massage has its roots in ancient China, shiatsu and Do-In, two forms that are becoming increasingly popular in the West, have come to us this century from Japan. As early as 2600 BC, the *Nei Ching*, the most original and interesting of the great Chinese medical classics, set out the theories on which shiatsu and Do-In, as well as the healing treatments, acupuncture and moxibustion, are based. The basic principle is that sickness is caused by a disharmony of the body's energy. This energy, or Ki (pronounced key), flows along 14 pathways in the body, known as meridians, ten corresponding to a particular organ, the other four being concerned with receiving, distributing and balancing the body's Ki. Along the meridians are points, known as tsubos, where this energy gathers and can be felt.

Ki should flow evenly along all the meridians; if it becomes blocked, ill-health results. There are many techniques, some laid out in the *Nei Ching*, for discovering where the Ki is blocked and what has caused the blockage, and there are also various methods of restoring the flow. For example, in acupuncture a needle is used to stimulate the tsubos, whereas in moxibustion, the stimulus is a quietly burning stick of concentrated mugwort (the moxa), held close to the skin.

The only tools used for diagnosis and treatment in shiatsu are the hands. The flow of Ki is encouraged by thumb pressure on the tsubos, or pressure from the whole palm; the practitioner may also cup a hand and gently tap it over the tsubo or tap his fingertips along the meridians. Treatment for some common problems, such as headaches, is standard and can be easily learnt without personal supervision (see page 235). Full diagnosis and appropriate treatment, however, involve detailed knowledge of tsubos and meridians, best learnt from an experienced teacher; the practitioner must be skilled in order to act effectively as a channel for Ki.

Do-In Pronounced 'doe-een', this could be described as do-it-yourself shiatsu: it's an invigorating self-massage, which doesn't involve specialized knowledge. Done briskly in the morning, it awakens and refreshes; practised quietly in the evening, it will help you to relax – but bear in mind the cautions on page 221.

Set aside about half an hour for your practice and choose a quiet, sunny room; or, if the weather's fine, practise outside. Spread a blanket or mat to sit or stand on and wear loose, comfortable clothes, take off your shoes and don't wear too many layers, as you'll warm up quickly. Remember to let all your movements in Do-In be loose and flexible. Focus on your breathing, making it slow, quiet and deep, but don't exaggerate it, as you may become dizzy. In general, you should breathe out as you apply pressure, relax as you breathe in, but where no instructions are given, breathe normally. If you feel any discomfort, exhaling as you work will be helpful. Repeat each movement once or, if it's a continuous motion, for a few moments, unless specific directions are given. Where a time-limit is suggested, it's intended only as a guide – there's no need to clock-watch.

Do-In massage

1 Begin by kneeling on your blanket with your back straight, knees the width of one fist apart, buttocks resting on your heels and your toes tucked under – this posture is known as 'seisa' by the Japanese. If it becomes uncomfortable, stand up, shake your legs and feet out vigorously and continue the massage standing, with your feet parallel and hip-width apart. Whether standing or sitting, make sure that you keep your back straight, as it's easy to start slumping forwards or to lean to one side.

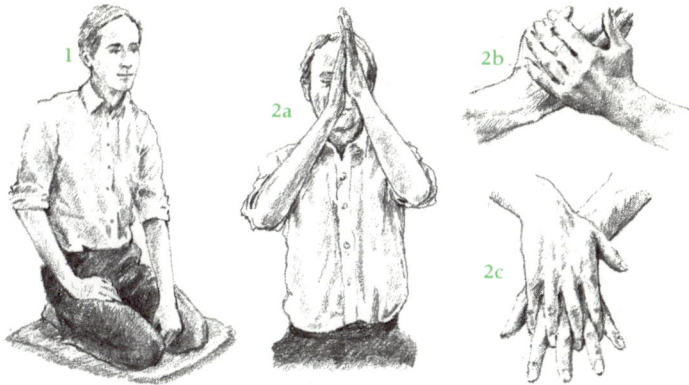

3 With your left hand on your thigh, use your right thumb and forefinger to pinch the fleshy webbing between each finger on your left hand, breathing out as you squeeze. Repeat on your right hand.

2 The first four stages of this massage are designed to charge your hands with Ki. Rub your hands together at forehead height, exerting as much pressure between the palms as possible but keeping your shoulders and wrists flexible (a). Keep this up for one minute and

4 With the right hand, firmly rotate the left thumb and each finger, taking them in a wide circle in both directions (a). Clench your fist round each finger and the thumb and give a hard squeeze and pull (b). Repeat with the other hand. Rub your hands together at forehead height, as in 2, for 30 seconds, and shake your hands out to your sides.

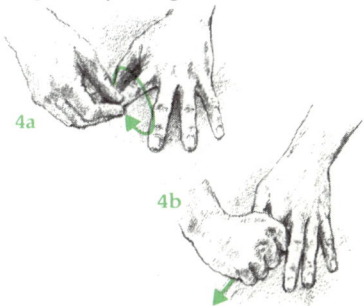

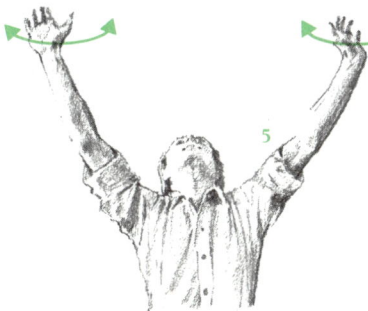

5 Without letting your shoulders tense up, stretch your arms up above you with the palms of your hands facing the ceiling, your fingers relaxed. Look upwards and rotate your wrists quickly from side to side, as if you were polishing the ceiling. Continue until your arms feel heavy, then relax and shake your arms and hands out to your

then shake your hands out vigorously from the wrists. Rub the back of each hand with the opposite palm for a few moments (b). Stretch your left hand open and, with your right hand, rub deeply in between the thumb and each finger (c). Repeat on your right hand.

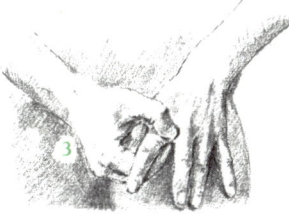

sides. Your hands should feel warm and tingly with Ki. If they become heavy or clay-like during the massage, shake them out and briefly repeat the rubbing at forehead height and imaginary polishing.

6 Tap lightly all over your scalp, first with the palms of your hands, then with your knuckles and lastly with your fingertips. If you keep your shoulders and wrists loose and flexible, you'll feel little discomfort. Run your hands down from the top of your head over your brow, cheeks and jaw. Repeat this smoothing down three times.

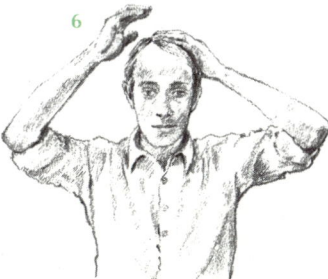

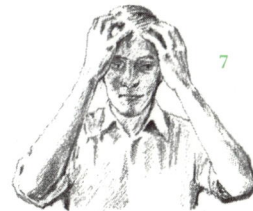

7 With the fingertips of both hands, rub hard into the forehead, just below the hairline, breathing out as you apply the pressure. Stroke deeply across the forehead with the palms of your hands.

231

▷

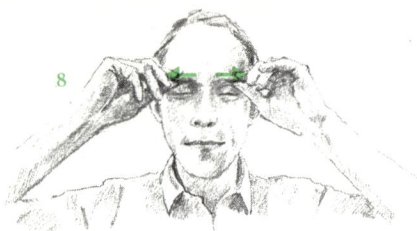

8 Grasp each eyebrow at the bridge of your nose between your thumb and forefinger, and, on an exhalation, squeeze along the length of the brows. Repeat three times.

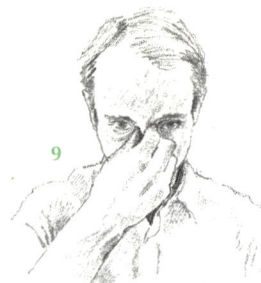

9 With your thumb and forefinger, squeeze deeply at either side of the nose near the corner of each eye.

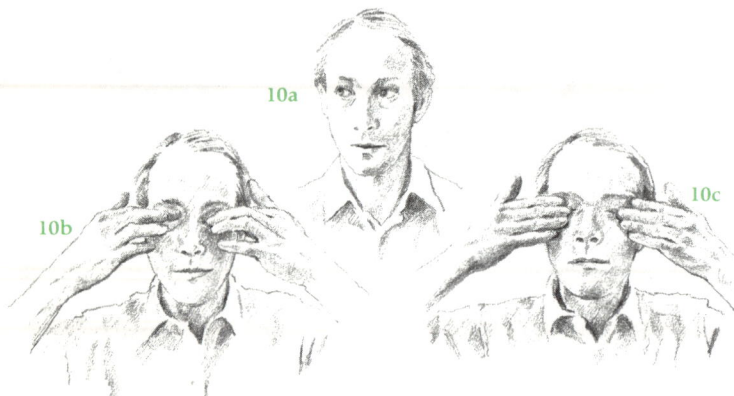

10 Swivel your eyes to look in a wide circle (a), changing direction after three rotations. Exaggerate the movement as much as possible, as this is excellent exercise for the eye muscles. Close your eyes and lightly rub over the lid with your fingertips (b). Blink vigorously for a few moments then close your eyes and, with your fingertips, stroke gently across your eyelids from your nose outwards (c).

11 Rub your cheeks up and down vigorously with the palms of your hands for 30 seconds (a). Using the middle three fingers of each hand, rub up and down either side of the nose for 30 seconds (b). Stop and breathe out. With the outer edges of your hands, quickly flick your ears forwards for 30 seconds (c).

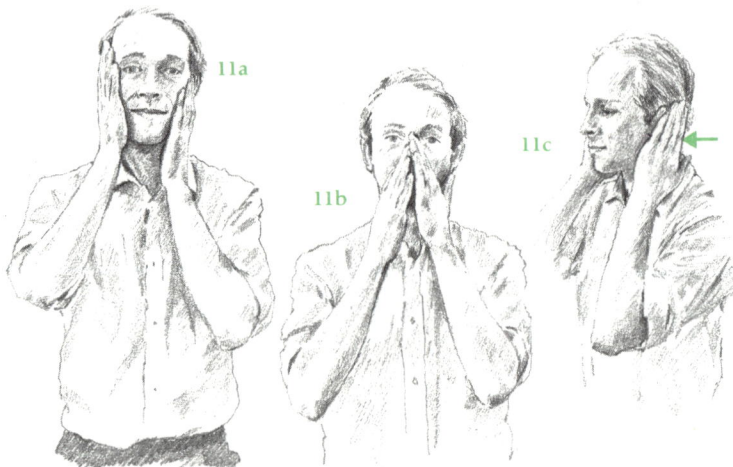

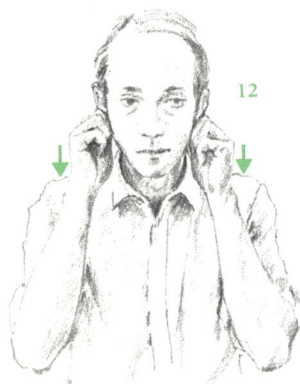

12 Take hold of each earlobe between your thumb and forefinger. As you exhale, let the weight of your arms pull your earlobes down.

13 Rotate your jaw in a wide circle, up towards your nose and down towards your chest. Do this ten times in each direction. Repeat, rotating your jaw forwards and backwards. Massage your gums by running your tongue along the inside of your top and bottom teeth. Repeat in both directions. With your fingertips, massage the outer edge of your gums, working from the centre of your teeth outwards. Keeping your tongue out of the way, chatter your teeth together for 30 seconds.

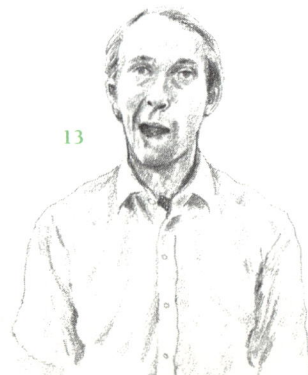

14a 14b

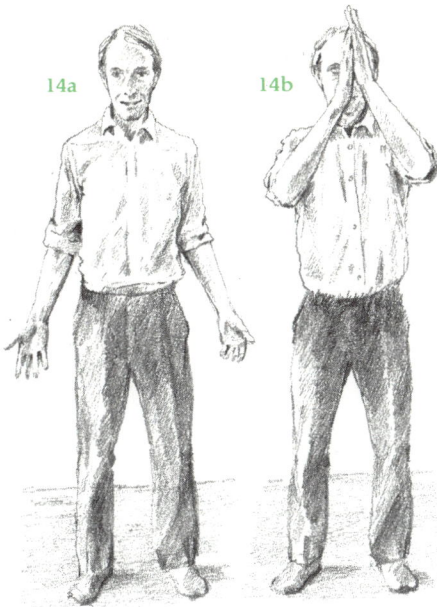

14 Stand up, your back straight, your feet the width of your hips apart, and shake your hands (a) and feet out well. Rub your hands together vigorously at forehead height, as in 2, for 30 seconds (b). Shake out again briefly.

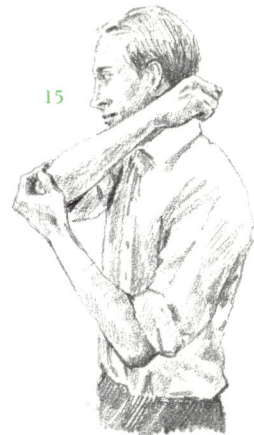

15 Clench your right fist and, keeping your arms and wrist flexible, pound on to the soft area of the left shoulder. To make this easier, support your elbow with the other hand. If you find a tender area, breathe out as you move over it. Repeat with the left fist.

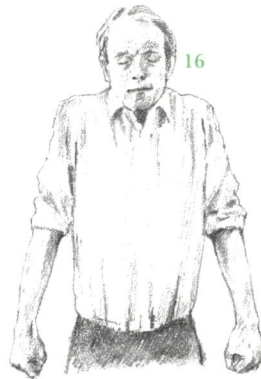

15

16 With your arms hanging comfortably by your sides, take a very slow and deep breath and, at the same time, tighten up all the muscles in your fists, forearms, shoulders, neck and face. Hold this posture for as long as you can. As you let go, exhale forcibly through your mouth and completely relax all the muscles that you tensed up. Repeat three times.

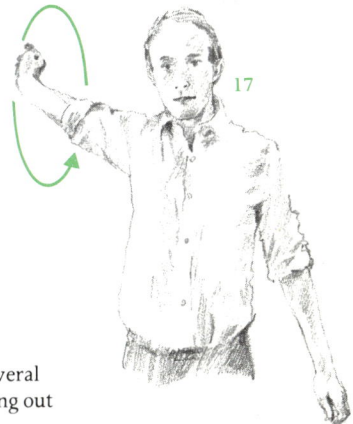

16

17 Swing your right arm in several full backward circles, breathing out as you press back. Repeat the movement with the left arm.

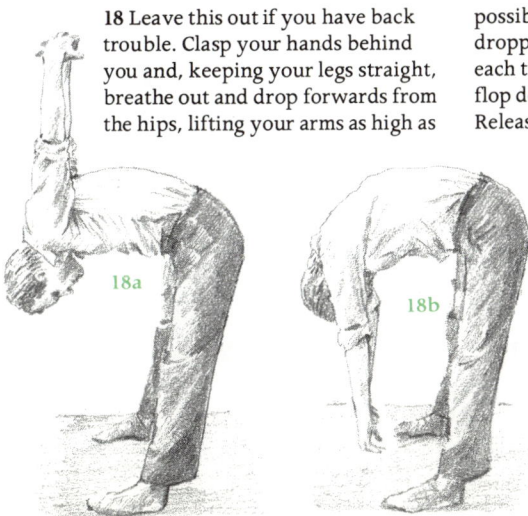

17

18 Leave this out if you have back trouble. Clasp your hands behind you and, keeping your legs straight, breathe out and drop forwards from the hips, lifting your arms as high as

possible (a). Hold for two minutes, dropping a little further forwards each time you exhale. Let your arms flop down (b) and hold briefly. Release and stand up.

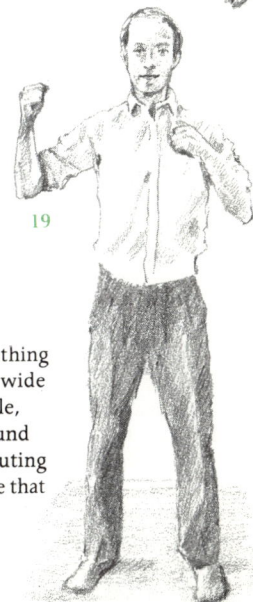

18a 18b

19 Clench your fists and, breathing in, stretch your arms high and wide above your head. As you exhale, bring your arms down and pound your chest with both fists, shouting 'aah'. Repeat twice, at a volume that won't upset your neighbours.

19

233
▷

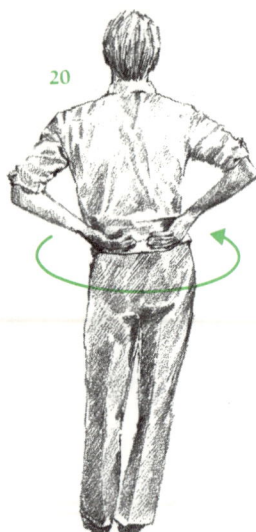

20

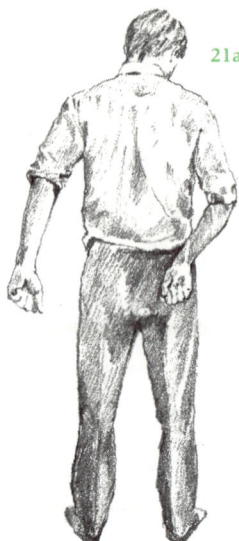

21a

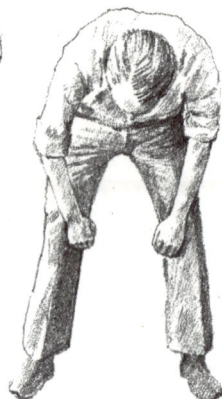

21b

20 Put your feet close together and place the palms of your hands, fingers pointing in, over the kidney area in the lower back. Rotate your hips *without* moving your head or shoulders. Circle six times and repeat in the opposite direction.

21 Before you start, make sure you don't have anything bulky in your back pockets. Clench your fists and pound your buttocks, keeping your wrists loose (a). This tends to be an area of stagnation in the body and may be quite tender – make sure you breathe out as you apply the pressure. Keeping your legs straight, pound down the outside of your legs (b) and up the inside towards the groin. Repeat three times.

22 Sit down with your right foot bare. Rub the right calf vigorously between the palms of your hands side to side from knee to ankle (a). Rest your right foot across your left knee and rub it between your hands (b). Shake out your hands and place your right foot on the floor. Rub well in between each of the toes, squeezing the flesh between them at the same time (c). Rotate each toe in both directions and give each a sharp pull, grasping either side of the nail with the thumb and forefinger (d). Rest your foot on your knee again and with one hand above your ankle, the other holding your toes, rotate your ankle firmly in both directions (e). With your leg out in front, knee bent, slam the sole of your foot several times on to the floor. Stretch both legs out in front and wiggle your toes. Repeat the sequence on your left leg and foot.

23 Sit comfortably in the seisa posture for a few moments and, to finish, place both hands, palms down, on the floor in front of you with the thumbs and forefingers touching. As you exhale, bend forwards and rest your forehead briefly on the floor, in the triangle created with your thumbs and forefingers. Breathe in and sit up again.

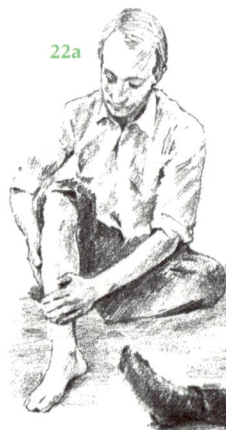

22a

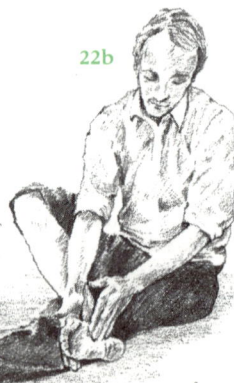

22b

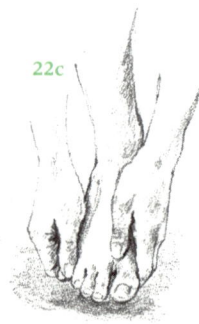

22c

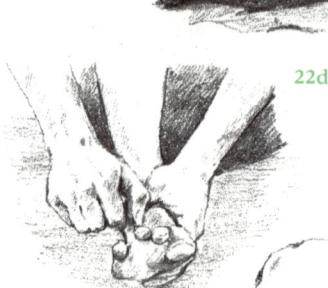

22d

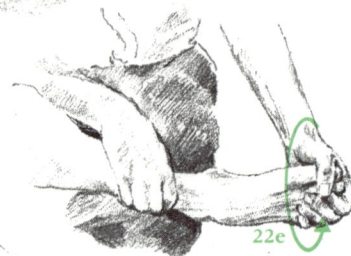

22e

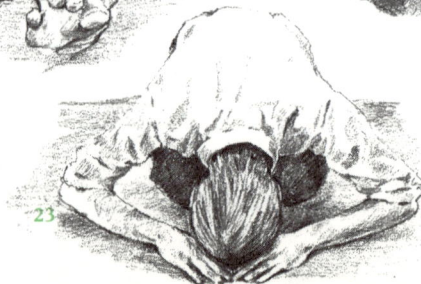

23

Shiatsu for specific problems

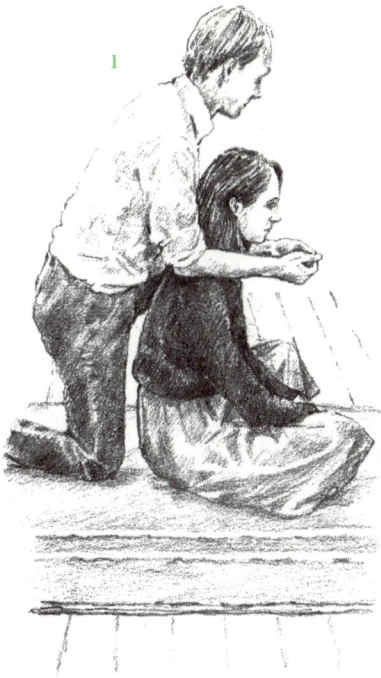

The following techniques help to relieve physical symptoms of tension. You'll need a partner for all the exercises, except the third – instructions are for the person giving the massage. Before you start, stimulate the Ki in your hands (see stages 2 to 5, page 231).

1 Exercises 1 and 2 help to bring relief when the neck and shoulders feel tight and stiff. During both, your partner should sit comfortably on the floor or in a hard, straight-backed chair.

Stand or kneel behind your partner and harmonize your breathing, so you both breathe in and out together. Place your forearms on your partner's shoulders, close in to the neck and, as you breathe out, gently drop your weight forwards, pressing down firmly on the shoulders. Relax as you inhale and press down as you exhale; continue for at least three minutes, increasing the pressure.

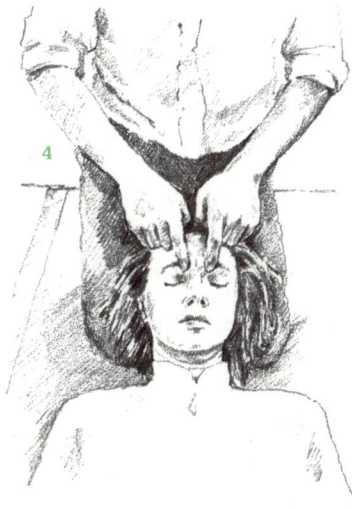

2 Ask your partner to relax the neck and let the chin drop forwards so the chin touches the chest. Supporting your partner's forehead in the palm of your left hand, massage either side of the neck at the base of the skull with your thumb and forefinger, using a slow, circular, kneading motion. Continue for two to three minutes.

3 Difficulties and discomfort experienced with the colon may be a symptom of stress. Although this massage can relieve the symptoms, appropriate diet and activity are more of a priority in the long term. Sit or lie on the floor; as you breathe out, apply firm thumb pressure to the fleshy part of the hand between the thumb and forefinger. Repeat, pressing as you exhale and releasing as you inhale, for two minutes. If this area is slightly painful when you apply pressure and swollen, this indicates digestive problems in the large intestine.

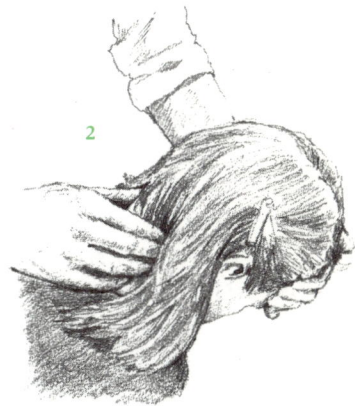

4 Exercises 4 and 5 help to relieve headaches. For both, have your partner lie facing up on the floor and sit just behind in the seisa posture, as on page 231, resting your partner's head on your knees.

Feel along the eyebrows with your forefingers until you find a hollow on either side of the nose that neatly fits your fingertips. As you both breathe out, hook your forefingers into these depressions and gently apply pressure by pulling your fingers towards you. Relax and breathe in. Repeat for three minutes.

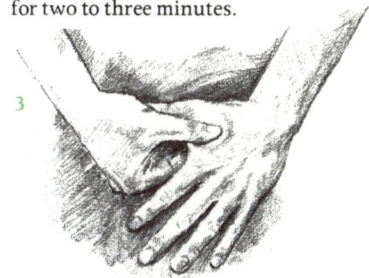

5 This is a pleasant way to finish and brings a quality of calm. Relax your arms and, cupping your hands round your partner's temples, put both your thumbs, one over the other, in the centre of the forehead. Do this for three minutes, pressing gently as you exhale and releasing as you breathe in.

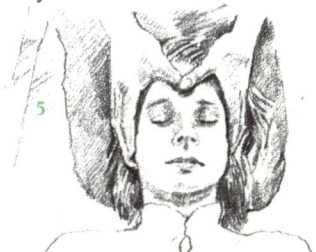

Hydrotherapy

There are a number of different forms of hydrotherapy or water treatment. Some are not generally available for regular use; some are extolled by only a few adherents; while others, such as the neutral bath, hot bath and cold pack, can not only be readily enjoyed at home but are also widely recommended in a holistic approach to health, and can be extremely effective in promoting relaxation. Anyone with a skin complaint, however, should always check with a doctor before embarking on any form of hydrotherapy.

Neutral bath

33·5 – 35·6 °C
[92 – 96 °F]

▶

◀ 30 minutes

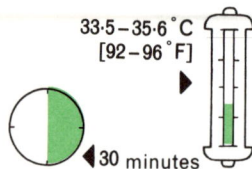

Water that is the same temperature as the body has a sedative effect on the nervous system and so the neutral bath is excellent for stress conditions. (Before the development of tranquillizing drugs, the most dependable method of quieting an agitated patient was the use of this type of bath.) The temperature of the water must be maintained at between 33.5 and 35.6°C [92 and 96°F]; you'll need a bath thermometer, available at chemists [druggists], for this. Also the air temperature of the bathroom should be high enough to avoid any sense of chilliness. Spend half an hour immersed in such a bath and it will have a sedative or even a soporific effect. The skin will pucker slightly but this temporary disadvantage is far outweighed by the bonus points. The neutral bath places no strain on the heart, circulation or nervous system and achieves muscular relaxation and a general vasodilatation (relaxation and expansion of the blood vessels), all of which are prerequisites of relaxation. For a further counter to stress, combine this treatment with meditation (see pages 238–39).

Hot bath

36·5 – 37 °C
[98 – 99 °F]

▶

5 – 10
◀ minutes

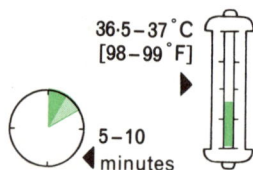

Some people find the hot bath more effective than the neutral one in achieving muscle, and so general, relaxation. In this type of bath the water temperature should be between 36.5 and 37°C [98 and 99°F]. Stay in it for no more than five minutes at first. If you don't experience any sensations of lightheadedness or other general symptoms of weakness, then increase the immersion time to ten minutes daily, a few minutes at a time. (There's no point in increasing the time beyond this. A short, hot bath is relaxing while a long, hot bath has the opposite effect.) Immersion in hot water acts not only on the surface nerves but also on the autonomic nervous system – that part that is normally outside our control – and on the hormone-producing glands, particularly the adrenal, making them less active.

In both types of bath, and in a jacuzzi (see opposite), herbs such as camomile, valerian and rosemary can have an added calming effect, chiefly through inhalation. Use 30 g [1 oz] of the dried herb to 600 ml [1 pint] of water. Boil, allow to stand for 15 minutes, then strain and add the liquid to the bath.

Cold pack

The overall effect of cold packs is a calming one. They can be slept in and, in fact, should help produce a deeper, more refreshing sleep. They improve local circulation, the initial application producing a reaction that draws fresh blood to the area; this warmth, being well

236

insulated, is retained, giving a warm continuous application, which gradually, over six to eight hours, bakes itself dry. Maximum benefit is gained in this way, but a cold pack applied for a minimum of two hours helps relaxation too.

You need a piece of cotton or linen, 38 to 45 cm [15 to 18 in] wide and long enough to be wrapped once around the body from just below the armpits to just above the hips; one piece of flannel or blanket material of about the same size; one plastic or rubber sheet to protect the bedding; large safety pins and a hot-water bottle. You'll also find it an advantage to have someone to help you apply the pack. Open out the flannel on top of the plastic sheet; soak the cotton material in very cold water, wring it out and place it on the flannel. Lie on this so that the dampened cotton and then the flannel can be folded round your body and pinned securely in place. The bedcovers should then be drawn up and a hot-water bottle provided. You may sweat quite heavily so wash the material well before re-using it. If you experience a sensation of damp cold, it's probably because the material is too wet or the insulation inadequate or too loose.

Larger, whole body packs can also be used but these definitely require assistance in application and in extrication.

Jacuzzi

33·5 – 37 °C
[92 – 99 °F]

10 – 20
minutes

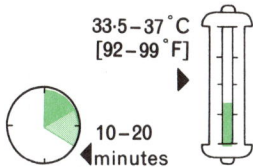

A jacuzzi, or whirlpool, bath combines heat and massage, both the temperature and agitation of the water being controlled by means of an electric agitator or jets of compressed air – so they're not the type of bath that the average person could afford to install at home, but they are available at many health clubs. For a relaxing effect the temperature needs to be maintained at a level between 33.5 and 37°C [92 to 99°F] and immersion time is 10 to 20 minutes.

Sauna

75 – 100 °C
[167 – 212 °F]

10 – 15
minutes

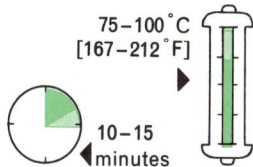

The dry, very hot atmosphere of the Finnish sauna was originally produced by hot coals but is often electrically controlled now. Adherents claim that sitting in this atmosphere for varying lengths of time has a relaxing effect. It is, however, more likely a mild state of exhaustion that they experience. The actual physiological stress involved in coping with temperatures of 75 to 100°C [167 to 212°F] is profound. Certainly there is a slight overall reduction in the metabolic rate after a sauna and a significant decrease in blood pressure in the majority of users, both of which indicate that the body is relaxing. However, in 12.5 per cent of users there is an overall increase in blood pressure, so saunas are advisable only for those in good health.

Turkish bath

40 – 50 °C
[104 – 122 °F]

10 – 20
minutes

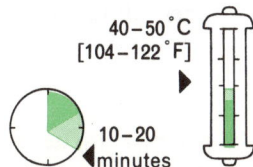

Turkish baths are different from saunas in as much as the humidity is far higher but the same general observations apply. These systems are tolerable for the healthy but are not advisable for anyone with a health problem and, in this regard, anyone under obvious stress must be considered as having a problem. When stressed, the body responds unpredictably and the addition of lengthy periods of intense heat can be seen only as a further stress factor.

Meditation

All meditation methods help to develop inner awareness or reflection and a fuller awareness of reality. Practising meditation brings various other benefits, enhancing, it is claimed, the creative and intuitive faculties and increasing overall mental efficiency. It leads not only to a more balanced and integrated personality but also to a marked reduction in stress symptoms. Claims that Transcendental Meditation can induce physiological and metabolic changes have long been made by its devotees, and have been confirmed by research undertaken by Dr. Herbert Benson, associate professor at Harvard Medical School. Indeed, Dr. Benson has found that other methods, like Buddhist or yoga meditation (see below), are equally effective in achieving these changes: slowing down the heart rate; raising skin resistance to electricity – the higher the resistance the more relaxed you are; lowering blood pressure – the lower rate being maintained long after the period of meditation; inducing alpha brainwave patterns, indicative of a calm mind; lowering blood lactate (lactate levels rise when you're anxious); and slowing down general metabolism, as evidenced by lower oxygen intake and carbon dioxide exhalation. In addition, meditation has been shown to lead, in the longer term, to shorter reaction time, enhanced perception and an overall improvement in health, with a corresponding reduction in the need for drugs.

To be effective, meditation requires: a focal point, passivity, a relaxed position, a quiet environment, and regular practice.

Focal point: this can be a sound (mantra), word or phrase that is silently or audibly repeated, or an object that is stared at or imagined, for instance a candle flame or black curtain. In some methods a thought or feeling, such as positive health or peace, or the concept of God, is visualized. The purpose is to shift the attention from logical external thought to a fixed, internally held object.

Passivity: meditation involves discipline in its regular application but not effort in its performance. If external thoughts intrude – and it's likely that they will for quite some time at first – don't let it worry you; just observe them gently and replace them by the object of thought required by the technique.

Relaxed position: lying, sitting or reclining are all acceptable, as long as they don't involve any muscular effort.

Quiet environment: there should be no external distractions, such as television, radio or music.

Regular practice: whatever the method, practise at least once, ideally twice, a day (allow a two hour gap after meals).

How to meditate

The synthesis of meditation systems, which Dr. Benson developed and has found to be effective, is as follows (the whole process should take at least 15 minutes):

1 Sit or lie quietly in a comfortable position.
2 Close your eyes.
3 Relax all your muscles, beginning at the feet and progressing up to the face. Keep them relaxed by repeating the procedure if necessary.

It helps to tense the muscles before relaxing them; see also pages 208–09. Don't worry about whether you're successful in achieving a deep level of relaxation; just be completely passive and let relaxation occur at its own pace.

4 Breathe through your nose. Become aware of your breathing. As you breathe out, say the word 'one', silently and slowly, to yourself. Breathe easily and naturally. Continue for 10 to 20 minutes. When distracting thoughts occur, try to ignore them by not dwelling on them and return to repeating 'one'.

5 When you finish, don't stand up immediately but sit or lie quietly for several minutes, first with your eyes closed, then open.

Dr. Benson calls the response to meditation methods 'the Relaxation Response', seeing it as the natural antidote to the stress response (see pages 175–79). He speculates that by focusing attention, separated from the thinking and perception processes, meditators are able to stay alert while being in a deeper state of relaxation than when they are asleep.

It should be emphasized that, although it's possible to learn to meditate by reading about it, it's better, to begin with, to go to a qualified teacher, who will ascertain the most suitable method for you; this is particularly true of the methods described below. Most people can learn a technique such as the one above after an hour of instruction, with a follow-up to check that they're doing it properly, and achieving the appropriate results.

Transcendental Meditation

The silent repetition of a mantra that has been specifically chosen for the meditator is the focus which, it is claimed, leads the meditator into a higher, or transcendental, state of consciousness. Two daily sessions of 20 minutes each are required.

Yoga and Buddhist meditation

These involve concentration on a single object or thought, usually accompanied by specific, sometimes complicated, breathing techniques. The meditator may also focus on his or her own mind, trying to watch thoughts and reactions without emotion, or observe the surroundings with heightened awareness but no bias or point of view. The eventual aim is to achieve a state known variously as *samadhi*, *nirvana* or *satori*, in which all perception of self and personal desire are lost in a sense of unity with the universe.

Active meditation

Of the numerous different forms, all with roots going back many hundreds of years, the following are among the most widespread: Rajneesh meditation, named after Bhagwan Rajneesh, who developed and popularized it, siddha yoga and subud, the latter originating in southeast Asia. All involve spontaneous movement, posturing, gesturing, rapid and deep breathing and facial contortions. Anything that wells up during practice can be incorporated. These methods seem to allow a cathartic expression of emotions, so they can be especially beneficial if you have a rigid or unexpressive personality.

239

Autogenics

Practising autogenics is a safe, simple and effective way to combat stress and nervous tension and promote rest and relaxation. Autogenics are a series of easy mental exercises based on auto- or self-suggestion. They have been found to slow down the heart rate and to have other physiological effects identical to those produced by meditation (see page 238); they can also prevent or relieve many stress-related disorders, ranging from high blood pressure, migraine, insomnia and asthma to nervous sweating and skin problems.

The technique was devised by a German neurologist, Dr. J. H. Schultz, and consists of a sequence of autogenic instructions (instructions made to yourself by yourself) used in conjunction with the passive focusing of meditation. These instructions are specific verbal messages that focus awareness on a particular area of the body: no effort is involved, simply a passive concentration on the sensations or emotions that might result from each exercise-message. Although it's possible to learn the technique simply by reading about it, it's best to have a short course of lessons from a properly trained instructor. Check his or her credentials as you would with a physical training instructor.

What follows is a basic guide to exercises that can safely be done at home. Exercises directed to heartbeat and the solar plexus, which form part of a more complete routine, have been omitted as they can produce adverse reactions, such as a rise in blood pressure, and should be done only under the supervision of a qualified practitioner.

Do the exercises in a comfortable reclining position in a quiet room – minimize external distracting sounds as far as possible. Practise them twice daily – it's best to allow a two hour gap after meals – for 20 minutes each time (as with any such technique, it will take a little time before you begin to reap the full benefit).

Begin by repeating to yourself several times 'I am relaxed and at peace with myself'. Then do the following exercises in sequence.

Exercise 1: Focus mentally on your right arm. Say to yourself 'My right arm is heavy'. After a few seconds, repeat the phrase several times, then proceed to the left arm, right leg, left leg, neck and shoulders, and back. Spend from half a minute to a minute on each.

Exercise 2: Again begin with the right arm, concentrating on it as you say to yourself 'My right arm is warm'. Repeat a number of times and proceed through the same body areas, pausing for some seconds to assess sensations that may become apparent. Such changes can't be controlled but happen when the mind is in a passive, receptive state.

Exercise 3: This focuses on the breathing cycle with the phrase 'My breathing is calm and regular'. Don't make a conscious effort to control your breathing; repeating the phrase slowly promotes deep, slow, regular breathing without effort.

Exercise 4: Repeat the phrase 'My forehead is cool' for several minutes; this is designed to produce both alertness and relaxation.

Exercise 5: Repeat the phrase 'I am alert and refreshed'. Then breathe deeply, have a really good allover stretch, and you are ready to continue the day's activities.

FOOD CHARTS

These charts contain information on the nutrients found in a range of common foods and liquids. The figures represent grams of the nutrient per 100 g serving, for alcoholic beverages grams per 100 ml. Cholesterol is given in mg per 100 g. Tr. indicates that only a trace of the nutrient is present. The total carbohydrate content of a food can be calculated by adding together the values for starch and sugar; where these figures are not available, the carbohydrate content is given, marked by a C. A dash indicates that the information for a particular category was not available. Vitamins and minerals are given where known; those that are shown are present in a significant quantity. They are abbreviated as follows: Ni = Nicotinic acid, Fo = Folic acid, Pa = Pantothenic acid, Bi = Biotin, Ca = Calcium, I = Iron, M = Magnesium, P = Potassium, S = Sodium, Z = Zinc.

per 100 g	Calories	Sugar g	Starch g	Protein g	Total fat g	Saturated fat g	Polyunsaturated fat g	Cholesterol mg	Dietary fibre g	Good sources of vitamins and minerals
VEGETABLES										
Artichokes, globe, boiled	7	1.2*	0	0.5	Tr.	–	–	0	–	Bi
Artichokes, Jerusalem, boiled	18	3.2*	0	1.6	Tr.	–	–	0	–	
Asparagus, boiled	9	0.6	0	1.7	Tr.	–	–	0	0.8	E
Aubergine [eggplant], boiled	19	4.1C	–	1.0	0.2	–	–	0	–	
Beans, broad, boiled	48	0.6	6.5	4.1	0.6	–	–	0	4.2	Ni, Pa, Bi; P
butter, raw	273	3.6	46.2	19.1	1.1	–	–	0	21.6	B_1, Ni, B_6, Fo, Pa; I, M, P, Z
French [string], boiled	7	0.8	0.3	0.8	Tr.	–	–	0	3.2	
haricot, raw	271	2.8	42.7	21.4	Tr.	–	–	0	25.4	B_1, Ni, B_6; Ca, I, M, P, Z
kidney, raw	272	3.0	42.0	22.1	1.7	–	–	0	25.0	B_1, B_2, Ni, B_6, Fo; Ca, I, M, Z
runner, boiled	19	1.3	1.4	1.9	0.2	0.0	0.1	0	3.4	
soya, raw	403	33.5C	–	34.1	17.7	–	–	0	–	B_1, B_2, Ni; Ca, I, P
Beetroot, boiled	44	9.9	0	1.8	Tr.	–	–	0	2.5	Fo; P
Broccoli tops, boiled	18	1.5	0.1	3.1	Tr.	–	–	0	4.1	A, B_2, B_6, C, E; P
Brussels sprouts, boiled	18	1.6	0.1	2.8	Tr.	–	–	0	2.9	B_6, C; P
Cabbage, red, raw	20	3.5	Tr.	1.7	Tr.	–	–	0	3.4	B_6, Fo, C; P
Savoy, boiled	9	1.1	Tr.	1.3	Tr.	–	–	0	2.5	B_6
white, raw	22	3.7	0.1	1.9	Tr.	–	–	0	2.7	B_6, Fo, C; P
Carrots, old, raw	23	5.4	0	0.7	Tr.	–	–	0	2.9	A, B_6, Fo; P
boiled	19	4.2	0.1	0.6	Tr.	–	–	0	3.1	A
young, boiled	20	4.4	0.1	0.9	Tr.	–	–	0	3.0	A; P
Cauliflower, raw	13	1.5	Tr.	1.9	Tr.	–	–	0	2.1	B_6, Fo, Bi, C; P
boiled	9	0.8	Tr.	1.6	Tr.	–	–	0	1.8	B_6, Bi, C
Celeriac, boiled	14	1.5	0.5	1.6	Tr.	–	–	0	4.9	B_6; P
Celery, raw	8	1.2	0.1	0.9	Tr.	–	–	0	1.8	B_6; P
boiled	5	0.7	0	0.6	Tr.	–	–	0	2.2	
Chicory, raw	9	1.5C	–	0.8	Tr.	–	–	0	–	Fo
Courgettes [zucchini], boiled	12	2.5C		1.0	0.1	–	–	0	–	
Cucumber, raw	10	1.8	0	0.6	0.1	0	0	0	0.4	Fo
Endive, raw	11	1.0	0	1.8	Tr.	–	–	0	2.2	A, Fo; I, P
Leeks, boiled	24	4.6	0	1.8	Tr.	–	–	0	3.9	B_6, Bi; I, P
Lentils, raw	304	2.4	50.8	23.8	1.0	–	–	0	11.7	B_1, B_2, Ni, B_6, Fo, Pa; I, M, P, Z
Lettuce, raw	12	1.2	Tr.	1.0	0.4	–	–	0	1.5	A, Fo; P
Marrow [squash], boiled	7	1.3	0.1	0.4	Tr.	0	0	0	0.6	
Mushrooms, raw	13	0	0	1.8	0.6	0.1	0.3	0	2.5	B_2, Ni, B_6, Fo, Pa; P
fried	210	0	0	2.2	22.3	–	–	–	4.0	B_2, Ni, Fo, Pa; P

*only 50% is usable

per 100 g	Calories	Sugar g	Starch g	Protein g	Total fat g	Saturated fat g	Polyunsaturated fat g	Cholesterol mg	Dietary fibre g	Good sources of vitamins and minerals
Onions, raw	23	5.2	0	0.9	Tr.	–	–	0	1.3	B_6, Fo
boiled	13	2.7	0	0.6	Tr.	–	–	0	1.3	
fried	345	10.1	0	1.8	33.3	–	–	–	4.5	P
spring, raw	35	8.5	0	0.9	Tr.	–	–	0	3.1	B_6, Fo, C; Ca, P
Parsnips, boiled	56	2.7	10.8	1.3	Tr.	–	–	0	2.5	E; P
Peas, chick [garbanzos], raw	320	10.0	40.0	20.2	5.7	–	–	0	15.0	B_1, B_2, Fo; Ca, I, M, P
garden, fresh, boiled	52	1.8	5.9	5.0	0.4	0.1	0	0	5.2	B_6
frozen, boiled	41	1.0	3.3	5.4	0.4	0.1	0	0	12.0	
split, dried, raw	310	1.9	54.7	22.1	1.0	0.4	0.1	0	11.9	B_1, B_2, Ni, B_6, Fo, Pa; I, M, P, Z
Peppers, green, raw	15	2.2	Tr.	0.9	0.4	0.1	0.2	0	0.9	B_6, C; P
boiled	14	1.7	0.1	0.9	0.4	0.1	0.2	0	0.9	B_6, C
red, raw	65	15.8C	–	2.3	0.4	–	–	0	–	A, B_2, Ni, C; P
Potatoes, new, boiled	76	0.7	17.6	1.6	0.1	0	0.1	0	2.0	B_6; P
old, baked, without skins	105	0.6	24.4	2.6	0.1	0	0.1	0	2.5	B_6; P
boiled	80	0.4	19.3	1.4	0.1	0	0.1	0	1.0	B_6; P
mashed	119	0.6	17.4	1.5	5.0	–	–	–	0.9	B_6; P
roast	157	27.3C	–	2.8	4.8	–	–	–	–	B_6; M, P
see also page 102 for chips [French fries]										
Radishes, raw	15	2.8	0	1.0	Tr.	–	–	0	1.0	B_6, Fo, C; P
Spinach, boiled	30	1.2	0.2	5.1	0.5	0.1	0.3	0	6.3	A, B_2, B_6, Fo, C, E; Ca, I, M, P
Spring greens, boiled	10	0.9	0	1.7	Tr.	–	–	0	3.8	A, B_2, E
Sweetcorn, on-the-cob, boiled	123	1.7	21.1	4.1	2.3	0.4	1.1	0	4.7	B_6, Fo; M, P
Sweet potatoes, boiled	85	9.1	11.0	1.1	0.6	0.2	0.2	0	2.3	A, B_6, E; P
Tomatoes, raw	14	2.8	Tr.	0.9	Tr.	–	–	0	1.5	B_6, Fo, Bi, C, E; P
Turnips, boiled	14	2.3	0	0.7	0.3	0	0.2	0	2.2	
Watercress, raw	14	0.6	0.1	2.9	Tr.	–	–	0	3.3	A, B_6, Fo, C, E; Ca, P
Canned vegetables										
Baked beans in tomato sauce	64	5.2	5.1	5.1	0.5	0.1	0.2	0	7.3	B_6; M, P, S
Carrots	19	4.4	Tr.	0.7	Tr.	0	0	0	3.7	A; S
Peas, garden	47	3.6	3.4	4.6	0.3	0.1	0	0	6.3	Ni, Fo; S
Sweetcorn, kernels	76	8.9	7.2	2.9	0.5	0.1	0.2	0	5.7	B_6, Fo; P, S
Tomatoes	12	2.0	Tr.	1.1	Tr.	0	0	0	0.9	B_6, Fo, Bi, E; P
Tomato purée	67	11.4	0	6.1	Tr.	0	0	0	–	A, B_2, Ni, B_6, Fo, Pa, Bi, C, E; I, M, P

FRUIT

All fruits are raw and whole, with pith, seeds, stones and skins unless otherwise stated

Apples, cooking, flesh only	37	9.2	0.4	0.3	Tr.	–	–	0	2.4	
eating	35	9.1	0.1	0.2	Tr.	–	–	0	1.5	
Apricots	25	6.2	0	0.5	Tr.	–	–	0	1.9	A; P
Avocado pears	223	1.8	Tr.	4.2	22.2	2.6	1.9	0	2.0	B_6, Fo, Pa, Bi, E; P
Bananas	47	9.6	1.8	0.7	0.2	0.1	0.1	0	2.0	B_6, Fo; P
Blackberries	29	6.4	0	1.3	Tr.	0	0	0	7.3	C, E; M, P
Blueberries	62	15.3C	–	0.7	0.5	–	–	0	–	
Cherries	41	10.4	0	0.5	Tr.	–	–	0	1.5	P
Cranberries	15	3.5	0	0.4	Tr.	–	–	0	4.2	
Currants, black	28	6.6	0	0.9	Tr.	–	–	0	8.7	Bi, C, E; P
red	21	4.4	0	1.1	Tr.	–	–	0	8.2	Bi, C; P
Figs, green	41	9.5	0	1.3	Tr.	–	–	0	2.5	B_6; P
Gooseberries, ripe	37	9.2	0	0.6	Tr.	–	–	0	3.5	C
Grapefruit	11	2.5	0	0.3	Tr.	–	–	0	0.3	C
Grapes, black	51	13.0	0	0.5	Tr.	–	–	0	0.3	P
white	63	16.1	0	0.6	Tr.	–	–	0	0.9	B_6; P
Greengages	45	11.2	0	0.7	Tr.	–	–	0	2.5	P
Lemons	15	3.2	0	0.8	Tr.	–	–	0	5.2	B_6, C; Ca

per 100 g	Calories	Sugar g	Starch g	Protein g	Total fat g	Saturated fat g	Polyunsaturated fat g	Cholesterol mg	Dietary fibre g	Good sources of vitamins and minerals
Lychees	64	16.0	0	0.9	Tr.	–	–	0	0.5	C
Mangoes, flesh only	59	15.3	Tr.	0.5	Tr.	–	–	0	1.5	A, C
Melon, cantaloupe	15	3.3	0	0.6	Tr.	–	–	0	0.6	A; P
honeydew	13	3.1	0	0.4	Tr.	–	–	0	0.6	
water	11	2.7	0	0.2	Tr.	–	–	0	–	Fo
Nectarines	46	11.4	0	0.9	Tr.	–	–	0	2.2	P
Olives, in brine	82	Tr.	0	0.7	8.8	1.2	1.0	0	3.5	S
Oranges	26	6.4	0	0.6	Tr.	–	–	0	1.5	Fo, C
Peaches	32	7.9	0	0.6	Tr.	–	–	0	1.2	P
Pears	29	7.6	0	0.2	Tr.	–	–	0	1.7	
Pineapple, flesh only	46	11.6	0	0.5	Tr.	–	–	0	1.2	Fo; P
Plums, dessert	36	9.0	0	0.5	Tr.	–	–	0	2.0	
Raspberries	25	5.6	0	0.9	Tr.	–	–	0	7.4	Bi, C; P
Rhubarb	6	1.0	0	0.6	Tr.	–	–	0	2.6	Fo; Ca, P
Strawberries	26	6.2	0	0.6	Tr.	–	–	0	2.2	Fo, Bi, C
Tangerines	23	5.6	0	0.6	Tr.	–	–	0	1.3	Fo, C
Canned fruit										
Apricots	106	27.7	0	0.5	Tr.	–	–	0	1.3	A; P
Fruit salad	95	25.0	0	0.3	Tr.	–	–	0	1.1	
Grapefruit	60	15.5	0	0.5	Tr.	–	–	0	0.4	Bi
Mandarin oranges	56	14.2	0	0.6	Tr.	–	–	0	0.3	
Peaches	87	22.9	0	0.4	Tr.	–	–	0	1.0	
Pears	77	20.0	0	0.4	Tr.	–	–	0	1.7	
Pineapple	77	20.2	0	0.3	Tr.	–	–	0	0.9	
Raspberries	87	22.5	0	0.6	Tr.	–	–	0	5.0	
Strawberries	81	21.1	0	0.4	Tr.	–	–	0	1.0	Fo, Bi, C
Dried fruit										
Apricots	182	43.4	0	4.8	Tr.	–	–	0	24.0	A, B_2, Ni, B_6, Fo; I, M, P
Currants	243	63.1	0	1.7	Tr.	–	–	0	6.5	B_6; M, P
Dates	213	54.9	0	1.7	Tr.	–	–	0	7.5	Ni, B_6, Fo; M, P
Figs	213	52.9	0	3.6	Tr.	–	–	0	18.5	B_6; Ca, I, M, P
Prunes	161	40.3	0	2.4	Tr.	–	–	0	16.1	A, B_2, B_6; I, P
Raisins	246	64.4	0	1.1	Tr.	–	–	0	6.8	B_6; M, P
Sultanas	250	64.7	0	1.8	Tr.	–	–	0	7.0	B_6; M, P

NUTS

All nuts are shelled.

per 100 g	Calories	Sugar g	Starch g	Protein g	Total fat g	Saturated fat g	Polyunsaturated fat g	Cholesterol mg	Dietary fibre g	Good sources of vitamins and minerals
Almonds	565	4.3	0	16.9	53.5	4.2	10.0	0	14.3	B_2, Ni, B_6, Fo, E; Ca, I, M, P, Z
Brazils	619	1.7	2.4	12.0	61.5	15.7	23.0	0	9.0	B_1, B_6, E; Ca, I, M, P, Z
Cashews	561	29.3C	–	17.2	45.7	–	–	0	–	B_1, B_2; I, P
Chestnuts	170	7.0	29.6	2.0	2.7	0.5	1.1	0	6.8	B_2, B_6, Bi; M, P
Coconut, desiccated	604	6.4	0	5.6	62.0	53.3	1.0	0	23.5	Fo; I, M, P
fresh	351	3.7	0	3.2	36.0	30.9	0.6	0	13.6	Fo; I, M, P
Hazelnuts [filberts]	380	4.7	2.1	7.6	36.0	2.6	3.7	0	6.1	B_6, Fo, Pa, E; M, P, Z
Peanuts, raw/roasted and salted	570	3.1	5.5	24.3	49.0	9.2	13.9	0	8.1	B_1, Ni, B_6, Fo, Pa, E; I, M, P, S (salted peanuts), Z
peanut butter	623	6.7	6.4	22.6	53.7	10.6	13.4	0	7.6	B_6, Fo, Pa, E; I, M, P, S, Z
Pecans	687	14.6C	–	9.2	71.2	–	–	0	–	B_1; I, P
Pistachios	594	19.0C	–	19.3	53.7	–	–	0	–	B_1; I, P
Walnuts	525	3.2	1.8	10.6	51.5	5.6	35.1	0	5.2	B_6, Fo, Bi; I, M, P, Z

MEAT

per 100 g	Calories	Sugar g	Starch g	Protein g	Total fat g	Saturated fat g	Polyunsaturated fat g	Cholesterol mg	Dietary fibre g	Good sources of vitamins and minerals
Bacon, rashers, back, fried	465	0	0	24.9	40.6	16.4	2.9	80	0	B_1, B_2, Ni, B_6, Bi; P, S, Z
grilled [broiled]	405	0	0	25.3	33.8	13.6	2.5	74	0	B_1, B_2, Ni, B_6, Bi; P, S, Z
rashers, streaky, fried	496	0	0	23.1	44.8	18.1	3.3	80	0	B_2, Ni, B_6; P, S, Z
grilled [broiled]	422	0	0	24.5	36.0	14.5	2.6	74	0	B_1, B_2, Ni, B_6, Bi; P, S, Z

per 100 g	Calories	Sugar g	Starch g	Protein g	Total fat g	Saturated fat g	Polyunsaturated fat g	Cholesterol mg	Dietary fibre g	Good sources of vitamins and minerals
Beef, minced [ground], cooked	229	0	0	23.1	15.2	6.4	0.6	82	0	B$_2$, Ni, B$_6$, B$_{12}$; I, P, S, Z
rumpsteak, fried	246	0	0	28.6	14.6	6.1	0.6	–	0	B$_2$, Ni, B$_6$, B$_{12}$; I, P, Z
fried, lean only	190	0	0	30.8	7.4	3.1	0.3	–	0	B$_2$, Ni, B$_6$, B$_{12}$; I, P, Z
grilled [broiled]	218	0	0	27.3	12.1	5.1	0.5	82	0	B$_2$, Ni, B$_6$, B$_{12}$; I, P, Z
grilled [broiled], lean only	168	0	0	28.6	6.0	2.5	0.2	82	0	B$_2$, Ni, B$_6$, B$_{12}$; I, P, Z
sirloin, roast	284	0	0	23.6	21.1	8.9	0.8	82	0	B$_2$, Ni, B$_6$, B$_{12}$; P, Z
roast, lean only	192	0	0	27.6	9.1	3.8	0.4	82	0	B$_2$, Ni, B$_6$, B$_{12}$; I, P, Z
stewing steak, stewed	223	0	0	30.9	11.0	4.6	0.4	82	0	B$_2$, Ni, B$_6$, B$_{12}$; I, P, S, Z
Chicken, boiled, dark meat	204	0	0	28.6	9.9	3.3	1.5	110	0	B$_2$, Ni, B$_6$, B$_{12}$, Pa, Bi; P, Z
boiled, light meat	163	0	0	29.7	4.9	1.6	0.7	80	0	Ni, B$_6$, Pa, Bi; P
fried, drumstick	235	1.0C	–	32.6	10.2	–	–	–	–	B$_2$, Ni; I
fried, wing	268	2.7C	–	29.0	14.8	–	–	–	–	B$_2$, Ni; I
roast, dark meat	155	0	0	23.1	6.9	2.3	1.0	120	0	B$_2$, Ni, B$_6$, B$_{12}$, Fo, Pa, Bi; P, Z
roast, light meat	142	0	0	26.5	4.0	1.3	0.6	74	0	Ni, B$_6$, Pa, Bi; P
Duck, roast, meat, fat and skin	339	0	0	19.6	29.0	7.9	3.5	–	0	B$_2$, Ni, B$_6$, Pa, Bi; I, P
roast, meat only	189	0	0	25.3	9.7	2.6	1.2	160	0	B$_2$, Ni, B$_6$, B$_{12}$, Pa, Bi; I, P, Z
Ham, mild cure, roast	289	0	0	20.9	22.1	–	–	70	0	B$_1$, B$_2$, Ni; I
Goose, roast	319	0	0	29.3	22.4	–	–	–	0	B$_6$; I, M, P
Lamb, leg, roast,	266	0	0	26.1	17.9	8.7	0.8	110	0	B$_2$, Ni, B$_6$, B$_{12}$, Bi; I, P, Z
roast, lean only	191	0	0	29.4	8.1	3.9	0.4	110	0	B$_2$, Ni, B$_6$, B$_{12}$, Bi; I, P, Z
loin chops, grilled [broiled]	355	0	0	23.5	29.0	14.1	1.4	110	0	B$_2$, Ni, B$_6$, B$_{12}$, Bi; P, Z
grilled [broiled], lean only	222	0	0	27.8	12.3	6.0	0.6	110	0	B$_2$, Ni, B$_6$, B$_{12}$, Bi; I, P, Z
Pork, leg, roast	286	0	0	26.9	19.8	7.8	1.5	110	0	B$_1$, B$_2$, Ni, B$_6$, B$_{12}$, Pa, Bi; P, Z
roast, lean only	185	0	0	30.7	6.9	2.7	0.5	110	0	B$_1$, B$_2$, Ni, B$_6$, B$_{12}$, Pa, Bi; P, Z
loin chops, grilled [broiled]	332	0	0	28.5	24.2	9.6	1.9	110	0	B$_1$, B$_2$, Ni, B$_6$, B$_{12}$, Pa, Bi; P, Z
grilled [broiled], lean only	226	0	0	32.3	10.7	4.2	0.8	110	0	B$_1$, B$_2$, Ni, B$_6$, B$_{12}$, Pa, Bi; P, Z
Rabbit, stewed	179	0	0	27.3	7.7	3.1	2.5	–	0	B$_2$, Ni, B$_6$, B$_{12}$, Bi; P
Spareribs, medium fat, cooked	440	0	0	20.8	38.9	–	–	110	0	B$_2$, Ni; I
Turkey, roast, dark meat	148	0	0	27.8	4.1	1.4	1.3	100	0	B$_2$, Ni, B$_6$, B$_{12}$, Fo, Bi; P, Z
roast, light meat	103	0	0	29.8	1.4	0.5	0.5	82	0	Ni, B$_6$, B$_{12}$, Fo, Bi; P, T
Veal, fillet, roast	230	0	0	31.6	11.5	4.8	0.5	–	0	B$_2$, Ni, B$_6$, B$_{12}$; P
Venison, roast	198	0	0	35.0	6.4	–	–	–	0	I, M, P
Offal [variety meats]										
Kidney, lamb, raw	90	0	0	16.5	2.7	0.9	0.4	400	0	A, B$_1$, B$_2$, Ni, B$_6$, B$_{12}$, Fo, Pa, Bi; I, P, S, Z
Liver, calf, raw	153	1.9C	–	20.1	7.3	2.2	1.9	370	–	A, B$_2$, Ni, B$_6$, B$_{12}$, Fo, Pa, Bi; I, P, Z
chicken, raw	135	0.6C	–	19.1	6.3	2.0	1.3	380	–	A, B$_2$, Ni, B$_6$, B$_{12}$, Fo, Pa, Bi; I, P, Z
lamb, raw	179	1.6C	–	20.1	10.3	3.2	1.5	430	–	A, B$_2$, Ni, B$_6$, B$_{12}$, Fo, Pa, Bi; I, P, Z
Sweetbread, lamb, raw	131	0	0	15.3	7.8	3.0	0.3	260	0	B$_2$, Ni, B$_{12}$, Fo, Pa, Bi; P
Meat products										
Burgers, fried	264	7.0C	–	20.4	17.3	7.3	0.7	68	–	B$_2$, Ni, B$_6$, B$_{12}$, Bi; I, P, S, Z
Corned beef, canned	217	0	0	26.9	12.1	5.1	0.5	85	0	B$_2$, Ni, B$_{12}$, Bi; I, S, Z
Frankfurters	274	3.0C	–	9.5	25.0	9.9	1.9	46	–	B$_{12}$, Bi; S
Ham, canned	120	0	0	18.4	5.1	1.9	0.5	33	0	B$_1$, B$_2$, Ni, B$_6$, Bi; P, S, Z
Liver sausage	310	4.3C	–	12.9	26.9	8.7	2.1	120	–	A, B$_2$, Ni, B$_6$, B$_{12}$, Fo, Pa, Bi; I, S, Z
Salami	491	1.9C	–	19.3	45.2	17.9	3.5	79	–	B$_2$, Ni, B$_6$, B$_{12}$, Bi; S
Sausages, beef, grilled [broiled]	265	15.2C	–	13.0	17.3	7.3	0.8	42	–	Ni, B$_{12}$, Bi; S

per 100 g	Calories	Sugar g	Starch g	Protein g	Total fat g	Saturated fat g	Polyunsaturated fat g	Cholesterol mg	Dietary fibre g	Good sources of vitamins and minerals
pork, grilled [broiled]	318	11.5C	–	13.3	24.6	9.7	1.9	53	–	B_2, Ni, B_{12}, Bi; P, S
Tongue, canned	213	0	0	16.0	16.5	–	–	110	0	B_2, Ni, B_{12}, Bi; I, S, Z

FISH AND SEAFISH

All fish are with bones, unless otherwise indicated.

per 100 g	Calories	Sugar g	Starch g	Protein g	Total fat g	Saturated fat g	Polyunsaturated fat g	Cholesterol mg	Dietary fibre g	Good sources of vitamins and minerals
Bass, striped, fried	196	6.7C	–	21.5	8.5	–	–	–	–	
Clams, meat and liquid, raw	53	2.5C	–	8.1	0.9	–	–	–	–	
Cod, fillets, fried in batter	199	7.5C	–	19.6	10.3	–	–	–	–	P
middle cut, steamed	83	0	0	18.6	0.9	0.2	0.3	60	0	B_6, B_{12}, Bi; P
Crab, in shell, boiled	25	0	0	4.0	1.0	0.1	0.3	100	0	
Flounder, baked	202	0	0	30.0	8.2	–	–	–	0	P, S
Haddock, fillets, fried	174	3.6C	–	21.4	8.3	–	–	–	–	Ca, M, P
middle cut, steamed	98	0	0	22.8	0.8	0.1	0.3	75	0	Ni, B_6, B_{12}, Bi; P
smoked, steamed	101	0	0	23.3	0.9	0.2	0.3	75	0	B_6, B_{12}; P, S
Halibut, middle cut, steamed	131	0	0	23.8	4.0	0.5	1.3	60	0	Ni, B_6, B_{12}, Bi, E; P
Herring, grilled [broiled]	135	0	0	13.9	8.8	1.8	1.5	80	0	Ni, B_6, B_{12}, Bi, D; P
Kipper, baked	111	0	0	13.8	6.2	1.2	1.1	80	0	Ni, B_6, B_{12}, Bi, D; P, S
Lobster, in shell, boiled	42	0	0	7.9	1.2	0.1	0.4	150	0	Bi
Mackerel, fried	138	0	0	15.7	8.3	–	–	90	0	B_2, Ni, B_6, B_{12}, Bi, D; P
Mussels, in shell, boiled	26	Tr.C	–	5.2	0.6	0.1	0.1	–	0	I, P
Oysters, in shell, raw	6	Tr.C	–	1.3	0.1	0	0	50	0	B_{12}, Bi; Z
Plaice, fillets, fried in batter	279	14.4C	–	15.8	18.0	–	–	–	–	B_2, Ni, B_6; P, S
steamed	93	0	0	18.9	1.9	0.3	0.4	90	0	Ni, B_6, B_{12}; P
Prawns [large shrimps], in shell, boiled	41	0	0	8.6	0.7	0.1	0.2	200	0	S
Salmon, steamed	160	0	0	16.3	10.5	2.6	2.7	80	0	Ni, B_6, B_{12}, Pa, Bi; P*
smoked	142	0	0	25.4	4.5	1.1	1.1	70	0	B_2, Ni; M, P, S*
Scallops, steamed	105	Tr.C	–	23.2	1.4	0.3	0.3	40	0	Fo; Ca, I, M, P, S
Scampi, fried	316	28.9C	–	12.2	17.6	–	–	110	–	M, P, S
Shrimps [small shrimps], in shell, boiled	39	0	0	7.9	0.8	0.1	0.2	200	0	Ca, M, S
Sole, lemon, fillets, fried	216	9.3C	–	16.1	13.0	–	–	–	–	P
steamed	91	0	0	20.6	0.9	0.1	0.3	60	0	Ni, B_{12}, Bi; P
Swordfish, grilled [broiled]	174	0	0	28.0	6.0	–	–	–	0	A, Ni
Trout, steamed	89	0	0	15.5	3.0	–	–	80	0	P
Whitebait, fried	525	5.3C	–	19.5	47.5	–	–	–	–	Ca, I, M, S

Canned fish and seafish

per 100 g	Calories	Sugar g	Starch g	Protein g	Total fat g	Saturated fat g	Polyunsaturated fat g	Cholesterol mg	Dietary fibre g	Good sources of vitamins and minerals
Crab	81	0	0	18.1	0.9	0.1	0.3	100	0	Ca, I, M, S, Z
Pilchards, in tomato sauce	126	0.7C	–	18.8	5.4	1.7	1.8	70	–	B_2, Ni, B_{12}, D; Ca, I, M, P, S
Salmon	155	0	0	20.3	8.2	2.0	2.1	90	0	B_2, Ni, B_6, B_{12}, D, E; M, P, S
Sardines, in oil, drained	217	0	0	23.7	13.6	2.7	2.7	100	0	B_2, Ni, B_6, Bi, D; Ca, I, M, P, S, Z
with oil	334	0	0	19.7	28.3	5.5	5.6	80	0	B_2, Ni, B_6, Bi, D, E; Ca, I, M, P, S, Z
in tomato sauce	177	0.5C	–	17.8	11.6	3.3	3.7	100	–	B_2, Ni, B_6, Bi, D; Ca, I, M, P, S, Z
Shrimps [small shrimps]	94	0	0	20.8	1.2	0.2	0.4	–	0	B_{12}, Bi; Ca, I, M, S, Z
Tuna, in oil	289	0	0	22.8	22.0	3.9	8.0	65	0	Ni, B_6, B_{12}, Bi, D, E; P, S
in water	127	0	0	28.0	0.8	–	–	–	0	Ni; P

DAIRY PRODUCTS

per 100 g	Calories	Sugar g	Starch g	Protein g	Total fat g	Saturated fat g	Polyunsaturated fat g	Cholesterol mg	Dietary fibre g	Good sources of vitamins and minerals
Butter, salted/unsalted	740	Tr.C	–	0.4	82.0	49.0	2.2	230	0	A, E; S (salted butter)
Cheese, Camembert	300	Tr.C	–	22.8	23.2	13.9	0.6	72	0	A, B_2, B_6, B_{12}, Pa, Bi; Ca, S, Z
Cheddar [American]	406	Tr.C	–	26.0	33.5	20.0	0.9	70	0	A, B_2, B_{12}, Bi; Ca, S, Z
cottage, creamed	96	1.4	0	13.6	4.0	2.4	0.1	13	0	B_2, B_{12}; S
cream	439	Tr.C	–	3.1	47.4	28.3	1.3	94	0	A, B_{12}; E; S
Danish blue	355	Tr.C	–	23.0	29.2	17.4	0.8	88	0	A, B_2, B_6, B_{12}, Pa, Bi; Ca, S

*these values are for Atlantic salmon; Pacific salmon has a high vitamin D content

per 100 g	Calories	Sugar g	Starch g	Protein g	Total fat g	Saturated fat g	Polyunsaturated fat g	Cholesterol mg	Dietary fibre g	Good sources of vitamins and minerals
Edam	304	Tr.C	–	24.4	22.9	13.7	0.6	72	0	A, B₂, B₁₂, Bi; Ca, S, Z
Parmesan	408	Tr.C	–	35.1	29.7	17.7	0.8	90	0	A, B₂, B₆, B₁₂, Bi; Ca, M, S, Z
processed	311	Tr.C	–	21.5	25.0	14.9	0.7	88	0	A, B₂, B₁₂; Ca, S, Z
Stilton	462	Tr.C	–	25.6	40.0	23.9	1.1	120	0	A, B₂, B₁₂, E; Ca, S
Cream, double [heavy]	447	2.0	0	1.5	48.2	28.8	1.3	140	0	A, E
single [light]	212	3.2	0	2.4	21.2	12.6	0.6	66	0	A, Bi
Eggs, whole	147	Tr.C	–	12.3	10.9	3.4	1.2	450	0	B₂, B₆, B₁₂, Fo, Pa, Bi, E
white	36	Tr.C	–	9.0	Tr.	0	0	0	0	B₂, Bi
yolk	339	Tr.C	–	16.1	30.5	9.6	3.3	1260	0	A, B₂, B₆, B₁₂, Fo, Pa, Bi, D, E; Ca, Z
Milk, fresh, skimmed [low fat]	33	5.0	0	3.4	0.1	0	0	2	0	B₂, Bi; Ca
whole	65	4.7	0	3.3	3.8	2.3	0.1	14	0	B₂, Bi; Ca
buttermilk	36	5.1C	–	3.6	0.1	–	–	0	0	B₂
condensed, whole, sweetened	322	55.5	0	8.3	9.0	5.4	0.2	34	0	A, B₂, Bi; Ca, P
dried, skimmed [low fat]	355	52.8	0	36.4	1.3	0.8	0	18	0	A, B₁, B₂, B₆, B₁₂, Fo, Pa, Bi; Ca, M, P, S, Z
whole	490	39.4	0	26.3	26.3	15.7	0.7	120	0	A, B₂, B₆, B₁₂, Fo, Pa, Bi; Ca, M, P, S, Z
evaporated, whole, unsweetened	158	11.3	0	8.6	9.0	5.4	0.2	34	0	B₂; Ca, P
longlife [UHT]	65	4.7	0	3.3	3.8	2.3	0.1	14	0	B₂; Ca
Yogurt, fruit	95	17.9	0	4.8	1.0	0.6	0	6	0	B₂; Ca, P
natural	52	6.2	0	5.0	1.0	0.6	0	7	0	B₂; Ca, P

CEREALS AND CEREAL PRODUCTS

per 100 g	Calories	Sugar g	Starch g	Protein g	Total fat g	Saturated fat g	Polyunsaturated fat g	Cholesterol mg	Dietary fibre g	Good sources of vitamins and minerals
Barley, pearl, raw	360	Tr.	83.6	7.9	1.7	0.3	0.8	0	6.5	Ni, B₆; Z
boiled	120	Tr.	27.6	2.7	0.6	0.1	0.3	0	2.2	
Bran, wheat	206	3.8	23.0	14.1	5.5	0.9	2.9	0	44.0	B₁, B₂, Ni, B₆, Fo, Pa, Bi, E; Ca, I, M, P, Z
Bread, brown	223	1.8	42.9	8.9	2.2	0.4	0.9	0	5.1	Ni, Fo, Bi; Ca, I, M, P, S
French	290	55.4C	–	9.1	3.0	1.0	Tr.	–	–	S
rye	243	52.1C	–	9.1	1.1	–	–	–	–	S
white	233	1.8	47.9	7.8	1.7	0.4	0.7	0	2.7	Bi; Ca, S
wholemeal [wholewheat]	216	2.1	39.7	8.8	2.7	0.5	1.2	0	8.5	Ni, B₆, Fo, Bi; I, M, P, S, Z
Buckwheat	335	72.9C	–	11.7	2.4	–	–	0	–	B₁, Ni; I, P
Cornflour	354	Tr.	92.0	0.6	0.7	0.1	0.3	0	–	
Crackers	440	Tr.	68.3	9.5	16.3	–	–	–	3.0	Fo; Ca, S
Crispbread, rye	321	3.2	67.4	9.4	2.1	0.3	1.0	–	11.7	B₆, Fo, Pa, Bi; I, M, P, S, Z
wheat, starch reduced	388	7.4	20.6	45.0	7.6	2.7	2.3	–	4.9	Ni, B₆; I, M, P, S, Z
Macaroni, dry	370	Tr.	79.2	13.7	2.0	0.3	0.9	0	–	Ni; M, P
boiled	117	Tr.	25.2	4.3	0.6	0.1	0.3	0	–	
Matzo	384	4.2	82.4	10.5	1.9	0.3	0.9	–	3.9	
Millet	327	72.9C	–	9.9	2.9	1.0	1.0	0	–	B₁, B₂, Ni; I, P
Noodles, egg, dry	388	72.0C	–	12.8	4.6	1.0	Tr.	0	–	Ni
boiled	125	23.3C	–	4.1	1.5	–	–	Tr.	–	
Oatcakes	441	3.1	59.9	10.0	18.3	3.9*	5.5*	–	4.0	B₆, Fo, Pa, Bi, E; I, M, P, S, Z
Oatmeal, raw	401	Tr.	72.8	12.4	8.7	1.5	3.5	0	7.0	B₁, B₆, Pa, Bi; I, M, P, Z
Pasta, wholemeal [wholewheat]	327	0.6	65.7	13.2	2.8	–	–	0	10.0	Bi, Ni; I
Pastry, flaky, raw	427	0.8	35.0	4.4	30.6	12.0	3.8	–	1.5	A, E; S
cooked	565	1.1	46.3	5.8	40.5	15.7	5.0	–	2.0	A, E; S
shortcrust, raw	455	1.0	47.2	5.9	27.8	10.9	3.5	–	2.0	A, Fo, Bi, E; S
cooked	527	1.2	54.6	6.9	32.2	12.6	4.1	–	2.4	A, Bi, E; Ca, S
Rice, brown, raw	360	77.4C	–	7.5	1.9	–	–	0	5.5	Ni; P
white, raw	361	Tr.	86.8	6.5	1.0	0.2	0.3	0	2.4	Bi
Rolls, brown, crusty	289	2.1	55.1	11.5	3.2	0.6	1.4	0	5.9	Ni, B₆, Fo, Bi; Ca, I, M, P, S
white, crusty	290	2.1	55.1	11.6	3.2	0.8	1.2	0	3.1	Bi; Ca, I, M, S

*composition varies according to fat used by manufacturer

per 100 g	Calories	Sugar g	Starch g	Protein g	Total fat g	Saturated fat g	Polyunsaturated fat g	Cholesterol mg	Dietary fibre g	Good sources of vitamins and minerals
Rye flour (100%)	335	Tr.	75.9	8.2	2.0	0.3	0.9	0	–	B₁, B₂, B₆, Fo, Pa, Bi; I, M, P, Z
Semolina	350	Tr.	77.5	10.7	1.8	0.3	0.8	0	–	B₆, Fo, Bi; M
Soya bean flour, full fat	447	11.2	12.3	36.8	23.5	3.3	13.3	0	11.9	B₁, B₂, Ni, B₆, Pa; Ca, I, M, P
low fat	352	13.4	14.8	45.3	7.2	1.0	4.1	0	14.3	B₁, B₂, Ni, B₆, Pa; Ca, I, M, P
Spaghetti, dry	378	2.7	81.3	13.6	1.0	0.1	0.4	0	–	Ni, Bi; M
boiled	117	0.8	25.2	4.2	0.3	0	0.1	0	–	
Wheat flour, wholemeal [wholewheat] (100%)	318	2.3	63.5	13.2	2.0	0.3	0.9	0	9.6	Ni, B₆, Fo, Bi, E; I, M, P, Z
brown (85%)	327	1.9	66.9	12.8	2.0	0.3	0.9	0	7.5	Ni, B₆, Fo, Bi; Ca, I, M, P, Z
white (72%), breadmaking	337	1.5	73.3	11.3	1.2	0.2	0.5	0	3.0	Ni, B₆, Bi; Ca, I, M
plain (all-purpose)	350	1.7	78.4	9.8	1.2	0.2	0.5	0	3.4	Ni, B₆, Bi; Ca, I
self-raising	339	1.4	76.1	9.3	1.2	0.2	0.5	0	3.7	B₆, B₁; Ca, I, M, S
Wheatgerm	347	16.0	28.7	26.5	8.1	1.1	3.6	0	–	B₁, B₂, Ni, B6, Fo, Pa, E; I, M, P
Breakfast cereals										
All-Bran	273	15.4	27.6	15.1	5.7	1.0	3.0	–	26.7	B₁, B₂, Ni, B₆, Fo, E; I, M, P, S, Z
Cornflakes	368	7.4	77.7	8.6	1.6	0.2	0.8	–	11.0	B₁, B₂, Ni; S
Muesli [health cereal]	368	26.2	40.0	12.9	7.5	1.3	3.0	–	7.4	B₂, Ni, B₆, Fo, E; Ca, I, M, P, Z
Porridge, made with water and salt	44	Tr.	8.2	1.4	0.9	0.1	0.4	0	0.8	Bi; S
Puffed Wheat	325	1.5	67.0	14.2	1.3	0.2	0.6	–	15.4	Ni, B₆, Fo, E; I, M, P, Z
Rice Krispies	372	9.0	79.1	5.9	2.0	0.5	0.7	–	4.5	B₁, B₂, Ni, B₆; M, S
Weetabix (U.K. only)	340	6.1	66.5	11.4	3.4	0.5	1.5	–	12.7	B₁, B₂, Ni, B₆, Fo, E; I, M, P, S, Z
Sweetened cereal products										
Biscuits [cookies], chocolate digestive (U.K. only)	493	28.5	38.0	6.8	24.1	12.0	1.6	–	3.5	E; I, M, P, S
gingernuts	456	35.8	43.3	5.6	15.2	7.1*	1.4*	–	2.0	Fo, E; Ca, I, P, S
semi-sweet	457	22.3	52.5	6.7	16.6	7.9*	1.7*	–	2.3	Fo, E; Ca, I, S
shortbread	504	17.2	48.3	6.2	26.0	15.2	1.0	–	2.1	A; S
wafers, filled	535	44.7	21.3	4.7	29.9	18.4*	0.9*	–	1.6	Fo, E
Cake, fruit, rich	332	46.7	11.6	3.7	11.0	9.3	0.8	–	3.5	A, B₆, Bi, E; P
iced [frosted]	407	54.0	14.8	3.8	14.9	3.9*	1.7*	50	2.4	M, S
sponge, fatless [angel cake]	301	30.9	22.7	10.0	6.7	2.1	0.8	260	1.0	B₂, Fo, Bi
Cheesecake	421	13.9	10.1	4.2	34.9	18.7	2.1	95	0.9	A; Ca, S
Eclairs	376	26.3	11.9	4.1	24.0	12.4	1.6	90	0	A, Bi, E
Gingerbread	373	31.8	30.9	6.1	12.6	4.5	1.9	60	1.3	A, Bi, E; Ca, I, M, P, S
Pies, custard	287	6.0	23.6	5.9	16.9	6.9	1.9	60	1.0	A, Bi; Ca, S
fruit	180	14.7	12.9	2.0	7.6	2.9	1.0	–*	2.2	
lemon meringue	323	24.8	21.6	4.5	14.6	5.5	1.9	90	0.7	A, Bi, E; S
SUGAR AND SUGAR PRODUCTS										
Boiled sweets [candies]	327	86.9	0.4	Tr.	Tr.	–	–	0	0	
Chocolate, milk	529	56.5	2.9	8.4	30.3	17.7	1.1	–	–	B₂, Fo, Bi; Ca, M, P
plain	525	59.5	5.3	4.7	29.2	17.4	0.9	–	–	Fo, Bi; I, M, P
Honey, jar	288	76.4	0	0.4	Tr.	–	–	0	–	
Ice cream, dairy	167	22.6	2.2	3.7	6.6	0	0	0	–	B₂, E; Ca
Jam, fruit with seeds	261	69.0	0	0.6	0	0	0	0	1.1	
stone fruit	261	69.3	0	0.4	0	0	0	0	1.0	
Marmalade	261	69.5	0	0.1	0	0	0	0	0.7	
Marzipan	443	49.2	0	8.7	24.9	2.0	4.7	35	6.4	B₂, Fo, Bi, E; Ca, I, M, P
Molasses, blackstrap	213	70.0C	–	–	–	–	–	0	–	B₂, Ni; Ca, I, P
Peppermints	392	102.2	0	0.5	0.7	–	–	–	0	
Sugar, demerara	394	104.5	0	0.5	0	0	0	0	0	
white	394	105.0	0	Tr.	0	0	0	0	0	
Syrup, golden	298	79.0	0	0.3	0	0	0	0	0	P, S
Toffees, mixed	430	70.1	1.0	2.1	17.2	–	–	–	–	P
Treacle, black	257	67.2	0	1.2	0	0	0	0	0	Ca, I, M, P, S

* composition varies according to fat used by manufacturer

OILS, FATS, SPREADS AND SAUCES

per 100 g	Calories	Sugar g	Starch g	Protein g	Total fat g	Saturated fat g	Polyunsaturated fat g	Cholesterol mg	Dietary fibre g	Good sources of vitamins and minerals
Chutney, apple	193	50.1	0.4	0.7	0.1	–	–	0	1.8	P
French dressing	658	0.2	0	0.1	73.0	10.3	8.1	–	0	E; S
Lard	891	0	0	Tr.	99.0	41.8	9.0	70	0	
Low fat spread	366	0	0	0	40.7	11.0	12.1	Tr.	0	A, E
Margarine	730	0.1C	–	0.1	81.0	as below		–*	0	A, E
hard, animal and vegetable oils	–	–	–	–	–	29.8	13.8	–	–	
vegetable oils	–	–	–	–	–	29.8	9.7	–	–	
polyunsaturated	–	–	–	–	–	19.1	60.1	–	–	
soft, animal and vegetable oils	–	–	–	–	–	24.5	15.8	–	–	
vegetable oils	–	–	–	–	–	25.6	17.9	–	–	
Mayonnaise	718	0.1	0	1.8	78.9	–	–	260	0	B$_6$, Fo, Pa, Bi, E; S
Oils	899	0	0	Tr.	99.9	as below		Tr.	0	
coconut	–	–	–	–	–	85.2	1.7	–	–	
corn [maize]	–	–	–	–	–	16.4	49.3	–	–	E
cottonseed	–	–	–	–	–	25.6	48.1	–	–	E
olive	–	–	–	–	–	14.0	11.2	–	–	E
palm	–	–	–	–	–	45.3	8.3	–	–	E
peanut	–	–	–	–	–	18.8	28.5	–	–	E
safflower	–	–	–	–	–	10.2	72.1	–	–	E
sunflower	–	–	–	–	–	13.1	49.9	–	–	E
Pickle, sweet	134	32.6	1.8	0.6	0.3	–	–	–	1.7	I, S
Tomato ketchup	98	22.9	1.1	2.1	Tr.	–	–	0	–	Bi; P, S
Vinegar	4	0.6	0	0.4	0	0	0	0	0	
Yeast extract	179	0	1.8	41.4	0.7	–	–	0	–	B$_1$, B$_2$, Ni, B$_6$, Fo; I, M, P, S, Z

SOUPS

per 100 g	Calories	Sugar g	Starch g	Protein g	Total fat g	Saturated fat g	Polyunsaturated fat g	Cholesterol mg	Dietary fibre g	Good sources of vitamins and minerals
Chicken noodle, dried, as served	20	0.6	3.1	0.8	0.3	–	–	–	–	S
Lentil, home-made	99	2.0	9.9	4.4	3.7	1.4	0.4	–	2.2	
Minestrone, dried, as served	23	1.2	2.5	0.8	0.7	–	–	–	0.5	S
Mushroom, cream of, canned, ready to serve	53	0.8	3.1	1.1	3.8	–	–	–	–	S
Tomato, cream of, canned, ready to serve	55	2.6	3.3	0.8	3.3	–	–	–	–	S

BEVERAGES

per 100 g	Calories	Sugar g	Starch g	Protein g	Total fat g	Saturated fat g	Polyunsaturated fat g	Cholesterol mg	Dietary fibre g	Good sources of vitamins and minerals
Blackcurrant cordial, undiluted	229	60.9	0	0.1	0	0	0	0	0	C
Cocoa, powder (U.K. only)	312	Tr.	11.5	18.5	21.7	12.8	0.6	–	–	Fo; Ca, I, M, P, S, Z
Coffee, infusion of grounds	2	Tr.	0.3	0.2	Tr.	–	–	0	–	
Cola drinks	39	10.5	Tr.	Tr.	0	0	0	0	0	
Drinking chocolate, powder [cocoa]	366	73.8	3.6	5.5	6.0	3.5	0.2	–	–	Fo; I, M, P, S
Grapefruit juice, canned, sweetened	38	9.7	Tr.	0.5	Tr.	–	–	0	0	Bi, C
unsweetened	31	7.9	Tr.	0.3	Tr.	–	–	0	0	Bi, C
Lemonade	21	5.6	0	Tr.	0	0	0	0	0	
Lime cordial, undiluted	112	29.8	Tr.	0.1	0	0	0	0	0	
Low calorie soft drinks	0	0	0	0	0	0	0	0	0	
Orange juice, fresh	38	9.4	0	0.6	Tr.	–	–	0	0	Bi, C
canned, sweetened	51	12.8	Tr.	0.7	Tr.	–	–	0	0	Bi, C
unsweetened	33	8.5	Tr.	0.4	Tr.	–	–	0	0	Bi, C

*depends on blend of fats used

per 100 g	Calories	Sugar g	Starch g	Protein g	Total fat g	Saturated fat g	Polyunsaturated fat g	Cholesterol mg	Dietary fibre g	Good sources of vitamins and minerals
frozen concentrate, unsweetened, dilute	45	10.7C	–	0.7	Tr.	–	–	0	0	
Pineapple juice, canned	53	13.4	Tr.	0.4	0.1	–	–	0	0	B_6
Root beer	41	10.5C	–	0	0	0	0	0	0	
Tea, herb (infusion)	0	0	0	0	0	0	0	0	0	
Indian (infusion)	1	Tr.	0	0.1	Tr.	–	–	0	–	
Tomato juice, canned	16	3.2	0.2	0.7	Tr.	–	–	0	–	B_6, Fo, Bi, C; P, S
Alcoholic beverages per 100 ml										
Beer, bitter	32	2.3	0	0.3	Tr.	–	–	0	0	
lager	29	1.5	0	0.2	Tr.	–	–	0	0	
Cider, dry	36	2.6	0	Tr.	0	0	0	0	0	
sweet	42	4.3	0	Tr.	0	0	0	0	0	
Liqueurs, cherry brandy	255	32.6	0	Tr.	0	0	0	0	0	
curaçao	311	28.3	0	Tr.	0	0	0	0	0	
Spirits, 70% proof	222	Tr.	0	Tr.	0	0	0	0	0	
Wine, red	68	0.3	0	0.2	0	0	0	0	0	
rosé	71	2.5	0	0.1	0	0	0	0	0	
white, dry	66	0.6	0	0.1	0	0	0	0	0	
sweet	94	5.9	0	0.2	0	0	0	0	0	
fortified, port	157	12.0	0	0.1	0	0	0	0	0	
sherry, dry	116	1.4	0	0.2	0	0	0	0	0	
sweet	136	6.9	0	0.3	0	0	0	0	0	
vermouth, dry	118	5.5	0	0.1	0	0	0	0	0	
sweet	151	15.9	0	Tr.	0	0	0	0	0	

Bibliography

★ **GENERAL**
Blackie, M. G. *The Patient, Not the Cure* (Woodbridge Press, Santa Barbara CA, 1978). Bricklin, M. *The Practical Encyclopaedia of Natural Healing* (Rodale Press Inc. Emmaus PA, 1976, and Aylesbury, 1977). Hill, A. (ed.) *The Visual Encyclopedia of Unconventional Medicine* (New English Library, London, 1979, and Crown, New York). Stanway, A. *Alternative Medicine: Guide to Natural Therapies* (Macdonald & Jane's, London, 1980).

★ **FIT FOR LIFE**
POSTURE AND MOVEMENT Mitchell, L. and Dale, B. *Simple Movement* (John Murray, London, 1980). Noble, E. *Essential Exercises for the Childbearing Years* (John Murray, London, 1980, and Houghton Mifflin, Boston MA, 1976). ORGANIZING THE ENVIRONMENT Murrell, K. F. H. *Ergonomics: Man in his Working Environment* (Chapman & Hall, London, 1979, and Methuen Inc., New York, 1969). Panero, J. and Zelnik, M. *Human Dimension and Interior Space* (Architectural Press, London, 1980, and Watson-Guptill, New York, 1979). Tutt, P. and Adler, D. (eds.) *New Metric Handbook* (Architectural Press, London, 1979). Published in U.S.A. as *VNR Metric Handbook of Architectural Standards* (Van Nostrand Reinhold, New York, 1980). WEIGHT-TRAINING Pearl, B. *Keys to the Inner Universe* (Physical Fitness Architects, Pasadena CA, 1979). FITNESS Morehouse, L. E. and Gross, L. *Total Fitness* (Granada, St. Albans, 1979, and Simon & Schuster, New York, 1975). Morehouse, L. E. and Gross, L. *Maximum Performance* (Hart-Davis, St. Albans, 1978, and Simon & Schuster, New York, 1977). Royal Canadian Air Force, *Physical Fitness* (Penguin, Harmondsworth, 1970). *Royal*

Bibliography

Canadian Air Force Exercise Plans for Physical Fitness (Pocket Books, New York, 1976).
ALEXANDER PRINCIPLE Alexander, F. M. *The Alexander Technique: Essential Writings of F. Matthias Alexander* (ed. Maisel, E.) (Thames & Hudson, London, 1974, and University Books, Secaucus NJ).
AEROBIC EXERCISE Cooper, K. *Aerobics, The Aerobics Way, Aerobics for Women, The New Aerobics* (Bantam, New York and London). Fixx, J. *The Complete Book of Running* (Chatto & Windus, London, 1979, and Random House, New York, 1977).
RELIEVING ACHES AND PAINS Rudinger, E. (ed.) *Avoiding Back Trouble* (Consumers' Association, London, 1975). Warmbrand, M. *Overcoming Rheumatism, Arthritis and Other Rheumatic Ailments* (Bachman & Turner, Maidstone, 1977, and Devin-Adair, Old Greenwich CT, 1975).

★ **EATING FOR LIFE**
FOOD INFORMATION Bingham, S. *Nutrition: Better Health Through Good Eating* (Barrie & Jenkins and Corgi, London, 1978). Davidson, S. etc. *Human Nutrition and Dietetics* (Churchill Livingstone, Edinburgh and New York, 7th ed. 1979). Medical Research Council *The Composition of Foods* (H.M.S.O., Norwich, and Elsevier-North Holland, New York, 4th rev. ed. 1978).
DIET AGAINST HEART DISEASE AND DIABETES Pritikin, N. and McGrady, P. M. *The Pritikin Program for Diet and Exercise* (Grosset & Dunlap, New York, 1979, and Bantam, New York and London, 1981).
EATING PATTERNS AND HEALTH Cleave, T. L. *Saccharine Disease* (John Wright, Bristol, 1974, and Keats, New Canaan CT, 1975). Mount, J. L. *The Food and Health of Western Man* (Charles Knight, Tonbridge, and Halsted Press, New York, 1975). Polunin, M. *The Right Way to Eat* (J. M. Dent, London, Melbourne and Toronto, 1978, and Granada, St. Albans, 1980).
NON-ANIMAL PROTEIN Lappé, F. M. *Diet for a Small Planet* (Friends of the Earth/ Ballantine Books, New York, 1971).
FIBRE Burkitt, D. P. *Don't Forget Fibre in Your Diet* (Martin Dunitz, London, 1979). Stanway, A. *Taking the Rough with the Smooth* (Souvenir Press and Pan, London, 1976, and International Scholarly Book Services, Forest Grove OR, 1978).
EATING NATURALLY Bircher-Benner, R. *Eating Your Way to Health* (Faber & Faber, London, 1966, and Penguin, New York, 1973). The Bircher-Benner *Diet Plan for . . .* series, by members of the Bircher-Benner family (C. W. Daniel, London, and Keats, New Canaan CT, 1977). Moule, T. W. *Nature Cure in a Nutshell* (Thorsons, Wellingborough, 3rd rev. ed. 1973). These last two give information on fasting.
FOOD ALLERGIES Coca, A. F. *The Pulse Test* (Arc Books, New York, 1979). Mackarness, R. *Not all in the Mind* (Pan, London, 1976).
HEALTH COOKERY Rose Elliot's books, *Simply Delicious, Not Just a Load of Old Lentils, The Bean Book, Your Very Good Health* (Fontana, London). Lo, K. *Chinese Food* (Penguin, Harmondsworth, 1972, and Peter Smith, Magnolia MA). McNeill, F. M. *The Scots Kitchen: Recipes* (Mayflower, St. Albans, 1974). Singh, D. *Indian Cookery (Penguin, Harmondsworth and Allen Lane, 1980) Things, Delicious Cheat (Mitchell Beazley, London, 1980).
LOW FAT GOURMET COOKING Guérard, M. *Cuisine Minceur* (Macmillan, London, 1977, Pan, London, 1978, and William Morrow, New York, 1976).

★ **MIND AND BODY**
SMOKING Royal College of Physicians of London *Smoking* OR *Health* (Pitman Medical, London, 1977).
ALCOHOL Miller, W. R. and Munoz, R. F. *How To Control Your Drinking* (Prentice-Hall, Englewood Cliffs NJ, 1976). Robinson, D. *Talking Out of Alcoholism. The Self-Help Process of Alcoholics Anonymous* (Croom Helm, London, and University Park Press, Baltimore, 1979). Royal College of Psychiatrists *Alcohol and Alcoholism* (Tavistock Publications, London, and Free Press, New York, 1979).
BIOFEEDBACK Cade, C. M. and Coxhead, N. *The Awakened Mind* (Wildwood House, London, 1980, Delacorte Press, New York, 1979, and Dell, New York, 1980).
RELAXATION Mitchell, L. *Simple Relaxation* (John Murray, London, 1977, and Atheneum, New York, 1979).
YOGA Iyengar, B. K. S. *Light on Yoga* (Allen & Unwin, London, 1968, Mandala Books, London, 1971, and Schocken, New York, rev. ed. 1977).
MASSAGE Tappan, F. M. *Healing Massage Techniques: a Study of Eastern and Western Methods* (Reston Publishing Co., Reston VA, 1980).
ALTERNATIVE VIEW OF HEALTH, ENERGY AND STRENGTH Tohei, K. *Ki in Daily Life* (Japan Publications, Hemel Hempstead and New York, 1978).

Index

Index prepared by Anne Hardy
Sub-divisions of a sub-entry appear
in italics

A

Index

Index

255

Acknowledgements

The Publishers wish to thank the following individuals and organizations for their assistance and advice:

A.S.H.
The British Osteopathic and
    Naturopathic College and Clinic
Cancer Research Campaign
Dr. Malcolm Carruthers M.D.,
    M.R.C. Path., M.R.C.G.P.
Professor Michael Day, Department
    of Anatomy, St. Thomas's
    Hospital, London
Christopher Robbins, Coronary
    Prevention Group
Dr. Valerie Spotswood L.R.C.P.,
    M.R.C.S., D.P.M., M.R.C. Psych.

John Bell and Croyden; Geoffrey Blundell, Audio Ltd.; John Davis, McCain Foods; East West Centre; The Controller of Her Majesty's Stationery Office for permission to reproduce material from McCance and Widdowson *The Composition of Foods* in the food charts; Lambton Squash Club; Ann Lloyd; Westside Health Centre.

Special thanks are due to illustrator Sheilagh Noble for her major contribution to the book. We would also like to thank Pedro Prá Lopez, Colin Salmon and Valerie Wright.

Artists
Alicia Durdos
63, 106, 138, 146–47, 149, 155
Tim Foster
187–88
Caroline Hillier
72–75
Andrew Macdonald
100, 102, 105, 109, 112
Sheilagh Noble
12–17, 19–21, 26–45, 60, 76–79,
81–82, 176, 204–05, 208–13, 222–35
Jennie Smith
53–55, 57–59, 83–88, 94, 96, 111,
125–26, 136–37, 140–44, 158, 164,
173, 203
Valerie Wright
64–65
Kathy Wyatt
23, 25, 46–51, 70–71, 114, 151,
157, 179, 192–93, 215–20

Special thanks are also due to Bob Aldridge for his patience and perfectionism in the make-up of this book.